NUTRITION almanac

NUTRITION SEARCH, INC.

JOHN D. KIRSCHMANN,
Director

McGraw-Hill Book Company

NEW YORK   KUALA LUMPUR   PARIS
ST. LOUIS   LONDON   SÃO PAULO
SAN FRANCISCO   MEXICO   SINGAPORE
AUCKLAND   MONTREAL   SYDNEY
DÜSSELDORF   NEW DELHI   TOKYO
JOHANNESBURG   PANAMA   TORONTO

Library of Congress Catalog Card Number: 75 1193

First McGraw-Hill Paperback Edition, 1975

ISBN   07-034847-2

8 9 MU MU 7 9 8

This book is dedicated to the purpose of increased harmony in the human body through a better understanding of nutrition. I wish to extend my appreciation to the many people who helped compile this book, especially to Jim Christianson for his editorial supervision of this revised, third edition, and to Mona Holte and Deborah DuBois for their enthusiastic assistance. Also, a special thank you to my daughter Lavon for her diligent efforts in compiling research for the first edition.

JOHN D. KIRSCHMANN

Suggestions for Using This Book

The system presented in this book can be employed in two ways. It can help the reader work out a total plan for personal nutrition, or it can quickly answer simple questions regarding food, nutrition, and health.

Nutrients (p. 11). This section discusses over 40 vitamins and minerals in terms of description, absorption and storage, dosage and toxicity, deficiency effects and symptoms, beneficial effect on ailments, human tests, and animal tests. A list of ailments for which the nutrients may be beneficial follows the discussion of each vitamin or mineral. In order to obtain a more complete understanding of the function of nutrients in relation to total health, the reader should refer to related sections of the book.

Nutrients That Function Together (p. 93). Many vitamins and minerals prove to be more or less effective when taken simultaneously with other nutrients. This section provides an easy-to-follow guide for understanding which nutrients are compatable or antagonistic.

Available Forms of Nutrient Supplements (p. 100). This section may be of interest to persons who wish to determine which supplements are best suited to their needs. All types of nutrient supplements are explained in terms of available forms, source—natural or synthetic, and an explanation of the source.

Ailments (p. 107). It is a proven fact that many common ailments and weight problems are a result of unbalanced intake of nutrients. In this section, common ailments are discussed and explained in layman's language. The discussion of each ailment is accompanied by a list of nutrients that have proven beneficial in treatment of the ailment. When quantities for a particular nutrient are given, it must be remembered that these quantities are *not prescriptive* but merely represent research findings. This section can be best utilized when cross-referenced with the "Nutrients" and "Foods" sections.

Foods, Beverages and Supplementary Foods (p. 171). The discussions of foods and supplemental foods give valuable information about specific foods or classes of foods and supplements. The list of "Rich Sources of Nutrients," beginning on page 181, shows at a glance what foods are good sources of the vitamins and minerals.

Table of Food Composition (p. 185). The "Table of Food Composition" gives the complete nutrient analysis of over 600 foods. This simple guide makes it possible for the reader to compare food values and analyze and prepare meals balanced in nutrients and calories.

Essential Amino Acid Contents of Some Foods (p. 221). One of the most important breakthroughs in understanding the balance and value of foods in terms of the protein quality they provide, this table lists the essential amino acid content of many foods together with the percentage of protein Recommended Dietary Allowance for a man and a woman of average body size which the foods provide.

Example of a Nutritionally Balanced Meal (p. 231). This section shows how the previously mentioned table can best be utilized by comparing the food value of a nutritionally balanced Chicken Kiev dinner and a typical restaurant dinner, the hot beef sandwich.

Nutrient Allowance Chart (p. 235). The "Nutrient Allowance Chart" gives a complete breakdown of the nutrient needs for each person in view of body size, metabolism, and calorie requirements.

Diet Analysis (p. 239). Nutrition Search provides a complete, individual dietary analysis to persons who wish to examine their average daily consumption of food. This service is an accurate indication of nutritional deficiencies and the ways they may be corrected.

In summary, this "Almanac" is not the type of book that one would read from front cover to back cover as one would a novel, but it can be a very useful tool if a reader takes time to understand the importance of the various sections. Like the individual B-complex vitamins, each section of this book is important in its own right; when used simultaneously, *all* sections have a much more beneficial effect.

NOTE: The information contained in this book is not intended to be prescriptive. Any attempt to diagnose and treat an illness should come under the direction of a physician who is familiar with nutritional therapy. It is possible that some individuals may suffer allergic reactions from the use of various dietary supplement preparations or the media in which they are contained; if such reactions occur, consult your physician. Nutrition Search, Inc., and the publisher assume no responsibility.

Contents

Nutrition and Health

Nutrition is the relationship of foods to the health of the human body. Proper nutrition implies receiving adequate foods and supplements to convey the nutrients required for optimal health. Without proper nutrition and exercise, optimal health and well-being cannot be attained.

Proper nutrition means that all the essential nutrients—that is, carbohydrates, fats, protein, vitamins, minerals, and water—are supplied and utilized in adequate balance to maintain optimal health and well-being. Nutritional deficiencies result whenever inadequate amounts of essential nutrients are provided to tissues that must function normally over a long period of time. Good nutrition is essential for normal organ development and functioning; for normal reproduction, growth, and maintenance; for optimum activity level and working efficiency; for resistance to infection and disease; and for the ability to repair bodily damage or injury.

No single substance will maintain vibrant health. Although specific nutrients are known to be more important in the functions of certain parts of the body, even these nutrients are totally dependent upon the presence of other nutrients for their best effects. Every effort should therefore be made to attain and maintain an adequate, balanced daily intake of all the necessary nutrients throughout life.

Fasting and vegetarianism are two situations in which adequate daily intake of all essential nutrients may not be achieved if care is not taken to ensure the mainte-nance of good health. Fasting, whether for reasons of health, social protest, religion, or economic or environmental factors, may last from 1 to 70 days. Some persons advocate consuming only pure water during a fast, while others advocate drinking fruit and vegetable juices. Although many nutrients may not be as efficiently absorbed without the presence of solid food, one should consider taking nutrient supplements when fasting.

Vegetarianism is essentially the practice of eating a meatless diet, although there are several types of vegetarians. *Ovo-lacto vegetarians* include some animal products such as eggs, milk, and cheese, in their diet, but exclude all flesh foods, whether meat, poultry, or fish. *Pure*, or *strict*, *vegetarians* abstain from the use of all foods of animal origin. *Vegans* avoid all foods of animal origin as well as any commercial products such as leather, which require taking the life of animals.

The main concern in a vegetarian diet is the sufficient intake of protein. This can be achieved by the combination of nonflesh foods that are low in certain amino acids with other foods that have high concentrations of the same amino acids. This system of combining "complementary proteins" is described in detail in the section on protein (p. 9) and should be fully understood by anyone considering adopting a vegetarian diet. Amino acid contents of foods are listed in Section VII—"Essential Amino Acid Contents of Some Foods" (pp. 221-229). No one should attempt to vary from a standard diet for an extended period of time without first consulting a physician or naturopath knowledgeable in the field of nutrition and without studying the available literature on the subject.

The foods eaten by humans are chemically complex. They must be broken down by the body into simpler chemical forms so that they can be taken in through the intestinal walls and transported by the blood to the cells. There they provide energy and the correct building materials to maintain human life. These are the processes of digestion, absorption, and metabolism.

DIGESTION, ABSORPTION, AND METABOLISM

DIGESTION

Digestion is a series of physical and chemical changes by which food, taken into the body, is broken down in preparation for absorption from the intestinal tract into the bloodstream. These changes take place in the digestive tract, which includes the mouth, pharynx, esophagus, stomach, small intestine, and large intestine.

The active materials in the digestive juices which cause the chemical breakdown of food are called "enzymes," complex proteins that are capable of inducing chemical changes in other substances without themselves being changed. Each enzyme is capable of breaking down only a single specific substance. For example, an enzyme capable of breaking down fats cannot break down proteins or carbohydrates, or vice versa. Enzymatic action originates in four areas of the body: the salivary glands, the stomach, the pancreas, and the wall of the small intestine.

Digestion actually begins in the mouth, where chewing breaks large pieces of food into smaller pieces. The salivary glands in the mouth produce saliva, a fluid that moistens food for swallowing and which contains ptyalin, the enzyme necessary for carbohydrate breakdown. The masticated food mass passes back to the pharynx under voluntary control, but from there on and through the esophagus, the process of swallowing is carried on by peristalsis, a slow wavelike motion occurring along the entire digestive tract, which moves the food into the stomach.

Active chemical digestion begins in the middle portion of the stomach, where the food is mixed with gastric juices containing hydrochloric acid, water, and enzymes that break up protein and other substances.

After one to four hours, depending upon the combination of foods ingested by the system, peristalsis pushes the food, now in the liquid form of chyme, out of the stomach and into the small intestine. Foodstuffs leave the stomach and enter the small intestine in the following order: carbohydrates, protein, and fat—which takes the longest to digest.

When chyme enters the small intestine, the pancreas secretes its digestive juices. If fats are present in the food, bile, an enzyme produced by the liver and stored in the gallbladder, is also secreted. Bile separates the fat into small droplets so that the pancreatic enzymes can break it down. The pancreas also secretes a substance that neutralizes the digestive acids in the food, and it secretes additional enzymes that continue the breakdown of proteins and carbohydrates.

The remaining undigested products enter the large intestine and eventually are excreted. No digestive enzymes are secreted in the large intestine, and little change occurs there except for the absorption of water.

ABSORPTION

Absorption is the process by which nutrients in the form of glucose (from carbohydrates), amino acids (from protein), and fatty acids and glycerol (from fats) are taken up by the intestines and passed into the bloodstream to facilitate cell metabolism.

Absorption takes place primarily in the small intestine. The lining of the small intestine is covered with small fingerlike projections called "villi." These villi contain lymph channels and tiny blood vessels called "capillaries" that are the principal channels of absorption, depending upon the type of nutrient. Fats and fat-soluble vitamins move through the blood to the cells. Other nutrients are carried away from the villi by the capillaries, which funnel them into the portal vein leading to the liver.

In the liver, many different enzymes help change the nutrient molecules into new forms for specific purposes. Unlike earlier changes, which prepared nutrients for absorption and transport, the reactions in the liver produce the products needed by individual cells. Some of the products are used by the liver itself, but the rest are held in storage by the liver, to be released into the body as needed. The remainder go into the bloodstream, where they are picked up by the cells and put to work. Water-soluble vitamins and minerals are also absorbed into the bloodstream in the small intestine.

METABOLISM

At this point the handling of food within the body has reached its final stage. The process of metabolism involves all the chemical changes that nutrients undergo from the time they are absorbed until they become a part of the body or are excreted from the body. Metabolism is the conversion of the digested nutrients into building material for living tissue or energy to meet the body's needs.

Metabolism occurs in two general phases that occur simultaneously, *anabolism* and *catabolism*. Anabolism involves all the chemical reactions that the nutrients undergo in the construction or building up of body chemicals and tissues, such as blood, enzymes, hormones, glycogen, and others. Catabolism involves the reactions in which various compounds of the tissues are broken down to supply energy. Energy for the cells is derived from the metabolism of glucose, which combines with oxygen in a series of chemical reactions to form carbon dioxide, water, and cellular energy. The carbon dioxide and water are waste products, carried away from the cells by the bloodstream. Energy can also be derived from the metabolism of essential fatty acids and amino acids, although the primary effect of the metabolism of amino acids is to provide material for growth and the maintenance and repair of tissues. The waste products of essential fatty acid and amino acid metabolism are also carried away from the cells by the bloodstream.

The process of metabolism requires that extensive systems of enzymes be maintained to facilitate the thousands of different chemical reactions and regulate the rate at which these reactions proceed. These enzymes often require the presence of specific vitamins and minerals to perform their functions.

FACTORS INHIBITING DIGESTION

The movements of the stomach are interfered with by nervousness and anxiety. Eating while agitated, fa-

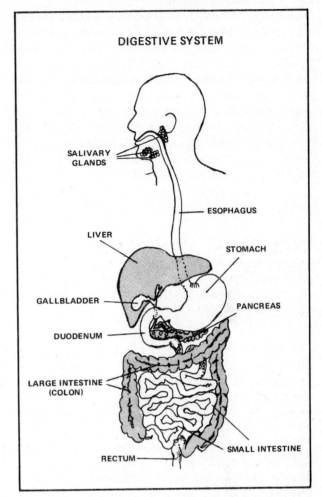

DIGESTIVE SYSTEM

SALIVARY GLANDS
ESOPHAGUS
LIVER
STOMACH
GALLBLADDER
PANCREAS
DUODENUM
LARGE INTESTINE (COLON)
SMALL INTESTINE
RECTUM

tigued, or worried may give rise to gastrointestinal disturbances. Hurried meals under tense conditions are not conducive to normal digestion. Weather variations and physical disorders such as diabetes or other illnesses may inhibit the proper digestion of foods.

EXERCISE

A healthy body is the result of proper nutrition combined with a regular pattern of physical exercise. Exercise imparts vigor and activity to all organs and secures and maintains healthful integrity of all their functions. Exercise improves the tone and quality of muscle tissue and stimulates the processes of digestion, absorption, metabolism, and elimination. It also strengthens blood vessels, lungs, and heart, resulting in improved transfer of oxygen to the cells and increased circulation of the blood and lymph systems. Exercise develops grace, poise, and symmetry of the body, helps in correcting defective development or injuries, and stimulates the mind.

The key to any type of exercise is a strong will and a sincere desire to improve one's physical condition. It is important to have a program that fits individual needs and capacities. A beginning exercise program should be light; it should increase in difficulty gradually as endurance increases. Exercise should not be done for at least an hour after eating because physical exertion may impede digestion. Exercise should be self-motivating and fun. An ideal exercise program may include many different forms of the following physical activities.

Calisthenics

Calisthenics consists of light exercises or gymnastics including sit-ups, push-ups, jumping jacks, etc., which promote grace and health. The emphasis of calisthenics is on building skeletal muscles.

Dancing

Dancing or rhythmic exercise is often an enjoyable way to exercise the body thoroughly and refresh the mind. Besides toning muscles, joints, glands, the respiratory system, and digestive organs, it gives everyday movements grace and poise.

Isometrics

Isometric exercise involves the pressure of a muscle or group of muscles against each other or against an immovable object. It is especially good for reducing because it can be applied to specific areas. Isometrics primarily tone and build the skeletal muscles.

Jogging

Jogging is a form of exercise that consists of alternately walking and running. It is an excellent exercise for improving the heart, lungs, and circulatory system by expanding their capacity to handle stress. It can help build muscle tone, reduce hips and thighs, redistribute weight, and flatten the abdomen.

Stretching

Stretching is natural exercise that should be practiced on a regular basis. A good habit to develop is stretching upon rising in the morning and throughout the day. Stretch exercises tend to increase both energy and en-

EXPENDITURE OF CALORIC ENERGY PER HOUR

Activity	Calories Expended per Hour
Ballroom dancing	330
Bed making	234
Bowling	264
Bricklaying	240
Carpentry	408
Desk work	132
Driving a car	168
Farm work in field	438
Golf	300
Handball	612
Horseback riding (trot)	480
Ironing (standing up)	252
Lawn mowing (hand mower)	462
Painting at an easel	120
Piano playing	150
Preparing a meal	198
Scrubbing of floors	216
Sitting and eating	84
Sitting and knitting	90
Sitting in a chair reading	72
Skiing	594
Sleeping (basal metabolism)	60
Standing up	138
Sweeping	102
Swimming (leisurely)	300
Walking (2.5 miles per hour)	216
Walking downstairs	312

durance for all parts of the body. Stretching tends to relieve many aches and pains; loosen up ligaments, joints, and muscles; and increase coordination and suppleness. Stretching stimulates circulation and alleviates the stiffness of contracted muscles.

Walking

Walking is one of the best overall exercises and helps the entire system function better. The metabolism is increased while walking; thus fat is burned up and weight loss is promoted. Blood pressure, blood cholesterol, and sugar levels tend to fall. Walking builds up the heart muscle and keeps the arteries clear and elastic. Walking helps increase the oxygen supply to the blood, thus bringing more oxygen to the heart. It also increases the capacity of the lungs, making more oxygen available to the circulatory system.

Weight Lifting

Weight lifting is a form of exercise involving the lifting of weights and is often used by athletes to strengthen muscle tone.

Above all, do not forget the recreational exercises, such as golf, tennis, riding, skating, skiing, etc. There are endless sports that can improve the functioning of the body. The important thing is to remember to exercise *regularly* and maintain a nutritionally balanced diet of good, healthy food.

Sources of Calories: Carbohydrates, Fats, and Protein

Carbohydrates, fats, and proteins are the primary sources of energy to the body because they supply fuel necessary for body heat and work. Their fuel potential is expressed in *calories*, a term that signifies the amount of chemical energy that may be released as heat when food is metabolized. Therefore foods that are high in energy value are high in calories, while foods that are low in energy value are low in calories. Fats yield approximately nine calories per gram, and carbohydrates and proteins yield approximately four calories per gram.

CARBOHYDRATES

Carbohydrates are the chief source of energy for all body functions and muscular exertion and are necessary to assist in the digestion and assimilation of other foods. Carbohydrates provide us with immediately available calories for energy by producing heat in the body when carbon in the system unites with oxygen in the bloodstream. Carbohydrates also help regulate protein and fat metabolism; fats require carbohydrates for their breakdown within the liver.

The principal carbohydrates present in foods are sugars, starches, and cellulose. Simple sugars, such as those in honey and fruits, are very easily digested. Double sugars, such as table sugar, require some digestive action, but they are not nearly as complex as starches, such as those found in whole grain. Starches require prolonged enzymatic action in order to be broken down into simple sugars (glucose) for digestion. Cellulose, commonly found in the skins of fruits and vegetables, is largely indigestible by humans and contributes little energy value to the diet. It does, however, provide the bulk necessary for intestinal action and aids elimination.

All sugars and starches are converted by the digestive juices to a simple sugar called "glucose." Some of this glucose, or "blood sugar," is used as fuel by tissues of the brain, nervous system, and muscles. A small portion of the glucose is converted to glycogen and stored by the liver and muscles; the excess is converted to fat and stored throughout the body as a reserve source of energy. When fat reserves are reconverted to glucose and used for body fuel, weight loss results.

Carbohydrate snacks containing sugars and starches provide the body with almost instant energy because

7

they cause a sudden rise in the blood sugar level. However, the blood sugar level drops again rapidly, creating a craving for more sweet food and possibly fatigue, dizziness, nervousness, and headache.

Overindulgence in starchy and sweet foods may crowd out other essential foods from the diet and can therefore result in nutritional deficiency as well as in obesity and tooth decay. Diets high in refined carbohydrates are usually low in vitamins, minerals, and cellulose. Such foods as white flour, white sugar, and polished rice are lacking in the B vitamins and other nutrients. Excessive consumption of these foods will perpetuate any vitamin B deficiency an individual may have. If the B vitamins are absent, carbohydrate combustion cannot take place, and indigestion, symptoms of heartburn, and nausea can result. Research continues as to whether or not such problems as diabetes, heart disease, high blood pressure, anemia, kidney disorders, and cancer can be linked to an overabundance of refined carbohydrate foods in the diet.

Carbohydrates can be manufactured in the body from some amino acids and the glycerol component of fats; therefore the National Research Council lists no specific requirement for carbohydrates in the diet.[1]

Differences in basal metabolism, amount of activity, size, and weight will influence the amount of carbohydrates the body needs to get from an outside source. However, a total lack of carbohydrates may produce ketosis, loss of energy, depression, and breakdown of essential body protein.

FATS

Fats, or lipids, are the most concentrated source of energy in the diet. When oxidized, fats furnish more than twice the number of calories per gram furnished by carbohydrates or proteins. One gram of fat yields approximately nine calories to the body.

In addition to providing energy, fats act as carriers for the fat-soluble vitamins, A, D, E, and K. By aiding in the absorption of vitamin D, fats help make calcium available to body tissues, particularly to the bones and teeth. Fats are also important for the conversion of carotene to vitamin A. Fat deposits surround, protect, and hold in place organs, such as the kidneys, heart, and liver. A layer of fat insulates the body from environmental temperature changes and preserves body heat. This layer also rounds out the contours of the body. Fats prolong the process of digestion by slowing down the stomach's secretions of hydrochloric acid. Thus fats create a longer-lasting sensation of fullness after a meal.

The substances that give fats their different flavors, textures, and melting points are known as the "fatty acids." There are two types of fatty acids, saturated and unsaturated. Saturated fatty acids are those that are usually hard at room temperature and which, except for coconut oils, come primarily from animal sources. Unsaturated fatty acids, including polyunsaturates, are usually liquid at room temperature and are derived from vegetable, nut, or seed sources, such as corn, safflowers, sunflowers, and olives. Vegetable shortenings and margarines have undergone a process called "hydrogenation" in which unsaturated oils are converted to a more solid form of fat. Other sources of fat are milk products, eggs, and cheese.

There are three "essential" fatty acids: linoleic, arachidonic, and linolenic, collectively known as vitamin F. They are termed "essential" because the body cannot produce them. They are unsaturated fatty acids necessary for normal growth and healthy blood, arteries, and nerves. Also, they keep the skin and other tissues youthful and healthy by preventing dryness and scaliness. Essential fatty acids may be necessary for the transport and breakdown of cholesterol.[2]

Cholesterol is a lipid or fat-related substance necessary for good health. It is a normal component of most body tissues, especially those of the brain and nervous system, liver, and blood. It is needed to form sex and adrenal hormones, vitamin D, and bile, which is needed for the digestion of fats. Cholesterol also seems to play a part in lubricating the skin.

Although a cholesterol deficiency is unlikely to occur, abnormal amounts of cholesterol may be stored throughout the body if fats are eaten excessively. Research continues, although it is yet inconclusive, as to the relationship of increased cholesterol storage to the devel-

[1] National Research Council, *Recommended Dietary Allowances* (Washington, D.C.: National Academy of Science, 1974), p. 34.

[2] Helen S. Mitchel et al., *Copper's Nutrition in Health and Disease,* 15th ed. (Philadelphia: J. B. Lippincott Co., 1968), p. 318.

opment of arteriosclerosis. Lecithin has been found to decrease cholesterol levels in some individuals.

Fat and fat-containing foods should be stored in covered containers, away from direct light, in a cool place to prevent rancidity caused by oxidation. Some protection from rancidity will be provided by vitamin E, a fat-soluble vitamin that is a natural antioxidant and is present in most fat-containing foods.

Although a fat deficiency rarely occurs in man, such a deficiency would lead to a deficiency in the fat-soluble vitamins. A deficiency of fatty acids may produce eczema or other skin disorders. An extreme deficiency could lead to severely retarded growth.

Excessive amounts of fat in the diet may lead to abnormal weight gain and obesity if more calories are consumed than are needed by the body. In addition to obesity, excessive fat intake will cause abnormally slow digestion and absorption, resulting in indigestion. If a lack of carbohydrates is accompanied by a lack of water in the diet, or if there is a kidney malfunction, fats cannot be completely metabolized and may become toxic to the body.

The National Research Council sets no Recommended Dietary Allowance for fats because of the widely varying fat content of the diet among individuals. Linoleic acid, however, should provide about 2 percent of the calories in the diet.[3] Vegetable fats, such as corn, safflower, and soybean oils, are high in linoleic acid. Nutritionists suggest that an intake of fat providing 25 to 30 percent of the calories is compatible with good health.[4]

PROTEIN

Next to water, protein is the most plentiful substance in the body. Protein is one of the most important elements for the maintenance of good health and vitality and is of primary importance in the growth and development of all body tissues. It is the major source of building mate-

rial for muscles, blood, skin, hair, nails, and internal organs, including the heart and the brain.

Protein is needed for the formation of hormones, which control a variety of body functions such as growth, sexual development, and rate of metabolism. Protein also helps prevent the blood and tissues from becoming either too acid or too alkaline and helps regulate the body's water balance. Enzymes, substances necessary for basic life functions, and antibodies, which help fight foreign substances in the body, are also formed from protein. In addition, protein is important in the formation of milk during lactation and in the process of blood clotting.

As well as being the major source of building material for the body, protein may be used as a source of heat and energy, providing 4 calories per gram of protein. However, this energy function is spared when sufficient fats and carbohydrates are present in the diet. Excess protein that is not used for building tissue or energy can be converted by the liver and stored as fat in the body tissues.

During digestion the large molecules of proteins are decomposed into simpler units called "amino acids." Amino acids are necessary for the synthesis of body proteins and many other tissue constituents. They are the units from which proteins are constructed and are the end products of protein digestion.

The body requires approximately twenty-two amino acids in a specific pattern to make human protein. All but eight of these amino acids can be produced in the adult body. The eight that cannot be produced are called "essential amino acids" because they must be supplied in the diet. In order for the body to properly synthesize protein, all the essential amino acids must be present simultaneously and in the proper proportions. If just one essential amino acid is missing, even temporarily, protein synthesis will fall to a very low level or stop altogether.[5] The result is that *all* amino acids are reduced in the same proportion as the amino acid that is low or missing.

Foods containing protein may or may not contain all the essential amino acids. When a food contains all the essential amino acids, it is termed "complete protein." Foods that lack or are extremely low in any one of the essential amino acids are called "incomplete protein." Most meats and dairy products are complete-protein

---

[3]Helen Andrews Guthrie, *Introductory Nutrition*, 2d ed. (St. Louis: C. V. Mosby Co., 1971), p. 46.

[4]Guthrie, *Introductory Nutrition*, p. 46.

[5]A. M. Altschul, *Proteins, Their Chemistry and Politics* (New York: Basic Books, 1965), p. 118.

foods, while most vegetables and fruits are incomplete-protein foods. To obtain a complete-protein meal from incomplete proteins, one must combine foods carefully so that those weak in an essential amino acid will be balanced by those adequate in the same amino acid.

The minimum daily protein requirement, the smallest amino acid intake that can maintain optimum growth and good health in man, is difficult to determine. Protein requirements differ according to the nutritional status, body size, and activity of the individual. Dietary calculations are usually based on the National Research Council's Recommended Dietary Allowances. The protein recommendations are considered to cover individual variations among most persons living in the United States under usual environmental stress. The National Research Council recommends that 0.42 gram of protein per day be consumed for each pound of body weight. To figure out individual protein requirements, simply divide body weight by 2, and the result will indicate the approximate number of grams of protein required each day. For example, a person weighing 120 pounds requires approximately 60 grams of protein daily. However, total daily protein needs in grams per pound will be reduced if the daily limited amino acid requirements are met. (See "Essential Amino Acid Contents of Some Foods," pp. 221-229.)

Protein deficiency may lead to abnormalities of growth and tissue development. The hair, nails, and skin especially will be affected, and muscle tone will be poor. A child whose diet is deficient in protein may not attain his potential physical stature. Extreme protein deficiency in children results in kwashiorkor, a disease characterized by stunted mental and physical growth, loss of hair pigment, and swelling of the joints. It is often fatal. In adults, protein deficiency may result in lack of vigor and stamina, mental depression, weakness, poor resistance to infection, impaired healing of wounds, and slow recovery from disease.

Loss of body protein occurs as a result of particular bodily stresses, such as surgery, hemorrhage, wounds, or prolonged illness. At times of stress, it is necessary to consume extra protein in order to rebuild or replace used or worn out tissues. However, excessive intake of protein may cause fluid imbalance.

Nutrients

Knowledge of the nutrients and their functions in the body is necessary for understanding the importance of good nutrition. The six nutrients—carbohydrates, fats, protein, vitamins, minerals, and water—are present in the foods we eat and contain chemical substances that function in one or more of three ways: they furnish the body with heat and energy, they provide material for growth and repair of body tissues, and they assist in the regulation of body processes.

Each nutrient has its own specific functions and relationship to the body, but no nutrient acts independently of other nutrients. All of the nutrients must be present in the diet in varying quantities in order for the body to maintain basic life processes. Although all persons have need for the same nutrients, the amounts of the nutrients required by an individual are influenced by age, sex, body size, environment, level of activity, and nutritional status. Processing, storage, and preparation of food may influence the nutritional value of food. Proper understanding of the nutrients and the means of balancing a diet of the foods that contain them will result in optimum health for the body and mind.

VITAMINS

All natural vitamins are organic food substances found only in living things, that is, plants and animals. There are about twenty substances that are believed to be active as vitamins in human nutrition. Each of these vitamins is present in varying quantities in specific foods, and each is absolutely necessary for proper growth and maintenance of health. With a few exceptions, the body cannot synthesize vitamins; they must be supplied in the diet or in dietary supplements.

Vitamins have no caloric or energy value but are important to the body as constituents of enzymes, which function as catalysts in nearly all metabolic reactions. As such, vitamins help regulate metabolism, help convert fat and carbohydrates into energy, and assist in forming bone and tissues. Vitamins are not components of major body structures but aid in the building of these structures.

Much work has been done to determine requirements of vitamins for various age groups and in circumstances of additional needs, such as pregnancy and lactation. The Recommended Dietary Allowances (RDA) of the nutrients mentioned in this book are based on the standards established by the Food and Nutrition Board of the National Research Council. Desirable levels for those vitamins whose requirements are known to be essential to healthy humans are based upon available scientific knowledge and are considered adequate to meet the known nutritional needs of practically all healthy persons. These levels are intended to apply to persons whose physical activity is considered "light" and who live in temperate climates, and they provide a safety margin for each vitamin above the minimum level that will maintain health.

To ensure that as yet unrecognized nutritional needs are met, one should obtain one's RDA from as varied a selection of foods as is practical: present knowledge of nutritional needs is incomplete. The human requirement for many nutrients has not been established. There is no way of actually predicting the requirements of specific individuals because of the variables of climate, sex, age, state of health, body size, genetic makeup, and amount of activity.

Where there is doubt that the requirements for certain nutrients are being met through the diet alone, supplements may be ingested to offset any deficiency. Vitamins taken in excess of the finite amount utilized in the metabolic processes are valueless and will be either excreted in the urine or stored in the body. Excessive ingestion of some nutrients may result in toxicity, and risks associated with ingestion of excessive quantities of nutrients are mentioned at appropriate points in the text.

Vitamins are usually distinguished as being water-soluble or fat-soluble. The water-soluble vitamins, B-complex vitamins, vitamin C, and the compounds termed "bioflavonoids," are usually measured in milligrams. The fat-soluble vitamins, A, D, E, and K, are measured in units of activity known as "International Units" (IU) or "United States Pharmacopoeia Units" (USP). (Vitamins A, D, E, and K are expressed in International Units (IU) throughout this book.) Generally, each unit represents the amount of any form of the vitamin needed to produce a specific change in the nutritional health of a laboratory animal.

MINERALS

Minerals are nutrients that exist in the body and in food in organic and inorganic combinations. Approximately seventeen minerals are essential in human nutrition. Although only 4 or 5 percent of the human body weight is mineral matter, minerals are vital to overall mental and physical well-being. All tissues and internal fluids of living things contain varying quantities of minerals. Minerals are constituents of the bones, teeth, soft tissue, muscle, blood, and nerve cells. They are important factors in maintaining physiological processes, strengthening skeletal structures, and preserving

the vigor of the heart and brain as well as all muscle and nerve systems.

Minerals act as catalysts for many biological reactions within the human body, including muscle response, the transmission of messages through the nervous system, digestion, and metabolism or utilization of nutrients in foods. They are important in the production of hormones.

Minerals help to maintain the delicate water balance essential to the proper functioning of mental and physical processes. They keep blood and tissue fluids from becoming either too acid or too alkaline and permit other nutrients to pass into the bloodstream. They also help draw chemical substances in and out of the cells and aid in the creation of antibodies.

All of the minerals known to be needed by the human body must be supplied in the diet. No RDAs have been established for minerals other than calcium, phosphorus, iodine, and iron. However, a varied and mixed diet of animal and vegetable origin which meets the energy and protein needs of healthy persons will also furnish adequate minerals.

Calcium, chlorine, phosphorus, potassium, magnesium, sodium, and sulfur are known as the "macro-minerals" because they are present in relatively high amounts in body tissues. They are measured in milligrams. Other minerals, termed "trace minerals," are present in the body only in the most minute quantities but are essential for proper body functioning. Trace minerals are measured in micrograms.

Although the minerals are discussed separately, it is important to note that their actions within the body are interrelated; no one mineral can function without affecting others. Physical and emotional stress causes a strain on the body's supply of minerals. A mineral deficiency often results in illness, which may be checked by the addition of the missing mineral to the diet.

HOW VITAMINS AND MINERALS ARE EXPLAINED IN THIS BOOK

Vitamins and minerals are explained in this book in terms of description, absorption and storage, dosage and toxicity, deficiency effects and symptoms, and beneficial effect on ailments. Human and animal tests are described at the end of some listed nutrients. A chart listing the ailments that are associated with a specific nutrient follows the discussion of each nutrient.

Description

The description of the vitamin or mineral defines the nutrient—whether or not it is water- or fat-soluble (if it is a vitamin) and its function in the body—and lists the major foods in which it is contained.

Absorption and Storage

The section on absorption and storage explains the places where the nutrient is absorbed and stored in the body, the synthesis of body processes, and if possible, the time factor involved. Any variables that may stimulate or interfere with absorption and storage of the nutrient are also mentioned together with the way the nutrient is excreted.

Dosage and Toxicity

Dosage is given in accordance with the Recommended Dietary Allowances as suggested by the National Research Council's Food and Nutrition Board. Symptoms and effects are given for those nutrients that may be toxic.

Deficiency Effects and Symptoms

If nutrient intake is insufficient to meet requirements for a prolonged period of time, the ability to respond to stress is lessened and depletion and deterioration eventually occur, despite the effectiveness of the various mechanisms that prolong survival. The effects and symptoms of a deficiency are stated for each nutrient.

Beneficial Effect on Ailments

Those ailments that have been successfully treated with a specific nutrient are mentioned here. Additional information, including dosages, is provided in the section "Ailments and Other Stressful Conditions." Dosages listed in the "Ailments" section should not be taken as prescriptive but merely as representations of research findings. In many instances, nutrients should not be taken alone: they are more beneficial when accompanied by other nutrients.

Human Tests

Examples of tests on humans, in clinical situations, are those involving nutritional therapy. Dosages used in these tests should not be taken as prescriptive but merely as examples of how specific nutrients affect some people. Nutritional therapy applied to one individual may not work as well on others. Sources of further information are provided.

Animal Tests

Before results are applied to humans, extensive animal tests are done. There are, however, many biological similarities between humans and animals in nutritional therapy.

Chart of Beneficial Effects on Ailments

A chart listing the ailments that are associated with a specific vitamin or mineral follows the discussion of each nutrient. These include ailments for which, according to nutritional studies, this particular nutrient may be beneficial.

VITAMINS

VITAMIN A

Description

Vitamin A is a fat-soluble nutrient that occurs in nature in two forms: preformed vitamin A and provitamin A, or carotene. Preformed vitamin A is concentrated only in certain tissues of animal products in which the animal has metabolized the carotene contained in its food into vitamin A.[1] One of the richest natural sources of preformed vitamin A is fish-liver oil, which is classified as a food supplement. Some animal products, such as cream and butter, may contain both preformed vitamin A and carotene.

Carotene is a substance that must be converted into vitamin A before it can be utilized by the body. Carotene is abundant in carrots, from which its name is derived, but it is present in even higher concentrations in certain green leafy vegetables, such as beet greens, spinach, and broccoli. If, due to any disorder, the body is unable to use carotene, a vitamin A deficiency may arise.

Vitamin A aids in the growth and repair of body tissues and helps maintain smooth, soft, disease-free

[1] Helen Andrews Guthrie, *Introductory Nutrition*, 2d ed. (St. Louis: C. V. Mosby Co., 1971), p. 196.

skin. Internally it helps protect the mucous membranes of the mouth, nose, throat, and lungs, thereby reducing susceptibility to infection. This protection also aids the mucous membranes in combating the effects of various air pollutants. The soft tissue and all linings of the digestive tract, kidneys, and bladder are also protected. In addition, vitamin A prompts the secretion of gastric juices necessary for proper digestion of proteins. Other important functions of vitamin A include the building of strong bones and teeth, the formation of rich blood, and the maintenance of good eyesight. It is essential in the formation of visual purple, a substance in the eye which is necessary for proper night vision.

Absorption and Storage

The upper intestinal tract is the primary area of absorption of vitamin A; it is here that the fat-splitting enzymes and bile salts convert carotene into a usable nutrient. This conversion is stimulated by thyroxine, an amino acid obtained from the thyroid gland. Once converted into vitamin A, carotene is absorbed in the same way as is the preformed vitamin. Vitamin A is carried through the bloodstream, readily accessible to tissues throughout the body. Preformed vitamin A as found in fish-liver oil or other animal products is absorbed by the body three to five hours after ingestion, whereas the conversion and absorption of carotene takes six to seven hours.[2]

The conversion of carotene into vitamin A is not 100 percent complete; approximately one-third of the carotene in food is converted into vitamin A. Less than one-fourth of the carotene in carrots and root vegetables undergoes conversion, and about one-half of the carotene in leafy green vegetables undergoes conversion.[3] Some unchanged carotene is absorbed into the circulatory system and stored in the fat tissues rather than in the liver. Unabsorbed carotene is excreted in the feces.

The ability of the body to utilize carotene varies with the food and the form in which the food is ingested. Cooking, pureeing, or mashing of vegetables ruptures the cell membranes and therefore makes the carotene more available for absorption.

Factors interfering with absorption of vitamin A and carotene include strenuous physical activity performed within four hours of consumption, intake of mineral oil, excessive consumption of alcohol, excessive consumption of iron, and the use of cortisone and other drugs. The intake of polyunsaturated fatty acids with carotene results in rapid destruction of carotene unless antioxidants also are present.[4] Even cold weather can hinder the transport and metabolism of both vitamin A and carotene. Diabetics cannot convert carotene into vitamin A.

Approximately 90 percent of the body's vitamin A is stored in the liver, with small amounts deposited in the fat tissues, lungs, kidneys, and retinas of the eyes. Under stressful conditions the body will use this reserve supply if it is not receiving enough vitamin A from the diet. Gastrointestinal and liver disorders, infections of any kind, or any condition in which the bile duct is obstructed may limit the body's capacity to retain and use vitamin A. Factors affecting absorption of vitamin A include the quantity given, influence of other substances present in the intestines, and amount of the vitamin stored in the body. For these reasons, the recommended dietary amounts vary for each individual.

Dosage and Toxicity

Recommended Dietary Allowances of vitamin A, as established by the National Research Council, are 1,500 International Units (IU) for infants, 3,000 IU for children one to eleven years of age, and 5,000 IU for adults. These amounts increase during disease, trauma, pregnancy, and lactation. Requirements vary for people who smoke, those who live in highly polluted areas, people who easily absorb vitamin A, and those who have had their stored supply of vitamin A depleted by pneumonia or nephritis. Increased intake of vitamins C and E will help prevent excessive oxidation of stored vitamin A.

Research indicates that no more than 50,000 IU per day can be utilized by the body except in therapeutic cases, where up to 100,000 IU is recommended. It has been suggested that the best level is somewhere between 25,000 and 50,000 IU.[5] If there is no vitamin deficiency, daily administration of 50,000 IU may be toxic. Dosages of 18,500 IU given daily for one to three months have been reported toxic for infants. Recommended amounts may be supplied through food sources;

[2] J. I. Rodale, *The Health Builder* (Emmaus, Pa.: Rodale Books, 1957), pp. 273-274.
[3] Rodale, *The Health Builder*, p. 196.

[4] Rodale, *The Health Builder*, p. 196.
[5] Paavo Airola, *How to Get Well* (Phoenix, Ariz.: Health Plus Pub., 1974), p. 260.

e.g., ½ pound of calf's liver contains approximately 74,000 IU preformed vitamin A, whereas a carrot contains 11,000 IU of carotene.

Toxicity symptoms include nausea, vomiting, diarrhea, dry skin, hair loss, headaches, appetite loss, sore lips, and flaky, itchy skin. Bone fragility, thickening of long bones, deep bone pain, enlargement of the liver and spleen, blurred vision, and skin rashes are symptoms of prolonged excessive intake. Excessive daily use of massive dosages of vitamin A also may lead to reduced thyroid activity and abnormalities in the skin, eyes, and mucous membranes. Vitamin A toxicity can occur when a person takes 100,000 IU of straight vitamin A daily for many months. If toxicity is detected, the symptoms will disappear in a few days if the vitamin is withdrawn. Vitamin C can help prevent the harmful effects of vitamin A toxicity.

Deficiency Effects and Symptoms

The eyes are well-known indicators of vitamin A deficiency. One of the first symptoms is night blindness, an inability of the eyes to adjust to darkness. Another eye-related deficiency symptom is xerosis, a disease in which the eyeball loses luster, it becomes dry and inflamed, and visual acuity is reduced.

Other signs of deficiency include rough, dry, or prematurely aged skin; loss of sense of smell; loss of appetite; frequent fatigue; skin blemishes; sties in the eye; and diarrhea. More severe symptoms are corneal ulcers and softening of bones and teeth. Deficiency of vitamin A leads to the rapid loss of vitamin C.

Vitamin A deficiency may occur when an inadequate dietary supply exists; when the body is unable to absorb or store the vitamin (as in ulcerative colitis, cirrhosis of the liver, and obstruction of the bile ducts); when an ailment interferes with the conversion of carotene to vitamin A (as in diabetes mellitus and hypothyroidism); and when any rapid bodily loss of the vitamin occurs (as in pneumonia, hyperthyroidism, chronic nephritis, scarlet fever, and some respiratory infections).

Beneficial Effect on Ailments

Many people are unaware of the importance of vitamin A in fighting infections. By giving strength to cell walls, it helps protect the mucous membranes against invading bacteria. People who live in environments with high air-pollution counts are more susceptible to infections and colds than are people who live in environments with cleaner air. If infection has already occurred, therapeutic doses of vitamin A will help keep it from spreading.

Vitamin A can be used successfully in treating several eye disorders, such as Bitot's spots (white, elevated, sharply outlined patches on the white of the eye), blurred vision, night blindness, cataracts, crossed eyes, and nearsightedness. Therapeutic dosages of vitamin A are necessary for treatment of glaucoma and conjunctivitis, an inflammation of the mucous membrane that lines the eyelids.

Administration of vitamin A has helped shorten the duration of communicable diseases—measles, scarlet fever, the common cold, and infections of the eye, middle ear, intestines, ovaries, uterus, and vagina. It also has been effective in reducing high cholesterol levels and atheroma, fatty degeneration or thickening of the wall of the larger arteries.

Vitamin A has proved successful in treating cases of bronchial asthma, chronic rhinitis, and dermatitis. Vitamin A has also been helpful in treating patients suffering from tuberculosis, cirrhosis of the liver, emphysema, gastritis, and hyperthyroidism. Patients with nephritis (inflammation of the kidney), migraine headaches, and tinnitus (ringing in the ear) have benefited from vitamin A therapy.

Externally, vitamin A is used in treating acne; when applied locally, it can clear up impetigo, boils, carbuncles, and open ulcers. Vitamin A applied directly to open wounds hastens the healing process in cases where healing has been retarded because cortisone has been used. It also stimulates the production of mucus, which in turn prevents scarring. A treatment using injections of vitamin A has proved effective in the removal of planter's warts.[6]

Human Tests

1. Vitamin A and Stress Ulcers. Dr. Merril S. Chernov and his associates, Dr. Harry W. Hale, Jr., and Dr. MacDonald Wood, did a two-part study of severely injured patients to determine whether administration of vitamin A would prevent formation of stress ulcers. According

[6] J. I. Rodale and Staff, *The Health Seeker* (Emmaus, Pa.: Rodale Books, 1967), p. 897.

to Chernov, serum vitamin A levels dropped "sharply and profoundly" in severely injured patients. (*Medical World News*, January 7, 1972.)

The first part of the study involved 35 patients suffering from burns covering more than 25 percent of their bodies or major injuries to two or more organs. Vitamin A levels in the serum fell dramatically in 29 of the patients within 24 to 72 hours after hospitalization.

In the second part of the study, 14 of 36 similarly stressed patients received 10,000 to 400,000 IU of water-soluble vitamin A daily. Their care was the same as that of the other 22 patients.

Results. Evidence of stress ulcers was seen in 15 of the 22 untreated patients in the second group (69 percent). Massive intestinal bleeding developed in seven of these patients, and serious intestinal bleeding developed in another seven. Of the fourteen patients treated with massive doses of vitamin A, upper gastrointestinal bleeding occurred in only two.

Dr. Chernov stated, "The sudden and marked depletion of vitamin A is directly related to the corresponding depression of the serum protein, and particularly that fragment of the serum protein involved in transport of vitamin A. This results initially in the development of superficial mucosal erosions followed later by frank ulceration and hemorrhage." The results of Dr. Chernov's study suggest that treatment with high doses of vitamin A reduced the risk of gastroduodenal ulceration in these severely stressed patients. (J. I. Rodale, ed., *Prevention*, April 1972.)

2. Vitamin A and Acne. 100 acne patients were given oral doses of 100,000 IU of vitamin A (halibut-liver oil) at bedtime.

Results. 36 patients were completely relieved of acne, and 43 were relieved except for an occasional pustule. In most cases, responses occurred in less than nine months. (Jon V. Straumfjord, M.D., Astoria, Oregon, reported in Rodale, ed., *Prevention*, November 1968.)

3. Vitamin A and Acne Lesions. 75 patients who failed to respond to other forms of treatment were given 100,000 IU of vitamin A per day.

Results. Disappearance of the lesions occurred for 30 patients in two and one-half months, for another 30 in three months, and for 10 more in five and one-half

months. All could be regarded as cured at the end of three months. Drawbacks stated: (1) treatment could take up to a year; (2) dosage given was very high and could have toxic effects. (Dr. K. D. Larharl, *Journal of the Indian Medical Association*, March 1954; reported in Rodale, ed., *Prevention*, November 1968.)

4. Vitamin A and Asthma. 5,000 cases suffering from bronchial dermatitis, bronchial asthma, and chronic rhinitis were treated with vitamins A and D and bone meal.

Results. There was success in relieving the symptoms of 75 percent of the patients, including 1,000 patients suffering from bronchial asthma. (Dr. Carl J. Reich, 1972; reported in Rodale, ed., *Prevention*, September 1970.)

5. Vitamin A and Premenstrual Symptoms. 24 patients were given large doses of vitamin A.

Results. There were improvements in premenstrual symptoms. Seventeen patients were partially relieved of symptoms, and all breast tenderness was eliminated. Three more noticed considerable improvement but had some distress. Four patients did not respond to the therapy. (Dr. Alexander Pou, *American Journal of Obstetrics and Gynecology*, June 1951.)

Animal Tests

1. Vitamin A and Tumors. Hamsters given high doses of vitamin A before being subjected to benzpyrene (a carcinogen in smoke) were protected against the appearance of squamous tumors on the lung. Hamsters given a similar high dosage after the development of lung cancer showed a complete block of the cancer process.

Results. Of the 60 treated animals, 5 developed tumors and 4 of these were noncancerous. Of the 53 untreated animals, 16 developed lung cancer. (Dr. Umberto Saffioto of the National Cancer Institute, Bethesda, Maryland, as reported in Rodale, ed., *Prevention*, December 1969.)

2. Vitamin A and Reproductive Processes. Bulls deficient in vitamin A suffered degeneration of their seminiferous tubules. They reportedly regained full potency after receiving strong doses of vitamin A. (J. L. Madsen, *Journal of Animal Science*, reported in Rodale, ed., *Prevention*, January 1971.)

VITAMIN A MAY BE BENEFICIAL FOR THE FOLLOWING AILMENTS*:

Body Member	Ailment or Other Stressful Condition*
Bladder	Cystitis
Blood/Circulatory system	Angina pectoris
	Arteriosclerosis
	Atherosclerosis
	Diabetes
	Hemophilia
	Jaundice
	Mononucleosis
	Stroke (cerebrovascular accident)
Bones	Fracture
	Osteomalacia
	Rickets
Bowel	Celiac disease
	Colitis
	Diarrhea
Brain/Nervous system	Alcoholism
	Epilepsy
	Meningitis
Ear	Ear infection
Eye	Amblyopia
	Bitot spots
	Cataracts
	Conjunctivitis
	Eyestrain
	Glaucoma
	Night blindness
Gallbladder	Gallstones
Glands	Cystic fibrosis
	Diabetes
	Goiter
	Hyperthyroidism
	Prostatitis
	Swollen glands
Hair/Scalp	Hair problems
Head	Fever
	Headache
	Sinusitis
Heart	Angina pectoris
	Arteriosclerosis
	Atherosclerosis

Body Member	Ailment or Other Stressful Condition*
	Congestive heart failure
	Myocardial infarction
Intestine	Celiac disease
	Constipation
	Hemorrhoids
	Worms
Joints	Arthritis
	Gout
Kidney	Kidney stones (renal calculi)
	Nephritis
Leg	Varicose veins
Liver	Cirrhosis of liver
	Hepatitis
	Jaundice
Lungs/Respiratory system	Allergies
	Asthma
	Bronchitis
	Common cold
	Croup
	Emphysema
	Hay fever (allergic rhinitis)
	Influenza
	Sinusitis
	Tuberculosis
Mouth	Canker sore
	Halitosis
Muscles	Muscular dystrophy
Nails	Nail problems
Reproductive system	Prostatitis
	Vaginitis
Skin	Abscess
	Acne
	Athlete's foot
	Bedsores
	Boil (furuncle)
	Burns
	Carbuncle
	Dandruff
	Dermatitis
	Dry skin
	Eczema
	Impetigo
	Psoriasis
	Shingles (herpes zoster)

*The word "ailment" used in subsequent tables of beneficial effects of nutrients is intended to include other stressful conditions.

Body Member	Ailment or Other Stressful Condition*
	Ulcers
	Warts
Stomach	Gastritis
	Gastroenteritis
	Stomach ulcer (peptic)
Teeth/Gums	Pyorrhea
	Tooth and gum disorders
General	Alcoholism
	Chicken pox
	Fatigue
	Fever
	Infection
	Kwashiorkor
	Measles
	Pregnancy
	Rheumatic fever
	Rhinitis
	Scurvy
	Stress

VITAMIN B COMPLEX

Description

All B vitamins are water-soluble substances that can be cultivated from bacteria, yeasts, fungi, or molds. *The known B-complex vitamins* are B_1 (thiamine), B_2 (riboflavin), B_3 (niacin), B_6 (pyridoxine), B_{12} (cyanocobalamin), B_{13} (orotic acid), B_{15} (pangamic acid), B_{17} (laetrile), biotin, choline, folic acid, inositol, and PABA (para-aminobenzoic acid). The grouping of these water-soluble compounds under the term "B complex" is based upon their common source distribution, their close relationship in vegetable and animal tissues, and their functional relationships.

The B-complex vitamins are active in providing the body with energy, basically by converting carbohydrates into glucose, which the body "burns" to produce energy. They are vital in the metabolism of fats and protein. In addition, the B vitamins are necessary for normal functioning of the nervous system and may be the single most important factor for health of the nerves. They are essential for maintenance of muscle tone in the gas-

trointestinal tract and for the health of skin, hair, eyes, mouth, and liver.

All the B vitamins except B_{17} are natural constituents of brewer's yeast, liver, or whole-grain cereals. Brewer's yeast is the richest natural source of the B-complex group. Another important source of the B vitamins is production by the intestinal bacteria. These bacteria grow best on milk sugar and small amounts of fat in the diet. Maintaining milk-free diets or taking sulfonamides and other antibiotics may destroy these valuable bacteria.

Absorption and Storage

Because of the water-solubility of the B-complex vitamins, any excess is excreted and not stored. Therefore, they must be continually replaced. All B vitamins mixed with salve absorb readily.

Sulfa drugs, sleeping pills, insecticides, and estrogen create a condition in the digestive tract which can destroy the B vitamins. Certain B vitamins are lost through perspiration.

Dosage and Toxicity

The most important thing to remember is that all the B vitamins should be taken together. They are so interrelated in function that large doses of any one of them may be therapeutically valueless or may cause a deficiency of others. For example, if extra B_6 is taken in 50-milligram potencies, it is important that a complete B complex accompany it. In nature, we find the B-complex vitamins in yeast, green vegetables, etc., but nowhere do we find a single B vitamin isolated from the rest. Natural forms of the B vitamins are preferable to the synthetic forms since the natural forms have all of the B factors, even those not yet known, plus valuable enzymes. Most preparations of single B vitamins are synthetic or, at least, no longer in their natural form. These synthetic B vitamins are used primarily to overcome severe deficiencies or serious physical conditions in which rapid results are needed. When taking supplements, it is very important to remember that the B vitamins exert many different effects upon each other; therefore excesses and insufficiencies may be harmful.

The need for the B-complex vitamins increases during infection or stress. Alcoholics and individuals who consume excessive amounts of carbohydrates require a higher intake of B vitamins for proper metabolism. Coffee uses up the B vitamins. Children and pregnant women need extra B vitamins for normal growth.

Deficiency Effects and Symptoms

The 13 or more B vitamins are so meagerly supplied in the American diet that almost every American lacks some of them. If a person is tired, irritable, nervous, depressed, or even suicidal, suspect a vitamin B deficiency. Gray hair, falling hair, baldness, acne, or other skin troubles indicate a lack of B vitamins. A poor appetite, insomnia, neuritis, anemia, constipation, or high cholesterol level is also an indicator of a vitamin B deficiency. Having an enlarged tongue (including the buds on each side) that is shiny, bright red, and full of grooves means B vitamins are needed. One reason there is so much B-vitamin deficiency in the American population is that Americans eat so many processed foods from which the B vitamins have often been removed. Another reason for widespread deficiency is the high amount of sugar consumed. *Sugar and alcohol destroy the B-complex vitamins.*

Beneficial Effect on Ailments

The B vitamins have been used in the treatment of barbiturate overdosage, alcoholic psychoses, and drug-induced delirium. An adequate dose has been found to control migraine headaches and attacks of Ménière's syndrome. Some heart abnormalities have responded to use of B complex because the nerves affecting the heart need the B-complex vitamins for smooth, quiet functioning. Massive dosages of the B-complex vitamins have been used to cure polio, to improve the condition of hypersensitive children who fail to respond favorably to drugs such as Ritalin, and to improve cases of shingles. Nervous individuals and persons working under tension can greatly benefit from taking larger than normal doses of B vitamins.

Postoperative nausea and vomiting, resulting from anesthesia, can be successfully treated with B vitamins. The amount of B vitamins needed seems to be related to the amount of female sex hormones available. Menstrual difficulty is often relieved with small doses. The B vitamins may also help these ailments: beriberi, pellagra, constipation, burning feet, tender gums, burning and drying eyes, fatigue, lack of appetite, skin disorders, cracks at the corner of the mouth, and anemia.

Human Tests

1. B Vitamins and Ménière's Syndrome. A person testified that the therapy of Dr. Mills Atkinson, which consisted of heavy intakes of the B-complex vitamins four times daily, reversed his case of Ménière's syndrome (see "Ailments," p. 147), which had lasted almost four months.

Results. Within two months the B-vitamin treatment relieved the dizziness, double vision, nausea, and inability to concentrate associated with this ailment. ("Migraine, Ménière's and Mealtime," Rodale, ed., *Prevention*, August 1971.)

2. B Vitamins and Senile Dementia (Deteriorative Mental State of the Aged). Patients in mental hospitals and convalescent homes who were suffering from senile dementia exhibited a dramatic improvement in their mental condition 24 to 48 hours after large doses of B vitamins were administered. (Bicknell and Prescott, *Vitamins in Medicine*, as reported in Linda Clark, *Know Your Nutrition*, 1973, p. 67.)

Animal Tests

1. B Complex; Natural versus Synthetic. Silver foxes were fed a synthetic diet so that each component of the diet could be known. The foxes were fed all of the known synthetic B vitamins as part of their rations, but the animals did not grow; their fur quality deteriorated, and finally they died. This condition was reversed with only one change in the diet fed to another group of foxes: B-complex foods—yeast and liver—were added.

Results. The animals in the second group grew normally, and the quality of the fur improved. (*Scandinavian Veterinary*, vol. 30, pp. 1121-1143, 1940, as reported in J. I. Rodale, ed., *The* Prevention *Method for Better Health*, Rodale Books, Emmaus, Pa., 1968, p. 568.)

2. B-Complex Vitamins and Hair. A group of mice were placed on a synthetic diet that included all necessary nutrients. They grew for a few days and then became stationary in weight. After 20 to 30 days they began to lose their hair and developed hunched backs. A similar group were placed on the same diet, with whole yeast added.

Results. When the natural products were added to their diet, the second group did not show the symptoms shown by the first group. (*Journal of Nutrition*, vol. 21, p. 609, 1941.)

3. B-Complex Vitamins and Fatigue. Three groups of rats were fed three different diets for 12 weeks. The first group ate a basic diet, fortified with nine synthetic and two natural vitamins. The second group was fed the same diet, vitamins and all, with a plentiful supply of vitamin B complex added. The third group was fed the original fortified diet, but instead of vitamin B complex, 10 percent desiccated liver was added to their ration.

Results. The first group showed the least amount of growth in 12 weeks. The second group experienced a little higher rate of growth in that 12-week period. The third group grew about 15 percent faster than the first group. (B. H. Ershoff, M.D., *Proceedings of the Society of Experimental Biology and Medicine*, July 1951, as reported in Rodale, ed., *The* Prevention *Method for Better Health*, p. 610.)

4. B-Complex Vitamins and Fatigue. This experiment is based on the same rats and their diets used in Test 3. These same rats were placed one by one into a drum of water from which they could not climb out.

Results. The rats on the original diet swam for an average of 13.3 minutes before they gave up. The second group of rats swam for 13.4 minutes before giving up. Of the third group, three swam for 63, 83, and 87 minutes, respectively. The rest of the rats in the third group were swimming vigorously at the end of two hours, when testing terminated. The rats that received desiccated liver (those in the third group) swam almost six times as long as did the others. (Rodale, ed., *The* Prevention *Method for Better Health*, p. 611.)

VITAMIN B COMPLEX MAY BE BENEFICIAL FOR THE FOLLOWING AILMENTS:

Body Member	Ailment
Bladder	Cystitis
Blood/Circulatory system	Anemia
	Angina pectoris
	Arteriosclerosis
	Atherosclerosis
	Cholesterol level, high
	Diabetes
	Hypertension
	Hypoglycemia
	Leukemia
	Stroke (cerebrovascular accident)
Bowel	Diarrhea
Brain/Nervous system	Alcoholism

Body Member	Ailment
	Bell's palsy
	Epilepsy
	Insomnia
	Meningitis
	Mental illness
	Multiple sclerosis
	Neuritis
	Parkinson's disease
	Stroke (cerebrovascular accident)
	Vertigo
Ear	Ménière's syndrome
Eye	Amblyopia
	Cataracts
	Conjunctivitis
	Eyestrain
	Glaucoma
	Night blindness
Gallbladder	Gallstones
Glands	Adrenal exhaustion
	Cystic fibrosis
	Hyperthyroidism
	Prostatitis
	Swollen glands
Hair/Scalp	Baldness
	Dandruff
	Hair problems
Head	Fever
	Headache
Heart	Angina pectoris
	Arteriosclerosis
	Atherosclerosis
	Congestive heart failure
	Hypertension
	Myocardial infarction
Intestine	Celiac disease
	Constipation
	Diverticulitis
	Hemorrhoids
	Indigestion (dyspepsia)
	Worms
Joints	Arthritis
	Bursitis
	Gout
Kidney	Nephritis

Body Member	Ailment
Leg	Leg cramp
	Phlebitis
	Sciatica
	Varicose veins
Liver	Cirrhosis of liver
	Hepatitis
Lungs/Respiratory system	Common cold
	Emphysema
	Hay fever (allergic rhinitis)
	Influenza
	Pneumonia
Mouth	Canker sore
	Halitosis
Muscles	Parkinson's disease
Nails	Nail growth
Reproductive system	Prostatitis
	Vaginitis
Skin	Abscess
	Acne
	Bedsores
	Bruises
	Burns
	Dandruff
	Dermatitis
	Eczema
	Psoriasis
	Shingles (herpes zoster)
	Ulcers
Stomach	Gastritis
	Gastroenteritis
	Indigestion (dyspepsia)
	Stomach ulcer (peptic)
Teeth/Gums	Pyorrhea
General	Aging
	Alcoholism
	Arthritis
	Backache
	Beriberi
	Cancer
	Edema
	Fatigue
	Fever
	Hypoxia
	Infection

Body Member	Ailment
	Overweight and obesity
	Pellagra
	Pregnancy
	Stress
	Stroke (cerebrovascular accident)

VITAMIN B$_1$ (THIAMINE)

Description

Thiamine or vitamin B$_1$ is a water-soluble vitamin that combines with pyruvic acid to form a coenzyme necessary for the breakdown of carbohydrates into glucose, or simple sugar, which is oxidized by the body to produce energy. Thiamine is vulnerable to heat, air, and water in cooking. Thiamine is a component of the germ and bran of wheat, the husk of rice, and that portion of all grains which is commercially milled away to give the grain a lighter color and finer texture.[7]

Known as the "morale vitamin" because of its relation to a healthy nervous system and its beneficial effect on mental attitude (see Human Test 4), thiamine is also linked with improving individual learning capacity.[8] It is necessary for consistent growth in children and for the improvement of muscle tone in the stomach, the intestines, and the heart. Thiamine is essential for stabilizing the appetite by improving food assimilation and digestion, particularly that of starches, sugars, and alcohol.

A diet rich in brewer's yeast, wheat germ, blackstrap molasses, and bran will provide the body with adequate thiamine and will help prevent undue accumulation of fatty deposits in the artery walls.

Absorption and Storage

Thiamine is rapidly absorbed in the upper and lower small intestine. It is then carried by the circulatory system to the liver, kidneys, and heart, where it may combine further with manganese and specific proteins to become active enzymes. These are the enzymes that break down carbohydrates into simple sugars.

Thiamine is not stored in the body in any great quantity and therefore must be supplied daily. It is excreted in the urine in amounts that reflect the intake and the quantity stored. Eating excessive amounts of sugar will

[7]J. I. Rodale, *The Complete Book of Vitamins* (Emmaus, Pa.: Rodale Books, 1968), pp. 179-184.
[8]Rodale, *The Complete Book of Vitamins*, p. 84.

cause a thiamine depletion, as will smoking and drinking alcohol. Thiamine can be destroyed by an enzyme present in raw clams and oysters.

Dosage and Toxicity

Individual thiamine needs are determined by body weight, the quantity of the vitamin synthesized in the intestinal tract, and daily calorie intake. As the calorie intake, especially of carbohydrates, increases, the proportion of thiamine ingested increases. The National Research Council recommends 0.5 milligram of thiamine per 1000 calories daily for all ages.[9] A thiamine intake of 1.4 milligrams daily is recommended during pregnancy and lactation. The need for additional B_1 increases during severe diarrhea, fever, stress, and surgery. There are no known toxic effects with thiamine.

Deficiency Effects and Symptoms

A deficiency of thiamine not only makes it difficult for a person to digest carbohydrates but also leaves too much pyruvic acid in the blood. This causes an oxygen deficiency that results in loss of mental alertness, labored breathing, and cardiac damage. First signs of a thiamine deficiency include easy fatigue, loss of appetite, irritability, and emotional instability. If the deficiency is not arrested, confusion and loss of memory appear, followed closely by gastric distress, abdominal pains, and constipation. Heart irregularities crop up, and finally, prickling sensations in the lower extremities, impaired vibratory sense, and tenderness of calf muscles will occur. A thiamine deficiency can also lead to inflammation of the optic nerve. Without thiamine, the function of the central nervous system, which depends upon glucose for energy, is impaired.

A thiamine deficiency affects the cardiovascular system as well. The heart muscles are weakened, and cardiac failure may occur. The gastrointestinal tract is also affected, and symptoms such as indigestion, severe constipation, anorexia (a loss of appetite), and gastric atony (loss of muscle tone in the stomach) may occur. "Some researchers believe that the lack of thiamine may be the first link in a chain leading by way of the liver and female hormones to cancer of the uterus."[10]

Beneficial Effect on Ailments

Thiamine is used in the treatment of beriberi, a deficiency disease associated with malnutrition.[11] Thiamine intake has improved the excretion of fluid stored in the body, decreased rapid heart rate, shrunken enlarged hearts, and normalized electrocardiograms.

Nutrients such as thiamine and niacin have been used together to treat multiple sclerosis patients. Dr. George Schumacher tells of his use of thiamine hydrochloride given intraspinally to two multiple sclerosis patients with noted improvement. Dr. Fredrick Klenner used large doses (100 milligrams) of B_1, B_3, and B_6 with reported success.[12]

Many other ailments have been aided by the administration of thiamine. Thiamine is essential in the manufacture of hydrochloric acid, which aids in digestion. It helps in eliminating nausea, especially that caused by air or sea sickness. It has improved people's dispositions by alleviating fatigue. Thiamine helps improve muscle tone in the stomach and intestines, which in turn relieves constipation. Herpes zoster, a painful clustering of blisters behind the ear, has been successfully treated with thiamine.[13]

Dentists have found B_1 useful. Dental postoperative pain is promptly and completely relieved in many patients by the administration of thiamine. Pain can often be prevented before the operation by administration of B_1 to the patient. Thiamine therapy has reduced the healing time of dry tooth sockets. Evidence shows that replacement of thiamine to injured and diseased nerves not only restores proper functioning but also relieves pain.[14]

Human Tests

1. Vitamin B_1 and Morale. Over several years, Horwitt and coworkers studied the psychological effects of thiamine deficiency on psychiatric patients in an institution. The subjects received varying amounts of thiamine in an adequate diet. They were tested for various deficiency effects.

[9]Marie V. Krause and Martha A. Hunscher, *Food, Nutrition and Diet Therapy* (Philadelphia: W. B. Saunders Co., 1972), p. 132.

[10]Ernest Ayre and W. A. G. Gauld, *Science*, April 12, 1946; also J. I. Rodale, *The Encyclopedia for Healthful Living* (Emmaus, Pa.: Rodale Books, 1970), p. 117.

[11]See "Beriberi," p. 116.

[12]J. I. Rodale and Staff, *Encyclopedia of Common Diseases* (Emmaus, Pa.: Rodale Books, 1969), pp. 786-787.

[13]Betty Lee Morales (ed.), *Cancer Control Journal*, vol. 2, no. 3, p. 13, June 1974.

[14]J. L. O. Bock, *U.S. Armed Forces Medical Journal*, March 1953.

Results. When approximately four-tenths milligram of thiamine was administered, specific conditions, including loss of inhibitory emotional control, paranoid trends, manic-depressive features, and confusion, were helped. (M. K. Horwitt et al., "Investigations of Human Requirements of B-Complex Vitamins," *National Research Council Bull.* 116, 1948.)

2. Vitamin B₁ and Herpes Zoster. 25 patients were given intramuscular injections of 200 milligrams of thiamine hydrochloride daily.

Results. Herpes zoster, a stubborn, painful clustering of small blisters near the ear, was successfully treated. (A. L. Oriz, *Medical World*, November 1958.)

3. Vitamin B₁ and Mental Ability. An experiment was conducted by Dr. Ruth Linn Harrell which involved 104 children from nine to nineteen years of age. Half of the children were given a vitamin B₁ pill each day, and the other half received a placebo. The test lasted six weeks.

Results. It was found by a series of tests that the group that was given the vitamin gained one-fourth more in learning ability than did the other group. (Dr. Ruth Flinn Harrell, "Effect of Added Thiamine on Learning," as reported in Rodale and Staff, *The Health Seeker*, pp. 18 and 19.)

VITAMIN B₁ MAY BE BENEFICIAL FOR THE FOLLOWING AILMENTS:

Body Member	Ailment
Blood/Circulatory system	Anemia
	Diabetes
Bowel	Constipation
	Diarrhea
Brain/Nervous system	Alcoholism
	Bell's palsy
	Mental illness
	Multiple sclerosis
	Neuritis
Ear	Ménière's syndrome
Eye	Amblyopia
	Night blindness
Head	Fever
	Headache
Heart	Congestive heart failure
Intestine	Worms
Leg	Leg cramp
	Sciatica
Lungs/Respiratory system	Influenza
Skin	Shingles (herpes zoster)
Stomach	Indigestion (dyspepsia)
General	Alcoholism
	Beriberi
	Pellagra
	Stress

VITAMIN B₂ (RIBOFLAVIN)

Description

Vitamin B₂, also known as riboflavin, is a water-soluble vitamin occurring naturally in those foods in which the other B vitamins exist. Riboflavin is stable to heat, oxidation, and acid although it disintegrates in the presence of alkali or light, especially ultraviolet light.

Riboflavin functions as part of a group of enzymes that are involved in the breakdown and utilization of carbohydrates, fats, and proteins. Riboflavin is necessary for cell respiration because it works with enzymes in the utilization of cell oxygen. It also is necessary for the maintenance of good vision, skin, nails, and hair.

The amount of B₂ found in most foods is so little that it normally is quite difficult to obtain a sufficient supply without supplementing the diet. Good sources of riboflavin are liver, tongue, and other organ meats. The richest natural source is brewer's yeast.

Absorption and Storage

Riboflavin is easily absorbed through the walls of the small intestine. It is then carried by the blood to the tissues of the body and excreted in the urine. The amount excreted depends upon the intake and relative need of the tissues and may be accompanied by a loss of protein from the body. Small amounts of riboflavin are found in the liver and kidneys, but it is not stored to any great degree in the body and therefore must be supplied regularly in the diet.[15]

[15] Krause and Hunscher, *Food, Nutrition and Diet Therapy*, p. 134.

Dosage and Toxicity

According to the National Research Council, the daily riboflavin requirements are related to body size, metabolic rate, and rate of growth. These factors are directly related to the protein and calorie intake of the individual. The Recommended Dietary Allowance is 1.6 milligrams for the adult male and 1.2 milligrams for the female. Pregnancy and lactation requirements are 1.5 and 1.7 milligrams, respectively.

There is no known toxicity of riboflavin. However, prolonged ingestion of large doses of any one of the B-complex vitamins, including riboflavin, may result in high urinary losses of other B vitamins. Therefore, it is important to take a complete B complex with any single B vitamin.

Deficiency Effects and Symptoms

Riboflavin deficiency is the most common vitamin deficiency in America. Deficiency may result from one or several of these factors: (1) long-established faulty dietary habits; (2) food idiosyncrasies ("I won't eat liver!"); (3) alcoholism; (4) arbitrarily selected diets for relief of symptoms of digestive trouble; and (5) prolonged following of a restricted diet in the treatment of a disease such as peptic ulcer or diabetes.[16]

The most common symptoms of a lack of B_2 are cracks and sores in the corners of the mouth; a red, sore tongue; a feeling of grit and sand on the insides of the eyelids; burning of the eyes; eye fatigue; dilation of the pupil; changes in the cornea; sensitivity to light; lesions of the lips; scaling around the nose, mouth, forehead, and ears; trembling; sluggishness; dizziness; dropsy; inability to urinate; vaginal itching; oily skin; and baldness. A vitamin B_2 deficiency can cause some types of cataracts.[17] Experimental studies have shown that some forms of cancer may be related to B_2 deficiency.[18]

A lack of stamina and vigor, retarded gorwth, digestive disturbances, impaired lactation, and pellagra are results of a riboflavin deficiency. Hair and weight losses also frequently result.

[16]Rodale and Staff, *The Complete Book of Vitamins*, pp. 194-195.
[17]Linda Clark, *Know Your Nutrition* (New Canaan, Conn.: Keats Publ., 1973), p. 78.
[18]Boris Sokoloff, *Cancer: New Approaches, New Hope* (New York: Devin-Adair).

Beneficial Effect on Ailments

Riboflavin plays an important role in the prevention of some visual disturbances, especially cataracts. Undernourished women during the end of pregnancy often suffer from conditions such as visual disturbances, burning sensations in the eyes, excessive watering of eyes, and failing vision. These conditions can be helped by supplementing the diet with large doses of B_2. Riboflavin has brought relief to children suffering from eczema.

Human Test

1. B_2 (Riboflavin) and Visual Disturbances. 47 patients suffered from a variety of visual disturbances. They were sensitive to light; they suffered from eyestrain, burning sensations in their eyes, and visual fatigue; and their eyes watered easily. Six of them had cataracts.

Results. Within 24 hours after the administration of riboflavin, symptoms began to improve. After two days, the burning sensations and other symptoms began to disappear. All disorders were gradually cured. When riboflavin was removed, the symptoms gradually appeared again and once again were cured with administration of riboflavin. (Dr. Syndensticker, as reported in Rodale, ed., *Prevention*, November 1970.)

VITAMIN B_2 MAY BE BENEFICIAL FOR THE FOLLOWING AILMENTS:

Body Member	Ailment
Blood/Circulatory system	Diabetes
Bowel	Diarrhea
Brain/Nervous system	Multiple sclerosis
	Neuritis
	Parkinson's disease
	Vertigo
Ear	Ménière's syndrome
Eye	Cataracts
	Conjunctivitis
	Glaucoma
	Night blindness
Glands	Adrenal exhaustion
Hair/Scalp	Baldness
Intestine	Worms
Joints	Arthritis

Body Member	Ailment
Kidney	Nephritis
Leg	Leg cramp
Lungs/Respiratory system	Influenza
Reproductive system	Vaginitis
Skin	Acne
	Bedsores
	Dermatitis
	Ulcers
Stomach	Indigestion (dyspepsia)
	Stomach ulcer (peptic)
General	Alcoholism
	Cancer
	Pellagra
	Retarded growth
	Stress

VITAMIN B$_6$ (PYRIDOXINE)

Description

Vitamin B$_6$ is a water-soluble vitamin consisting of three related compounds: pyridoxine, pyridoxinal, and pyridoxamine. It is required for the proper absorption of vitamin B$_{12}$ and for the production of hydrochloric acid and magnesium. It also helps linoleic acid function better in the body. Pyridoxine plays an important role as a coenzyme in the breakdown and utilization of carbohydrates, fats, and proteins. It must be present for the production of antibodies and red blood cells. The release of glycogen for energy from the liver and muscles is facilitated by vitamin B$_6$. It also aids in the conversion of tryptophan, an essential amino acid, to niacin and is necessary for the synthesis and proper action of DNA and RNA.

Vitamin B$_6$ helps maintain the balance of sodium and potassium which regulates body fluids and promotes the normal functioning of the nervous and musculoskeletal systems. The best sources of vitamin B$_6$ are meats and whole grains. Desiccated liver and brewer's yeast are the recommended supplemental sources.

Absorption and Storage

A daily supply of vitamin B$_6$, together with the other B-complex vitamins, is necessary because it is excreted in the urine within eight hours after ingestion and is not stored in the liver. Fasting and reducing diets can deplete the body's supply of vitamin B$_6$ if proper supplements are not taken.

Dosage and Toxicity

Vitamin B$_6$ seems to be another B vitamin that, if administered alone, can cause an imbalance or deficiency of other B vitamins. The Recommended Dietary Allowance of vitamin B$_6$ is determined by an individual's daily protein intake. Adults need 2 milligrams of pyridoxine per 100 grams of protein per day, and children need 0.6 to 1.2 milligrams per 100 grams of protein per day. The need for vitamin B$_6$ increases during pregnancy, lactation, exposure to radiation, cardiac failure, aging, and use of oral contraceptives. Intravenous doses of 200 milligrams have proved nontoxic, and daily oral doses of 100 to 300 milligrams have been administered to alleviate drug-induced neuritis without side effects.[19]

Deficiency Effects and Symptoms

In cases of B$_6$ deficiency there is low blood sugar and low glucose tolerance, resulting in a sensitivity to insulin. Deficiency may also cause loss of hair, water retention during pregnancy, cracks around the mouth and eyes, numbness and cramps in arms and legs, slow learning, visual disturbances, neuritis, arthritis, heart disorders involving nerves, temporary paralysis of a limb, and an increase in urination.

If a vitamin B$_6$ deficiency is allowed to continue through late pregnancy, stillbirths or postdelivery infant mortality may result. Certain types of anemia may also be related to a B$_6$ deficiency.

Symptoms of a B$_6$ deficiency are similar to those seen in niacin and riboflavin deficiencies and may include muscular weakness, nervousness, irritability, depression, and dermatitis. Tingling hands, shoulder-hand syndrome, wrist-hand syndromes and arthritis associated with menopause also may be present.

Beneficial Effect on Ailments

There is evidence that suggests a relationship between vitamin B$_6$ and cholesterol metabolism; therefore B$_6$

[19] National Academy of Sciences, *Toxicants Occurring Naturally in Foods* (Washington, D.C.: National Research Council, 1973), p. 246.

may be involved in the control of atherosclerosis. Vitamin B_6 has been used in the treatment of nervous disorders and in the control of nausea and vomiting during pregnancy.

Vitamin B_6 has been successfully used to help treat a form of anemia in which red blood cells are too small; also male sexual disorders, eczema, thinning and loss of hair, elevated cholesterol level, diarrhea, hemorrhoids, pancreatitis, ulcers, muscular weakness, some types of heart disturbances, burning feet, some types of kidney stones, acne, tooth decay, and diabetes. It is needed to prevent and treat shoulder-hand syndrome. Administration of B_6 to mentally retarded children has helped relieve convulsize seizures. It also appears to be beneficial in treating stress.

As a natural diuretic, vitamin B_6 aids in the prevention of water buildup in the tissues. It has helped women who suffer from temporary premenstrual changes such as edema and may be effective in helping problems of overweight caused by water retention.

Human Tests

1. Vitamin B_6 and Parkinson's Disease. It was found that Parkinson's disease, a nervous disorder that causes trembling hands, responded to B_6 treatments. A case of the disease which had existed for 25 years responded to B_6 injections within 2 months. This is one of the unexpected results of B_6—whereas it may take a long time to derive benefits from some vitamins, B_6 seems to bring results quickly and dramatically. (Dr. Douw G. Stern, University of South Africa, as reported in Clark, *Know Your Nutrition*, p. 91.)

2. Vitamin B_6 and Painful Finger Joints. Vitamin B_6 was given to women and men near the age of menopause who had developed painful spurs or knots on the sides of their finger joints.

Results. There was a dramatic change after the administration of B_6. Finger joints ceased to be painful, and finger sensitivity and hand flexion improved within six weeks. (John M. Ellis, "The Doctor Who Looked at Hands," as reported in Clark, *Know Your Nutrition*, p. 91.)

Animal Tests

1. Vitamin B_6 and Cleft Palates. Cleft palates developed in 85 percent of the offspring of mice injected with cortisone four times daily during pregnancy.

Results. When pyridoxine was injected along with the cortisone, such abnormalities were reduced to 45 percent, and the addition of folic acid reduced the occurrence of cleft palate to 20 percent. On the basis of these experiments, folic acid and pyridoxine were given to human mothers who had previously borne cleft palate children, and all children subsequently born to these mothers were normal. (Dr. Lyndon A. Peer, 22d Annual Meeting of International College of Surgeons, as reported in Rodale, *The Health Seeker*, p. 194.)

VITAMIN B_6 MAY BE BENEFICIAL FOR THE FOLLOWING AILMENTS:

Body Member	Ailment
Blood/Circulatory system	Anemia
	Cholesterol level, high
	Diabetes
	Hypoglycemia
	Jaundice
	Pernicious anemia
Bladder	Cystitis
Bowel	Colitis
	Diarrhea
Brain/Nervous system	Bell's palsy
	Epilepsy
	Insomnia
	Mental illness
	Multiple sclerosis
	Neuritis
	Parkinson's disease
Ear	Dizziness
Eye	Conjunctivitis
Glands	Prostatitis
Hair/Scalp	Baldness
	Dandruff
Head	Headache
Intestine	Celiac disease
	Hemorrhoids
	Worms

Body Member	Ailment
Joints	Arthritis
Kidney	Kidney stones (renal calculi)
Lungs/Respiratory system	Asthma
	Common cold
	Influenza
	Tuberculosis
Mouth	Halitosis
Muscles	Muscular dystrophy
	Rheumatism
Reproductive system	Prostatitis
	Vaginitis
Skin	Acne
	Dandruff
	Dermatitis
	Eczema
	Psoriasis
	Shingles (herpes zoster)
Stomach	Gastritis
	Indigestion (dyspepsia)
	Nausea of pregnancy
Teeth/Gums	Pyorrhea
General	Alcoholism
	Edema
	Overweight and obesity
	Stress

VITAMIN B_{12}

Description

Vitamin B_{12}, a water-soluble vitamin, is unique in being the first cobalt-containing substance found to be essential for longevity, and it is the only vitamin that contains essential mineral elements. It cannot be made synthetically but must be grown, like penicillin, in bacteria or molds. Animal protein is almost the only source in which B_{12} occurs naturally in foods in substantial amounts. Liver is the best source; kidney, muscle meats, fish and dairy products are other good sources.

Vitamin B_{12} is necessary for normal metabolism of nerve tissue and is involved in protein, fat, and carbohydrate metabolism. B_{12} is closely related to the actions of four amino acids, pantothenic acid, and vitamin C. It also helps iron function better in the body and aids folic acid in the synthesis of choline.

Absorption and Storage

Vitamin B_{12} is prepared for absorption by two gastric secretions. It is poorly absorbed from the gastrointestinal tract unless the "intrinsic factor," a mucoprotein enzyme, is present. B_{12} needs to be combined with calcium during absorption to benefit the body properly. The presence of hydrochloric acid aids in the absorption of B_{12} given orally, and a properly functioning thyroid gland also helps B_{12} to be better absorbed.

After absorption, B_{12} is bound to serum protein (globulins) and is transported in the bloodstream to various tissues. The highest concentrations of B_{12} are found in the liver, kidneys, heart, pancreas, testes, brain, blood, and bone marrow. These body members are all related to red blood cell formation.

People deficient in B_{12} usually lack one or more gastric secretions necessary for its absorption. Many people lack the ability to absorb it at all.

Absorption of B_{12} appears to decrease with age and with iron, calcium, and B_6 deficiencies; absorption increases during pregnancy. The use of laxatives depletes the storage of B_{12}.

Dosage and Toxicity

Human requirements are minute but essential. The Recommended Dietary Allowance of vitamin B_{12} is 3 micrograms for adults and 4 micrograms for pregnant and lactating women. Infants require a daily intake of 3 micrograms, and growing children need 1 to 2 micrograms. A vegetarian diet frequently is low in vitamin B_1 and high in folic acid, which may mask a vitamin B_{12} deficiency. No cases of vitamin B_{12} toxicity have been reported, even with large doses.

Deficiency Effects and Symptoms

Symptoms of a vitamin B_{12} deficiency may take five or six years to appear, after the body's supply from natural sources has been restricted.[20] A deficiency of vitamin B_{12} is usually due to an absorption problem caused by a lack of the intrinsic factor. A deficiency begins with changes in the nervous system such as soreness and weakness in the legs and arms, diminished reflex re-

[20] Krause and Hunscher, *Food, Nutrition and Diet Therapy*, p. 141.

sponse and sensory perception, difficulty in walking and speaking (stammering), and jerking of limbs.

Lack of B_{12} has been found to cause a type of brain damage resembling schizophrenia. This brain damage may be detected by the following symptoms: sore mouth, numbness or stiffness, a feeling of deadness, shooting pains, needles-and-pins, or hot-and-cold sensations. The *British Medical Journal* (March 26, 1966) stated editorially, "It is true that vitamin B_{12} deficiency may cause severe psychotic symptoms which may vary in severity from mild disorders of mood, mental slowness, and memory defect to severe psychotic symptoms . . . occasionally, these mental disturbances may be the first manifestations of B_{12} deficiency. . . ."

Vitamin B_{12} deficiency also manifests itself in nervousness, neuritis, unpleasant body odor, menstrual disturbances, and difficulty in walking. If a deficiency is not detected in early stages, it *may* result in permanent mental deterioration and paralysis. When symptoms become serious, do not try to treat them yourself. Consult a doctor.

Beneficial Effect on Ailments

Injections of B_{12} can be used to treat patients suffering from pernicious anemia, an ailment characterized by insufficient red blood cells in the bone marrow. Injections rather than oral doses of B_{12} are used to bypass the absorption defect in pernicious anemic patients. B_{12} helps the red blood cells to mature up to a certain point, and, after that, protein, iron, vitamin C, and folic acid help to finish the development of the cells so that they can mature.[21] Like folic acid, vitamin B_{12} has been effective in the treatment of the intestinal syndrome sprue.

The *Medical Press* reported remarkable results in the treatment of osteoarthritis, a degenerative joint disease, and osteroporosis, a softening of the bone, with vitamin B_{12} (see Human Tests). The condition known as "tobacco amblyopia," a dimness of vision or a loss of vision due to poisoning by tobacco, has been improved with injections of vitamin B_{12} whether or not the patient stopped smoking. Symptoms are blackouts, headaches, and farsightedness.

B_{12} has provided relief of the following symptoms: fatigue, increased nervous irritability, mild impairment in memory, inability to concentrate, mental depression, insomnia, and lack of balance.[22] B_{12} also has been used

[21] Rodale and Staff, *The Encyclopedia of Common Diseases*, p. 451.
[22] Rodale and Staff, *The Complete Book of Vitamins*, p. 101.

successfully in the treatment of hepatitis, bursitis, and asthma.

Human Tests

1. Vitamin B_{12} and Cancer. Cancerous children were treated with B_{12} so that it could be shown that B_{12} could reduce the growth rate of cancer of the nervous system in children.

Results. Among 82 children who were treated with B_{12}, 32 (39 percent) survived up to 12 years. With conventional treatment, 8 out of 25 (32 percent) survived. (*Archives of Disease in Childhood*, December 1963, as reported in *Cancer*, March 28, 1964.)

2. Vitamin B_{12} and Osteoarthritis and Osteoporosis. 33 cases of osteoarthritis and two cases of osteoporosis were treated with vitamin B_{12}. The injected dosages varied between 30 and 900 micrograms, but the optimum dose was 100 micrograms per week.

Results. 20 patients benefited from the treatment within the first week; 7 obtained complete relief. At the end of the second week, four more showed partial relief. By the end of the third week, all but three of the patients showed some benefit. Three cases of rheumatoid arthritis did not react at all to the vitamin. (*Medical Press*, March 12, 1952, as reported in Rodale, *The Encyclopedia for Healthful Living*, p. 942.)

3. Vitamin B_{12} and Mental Confusion. A seventy-six-year-old patient was suffering from ailments relating to a poor system of blood vessels and heart. He was unable to walk without pain in his legs, and he showed signs of extreme depression and mental confusion. Finally he came down with a siege of pneumonia and sciatica, severe pain leg. Dr. Grabner prescribed 400 micrograms daily of injected vitamin B_{12}.

Results. After the fourth injection the patient exhibited a more pleasant attitude, and his state of confusion had improved. After two weeks, the dosage was reduced to 200 micrograms daily; then that was cut to every other day; and finally the patient was receiving 200 micrograms twice weekly. The doctor described his condition as healthy and completely normal mentally. (Dr. Grabner, "*Munchener Medizenische Wochenschrift*," *Munich Medical Weekly*, October 31, 1958, as reported in Rodale, *The Encyclopedia for Healthful Living*, 1970, p. 946.)

4. Vitamin B$_{12}$ and Bursitis. Injections of 1,000 micrograms of vitamin B$_{12}$ were given to subjects suffering from all types of bursitis. They were given the doses daily for three weeks, then once or twice a week for two or three weeks depending upon clinical observations.

Results. Rapid relief was achieved in all cases. Calcium deposits, if present, were absorbed, and there were no side effects or toxicity. Dr. Klemes reported that over a five-year period, only three patients failed to respond to vitamin B$_{12}$ therapy for treatment of bursitis. (Dr. I. S. Klemes, *Industrial Medicine and Surgery*, June 1957, as reported in Rodale, *The Encyclopedia for Healthful Living*, pp. 108-110.)

VITAMIN B$_{12}$ MAY BE BENEFICIAL FOR THE FOLLOWING AILMENTS:

Body Member	Ailment
Blood/Circulatory system	Anemia
	Angina pectoris
	Arteriosclerosis
	Atherosclerosis
	Diabetes
	Hypoglycemia
	Pernicious anemia
Bones	Osteoporosis
Brain/Nervous system	Epilepsy
	Insomnia
	Multiple sclerosis
	Neuritis
	Vertigo
Glands	Adrenal exhaustion
Heart	Angina pectoris
	Arteriosclerosis
	Atherosclerosis
Intestine	Celiac disease
	Worms
Joints	Arthritis
	Bursitis
Liver	Cirrhosis of liver
Lungs/Respiratory system	Allergies
	Asthma
	Tuberculosis
Muscles	Muscular dystrophy
Skin	Pellagra
	Psoriasis
	Shingles (herpes zoster)
	Ulcers

Body Member	Ailment
Stomach	Gastritis
	Stomach ulcer (peptic)
General	Alcoholism
	Overweight and obesity

VITAMIN B$_{13}$ (OROTIC ACID)

Description

Vitamin B$_{13}$, orotic acid, is not yet available in the United States but has been synthesized in Europe and used to treat multiple sclerosis. Orotic acid is found in natural sources such as organically grown root vegetables and whey, the liquid portion of soured or curdled milk.

Orotic acid is utilized by the body in the metabolism of folic acid and vitamin B$_{12}$. Orotic acid is also vital for aiding the replacement or restoration of some cells.[23]

Absorption and Storage

No available information.

Dosage and Toxicity

Dietary requirements are not known. This nutrient is available in supplemental form as calcium orotate.

Deficiency Effects and Symptoms

Deficiency symptoms are not known, but is believed that a deficiency may lead to liver disorders, cell degeneration, and premature aging.[24] A deficiency of vitamin B$_{13}$ also may lead to degenerative symptoms in multiple sclerosis patients.

Beneficial Effects on Ailments

Dr. J. Evers, from West Germany, has produced successful results in treating multiple sclerosis patients with vitamin B$_{13}$.[25]

VITAMIN B$_{13}$ MAY BE BENEFICIAL FOR THE FOLLOWING AILMENT:

Body Member	Ailment
Brain/Nervous system	Multiple sclerosis

[23] Airola, *How to Get Well*, p. 267.
[24] Airola, *How to Get Well*, p. 267.
[25] "Multiple Sclerosis," *Cancer Control Journal*, vol. 2, no. 3, p. 8, May-June 1971.

BIOTIN

Description

Biotin is a water-soluble B-complex vitamin. As a co-enzyme, it assists in the making of fatty acids and in the oxidation of fatty acids and carbohydrates. Without biotin the body's fat production is impaired. Biotin also aids in the utilization of protein, folic acid, pantothenic acid, and vitamin B_{12}.

Biotin is an essential nutrient that appears in trace amounts in all animal and plant tissue. Some rich sources of biotin are egg yolk, beef liver, unpolished rice, and brewer's yeast.

Absorption and Storage

Biotin is synthesized by the intestinal bacteria; thus, man is not dependent upon dietary sources to ensure an adequate supply. Raw egg white contains the protein avidin, which binds with biotin in the intestine and prevents its absorption by the body. However, since eggs are usually eaten in a cooked form and avidin is inactivated by heat, there is no real danger of a deficiency resulting from the ingestion of a cooked egg.

Dosage and Toxicity

The National Research Council indicates that 150 to 300 micrograms of biotin will meet the body's daily needs. Additional amounts are required during pregnancy and lactation. There are no known toxic effects of this nutrient.

Deficiency Effects and Symptoms

Deficiency states have been reported in man only when the diet contained large amounts of raw egg white. A deficiency of biotin in man causes muscular pain, poor appetite, dry skin, lack of energy, sleeplessness, and a disturbed nervous system. Dermatitis, grayish skin color, and depression are other symptoms of a biotin deficiency. In severe deficiency there may be impairment of the body's fat metabolism.

Beneficial Effect on Ailments

Dermatitis has shown improvement when treated with biotin. The use of biotin has been beneficial in treating baldness.

Human Tests

1. Biotin and Seborrheic Dermatitis and Leiner's Disease. Nine cases of seborrheic dermatitis and two cases of Leiner's disease in infants were given 5 milligrams of biotin injected intramuscularly daily for seven to fourteen days. Milder cases were given 2 to 4 milligrams orally for two to three weeks.

Results. Both ailments showed marked improvement when treated with biotin. (*Journal of Pediatrics*, November 1957.)

2. Biotin and Biotin Deficiency Symptoms. Persons who were suffering from dermatitis, a grayish pallor of the skin and mucous membranes, diminuation of hemoglobin, a striking rise in serum cholesterol, depression, and muscle pain were given 150 or more milligrams of biotin, injected intravenously daily. The excretion of biotin in the urine was much below that of a person on a normal diet.

Results. After the injections the symptoms became less evident. The ashy pallor disappeared in four days, serum cholesterol was reduced, and urinary excretion of biotin increased. (Margaret S. Chaney and Margaret L. Ross, *Nutrition*, Houghton Mifflin Co., Boston, 1971, p. 307.)

BIOTIN MAY BE BENEFICIAL FOR THE FOLLOWING AILMENTS:

Body Member	Ailment
Hair/Scalp	Baldness
Muscles	Muscle pains
Skin	Dermatitis
	Eczema
	Infant dermatitis
General	Depression

CHOLINE

Description

Choline is considered one of the B-complex vitamins. It functions with inositol as a basic constituent of lecithin. It is present in the body of all living cells and is widely distributed in animal and plant tissues. The richest source of choline is lecithin, but other rich dietary sources include egg yolk, liver, brewer's yeast, and wheat germ.

Choline appears to be associated primarily with the utilization of fats and cholesterol in the body. It prevents fats from accumulating in the liver and facilitates the movement of fats into the cells. Choline combines with fatty acids and phosphoric acid within the liver to form lecithin. It is essential for the health of the liver and kidneys.

Choline is also essential for the health of the myelin sheaths of the nerves; the myelin sheaths are the principal component of the nerve fibers. It plays an important role in the transmission of the nerve impulses.[26] It also helps to regulate and improve liver and gallbladder functioning[27] and aids in the prevention of gallstones.

Absorption and Storage

Choline is synthesized by the interaction of B_{12} and folic acid with the amino acid methionine.

Dosage and Toxicity

Daily requirements for choline are not known. The average diet has been estimated to contain 500 to 900 milligrams of choline per day, according to the 1968 revision of the *Recommended Dietary Allowances.*[28] Dr. Paavo Airola has estimated the daily dietary intake to be 1,000 or more milligrams.[29] Usual therapeutic daily doses range from 500 to 6,000 milligrams; prolonged ingestion of massive doses of isolated choline may induce a deficiency of vitamin B_6.[30] It is important to remember that the B-complex vitamins function better when all are taken together.

Deficiency Effects and Symptoms

A choline deficiency is associated with fatty deposits in the liver, resulting in bleeding stomach ulcers, heart trouble, and blocking of the tubes of the kidneys. Insufficient supplies of choline may cause hemorrhaging of the kidneys. A deficiency can also result when too

little protein is in the diet.[31] Prolonged deficiencies may cause high blood pressure, cirrhosis and fatty degeneration of the liver, atherosclerosis, and hardening of the arteries.[32]

Beneficial Effect on Ailments

Choline has been successful in reducing high blood pressure because it strengthens weak capillary walls.[33] Symptoms such as heart palpitation, dizziness, headaches, ear noises, and constipation have been relieved or removed entirely within five to ten days after administration of choline treatments. Insomnia, visual disturbances, and blood flow to the eyes have also benefited from choline therapy.

Because choline is a fat and cholesterol dissolver, it is used to treat atherosclerosis and hardening of the arteries. It can be used to treat fatty livers, liver damage, cirrhosis of the liver, and hepatitis. Choline is also used in kidney damage, hemorrhaging of the kidneys, and nephritis, as well as for eye conditions such as glaucoma.

Human Tests

1. Choline and Atherosclerosis. 230 patients were hospitalized for atherosclerosis. Half the patients were given conventional medication but no choline after discharge from the hospital; the other half received choline daily for one to three years.

Results. Among the untreated patients, the three-year death rate was nearly 30 percent. Only 12 percent of the choline-treated patients died. (Dr. L. M. Morrison and W. F. Gonzalez, *Proceedings of the Society of Biology and Medicine*, vol. 73, pp. 37-38, 1950, as reported in Rodale, *The Encyclopedia for Healthful Living*, pp. 457 and 458.)

CHOLINE MAY BE BENEFICIAL FOR THE FOLLOWING AILMENTS:

Body Member	Ailment
Blood/Circulatory system	Angina pectoris
	Cholesterol level, high
	Hepatitis

[26] Krause and Hunscher, *Food, Nutrition and Diet Therapy,* p. 144.
[27] Airola, *How to Get Well*, p. 266.
[28] Krause and Hunscher, *Food, Nutrition and Diet Therapy,* p. 145.
[29] Airola, *How to Get Well*, p. 266.
[30] Airola, *How to Get Well*, p. 266.

[31] *The Vitamins Explained Simply* (Melbourne: Science of Life Books, PTY., 1972), p. 32.
[32] Airola, *How to Get Well*, p. 266.
[33] Clark, *Know Your Nutrition*, p. 110.

Body Member	Ailment
	Hypoglycemia
	Stroke (cerebrovascular accident)
Brain/Nervous system	Dizziness
	Multiple sclerosis
Eye	Glaucoma
Glands	Hyperthyroidism
Hair/Scalp	Hair problems
Heart	Arteriosclerosis
	Atherosclerosis
	Hypertension
Intestine	Constipation
Liver	Cirrhosis of liver
Lungs/Respiratory system	Asthma
Muscles	Muscular dystrophy
Skin	Eczema
General	Alcoholism

FOLIC ACID (FOLACIN)

Description

Folic acid is part of the water-soluble vitamin B complex and functions as a coenzyme, together with vitamins B_{12} and C, in the breakdown and utilization of proteins. Folic acid performs its basic role as a carbon carrier in the formation of heme, the iron-containing protein found in hemoglobin, necessary for the formation of red blood cells. It also is needed for the formation of nucleic acid, which is essential for the processes of growth and reproduction of all body cells. It also increases the appetite and stimulates the production of hydrochloric acid, which helps prevent intestinal parasites and food poisoning. In addition, it aids in performance of the liver. Folic acid is easily destroyed by high temperature, exposure to light, and being left at room temperature for long periods of time. The best sources of folic acid are green leafy vegetables, liver, and brewer's yeast.

Absorption and Storage

Folic acid is absorbed in the gastrointestinal tract by active transport and diffusion and is stored primarily in the liver. Sulfa drugs may interfere with the bacteria in the intestine which manufacture folic acid. Aminoperin and streptomycin destroy folic acid.

Dosage and Toxicity

The Recommended Dietary Allowance of folic acid is 400 micrograms for adults, 800 micrograms during pregnancy, and 600 micrograms during lactation. Stress and disease increase the body's need for folic acid, as does the consumption of alcohol. There is no known toxicity of this vitamin, although an excessive intake of folic acid can mask a vitamin B_{12} deficiency. A prescription is required for dosages higher than 400 micrograms per tablet.

Deficiency Effects and Symptoms

Deficiency of folic acid results in poor growth, graying hair, glossitis (tongue inflammation), and gastrointestinal-tract disturbances arising from inadequate dietary intake, impaired absorption, excessive demands by tissues of the body, and metabolic disturbances. Because of the role folic acid plays in the formation of red blood cells, a deficiency could lead to anemia that cannot be corrected by supplementary iron.[34] In the past few years there have been a number of studies implicating folic acid deficiency as a contributing factor in mental illness. Almost any interference with the metabolism of folic acid in the fetus encourages deformities such as cleft palate, brain damage, or slow development and poor learning ability in the child.[35] In addition, deficiency of folic acid may lead to toxemia, premature birth, after-birth hemorrhaging, and megaloblastic anemia in both mother and child.

Beneficial Effect on Ailments

Folic acid is not limited to treatment of anemia. It is beneficial in treating diarrhea, sprue, dropsy, stomach ulcers, menstrual problems, leg ulcers, and glossitis. Circulation may be improved in patients suffering from atherosclerosis. Folic acid may prevent the graying of hair when used with PABA and pantothenic acid.[36] During pregnancy, folacin-rich foods should be stressed in the diet so that the fetal and maternal needs are met and megaloblastic anemia is prevented.

Human Tests

1. **Folic Acid and Toxicity.** 20 healthy young adults were given 15 milligrams of folic acid daily for one month and were matched with a control group given placebos.

[34] Clark, *Know Your Nutrition*, p. 103.
[35] Rodale Press Editors, *Be a Healthy Mother, Have a Healthy Baby* (Emmaus, Pa.: Rodale Press, 1973), p. 29.
[36] Adelle Davis, *Let's Get Well* (New York: Harcourt, Brace & World, 1965), p. 166.

Results. No ill effects were detected. Physicians have given 150 milligrams of folic acid to children and 450 milligrams to adults, both daily, with no report of toxicity. (Davis, *Let's Get Well.*)

2. Folic Acid and Megaloblastic Anemia. A sixty-nine-year-old woman was suffering from megaloblastic anemia. She was brought to the hospital with a history of pallor, fatigue, forgetfulness, and lack of energy. According to tests, she lacked vitamin B_{12}, and some was administered before she came to the hospital. She was then given folic acid.

Results. Her condition improved immediately, and she was soon discharged from the hospital. Tests six months later showed her in good health; all symptoms of megaloblastic anemia had disappeared. (*Journal of the American Medical Association*, July 31, 1972.)

3. Folic Acid and Atherosclerosis. 17 elderly patients were treated with 5 to 7.5 milligrams of folic acid daily.

Results. 15 patients responded with increased capillary blood flow, resulting in improved vision due to better blood supply to the retina. In many cases there was increased skin temperature. (Roger J. Williams, *Nutrition Against Disease,* Pitman Publ., New York, 1971, pp. 75–76.)

Animal Tests

1. Folic Acid and Cleft Palate. Pregnant mice were first injected with cortisone, which can cause interference with vital life chemistry, four times daily. Cleft palates developed in 85 percent of their offspring. Pyridoxine and folic acid were separately injected with the cortisone.

Results. When pyridoxine was injected, the abnormalities were reduced to 45 percent; the folic acid in the combination reduced the cleft palate cases to 20 percent. (Dr. Lyndon A. Peer, *Chicago Daily Tribune*, September 11, 1957.)

FOLIC ACID MAY BE BENEFICIAL FOR THE FOLLOWING AILMENTS:

Body Member	Ailment
Blood/Circulatory system	Anemia
	Leukemia
	Pernicious anemia

Body Member	Ailment
Bowel	Diarrhea
Brain/Nervous system	Alcoholism
	Mental illness
Glands	Adrenal exhaustion
Hair/Scalp	Baldness
Heart	Arteriosclerosis
	Atherosclerosis
Intestine	Celiac disease
	Diverticulitis
Joints	Arthritis
Lungs/Respiratory system	Emphysema
Nails	Nail problems
Skin	Psoriasis
	Ulcers
Stomach	Gastritis
	Indigestion (dyspepsia)
General	Alcoholism
	Anemia
	Bruises
	Fatigue
	Kwashiorkor
	Pellagra
	Scurvy
	Stress
	Tonsilitis

INOSITOL

Description

Inositol is recognized as part of the vitamin B complex and is closely associated with choline and biotin. Like choline, inositol is found in high concentrations in lecithin.

Both animal and plant tissues contain inositol. In animal tissues it occurs as a component of phospholipids, substances containing phosphorus, fatty acids, and nitrogenous bases. In plant cells it is found as phytic acid, an organic acid that binds calcium and iron in an insoluble complex and interferes with their absorption.[37] Inositol is found in unprocessed whole grains, citrus fruits, brewer's yeast, crude unrefined molasses, and liver.

Inositol is effective in promoting the body's production of lecithin. Fats are moved from the liver to the

[37] Guthrie, *Introductory Nutrition*, p. 276.

cells with the aid of lecithin; therefore inositol aids in the metabolism of fats and helps reduce blood cholesterol.[38] In combination with choline, it prevents the fatty hardening of arteries and protects the liver, kidneys, and heart.

Inositol is also found to be helpful in brain cell nutrition. It is needed for the growth and survival of cells in bone marrow, eye membranes, and the intestines.[39] It is vital for hair growth and can prevent thinning hair and baldness.

Absorption and Storage

The body is able to synthesize sufficient amounts of inositol from glucose to meet its needs.[40] About seven percent of ingested inositol is converted to glucose; inositol is only one-third as effective as glucose in alleviating ketosis, the complete metabolism of fatty acids.[41]

There is some disagreement as to whether inositol is synthesized by the intestinal flora. One reliable source indicates it is,[42] while another claims that synthesis occurs within the individual cell rather than by intestinal organisms.[43] The amount the body excretes daily in the urine is small, averaging 37 milligrams. The diabetic excretes more inositol than does the nondiabetic.[44] Large amounts of coffee may deplete the body's storage of inositol.

Dosage and Toxicity

The Recommended Dietary Allowance has not yet been established, but most authorities recommend consuming the same amount of inositol as choline. The daily consumption of inositol in food is about one gram. The human body contains more inositol than any other vitamin except niacin. One tablespoon of yeast provides approximately forty milligrams each of choline and inositol. Therapeutic doses range from 500 to 1,000 milligrams daily.[45] There is no known toxicity of inositol.

[38]Airola, *How to Get Well*, p. 266.
[39]Clark, *Know Your Nutrition, p. 113.*
[40]Guthrie, *Introductory Nutrition*, p. 276.
[41]Robert Goodhart and Maurice Shils, *Modern Nutrition in Health and Disease* (Philadelphia: Lea and Febiger, 1973), p. 264.
[42]Rodale and Staff, *The Health Seeker*, p. 869.
[43]John Hoover (ed.), *Remington's Pharmaceutical Sciences* (Easton, Pa.: Mack Pub. Co., 1970), p. 1029.
[44]Krause and Hunscher, *Food, Nutrition and Diet Therapy*, p. 145.
[45]Airola, *How to Get Well*, p. 266.

Deficiency Effects and Symptoms

Caffeine may create an inositol shortage in the body. An inositol deficiency may cause constipation, eczema, and abnormalities of the eyes. The deficiency contributes to hair loss and a high blood cholesterol level, which may result in artery and heart disease.

Beneficial Effect on Ailments

Inositol is beneficial in the treatment of constipation because it has a stimulating effect on the muscular action of the alimentary canal. It also is recommended for men who are becoming bald and is vital in helping to lower cholesterol levels in the blood. Inositol aids in eliminating liver fats from patients about to be operated on for stomach cancer.

Animal Tests

1. Inositol and Cholesterol. Two groups of rabbits were fed a capsule of cholesterol daily. One group of rabbits received just cholesterol and a regulation diet. The other group of rabbits received a capsule of inositol in addition to the cholesterol.

Results. At the end of the feeding period, the first group of rabbits showed an increase of 337 percent in the cholesterol content in their blood. Those who had received inositol showed a cholesterol increase of only 181 percent. (*Newsweek*, September 11, 1950, Dr. Louis B. Potte, Dr. William C. Felch, and Stephanie J. Ilka of St. Luke's Hospital, New York; reported in Rodale, *The Encyclopedia for Healthful Living.*)

INOSITOL MAY BE BENEFICIAL FOR THE FOLLOWING AILMENTS:

Body Member	Ailment
Blood/Circulatory system	Arteriosclerosis
	Atherosclerosis
	Cholesterol level, high
	Stroke (cerebrovascular accident)
Bowel	Constipation
Brain/Nervous system	Dizziness
Eye	Glaucoma
Hair/Scalp	Baldness
Intestine	Constipation
Liver	Cirrhosis of the liver
Lungs/Respiratory system	Asthma

Body Member	Ailment
Stomach	Gastritis
General	Overweight and obesity

LAETRILE (VITAMIN B_{17}, AMYGDALIN, NITRILOSIDES)

Description

Laetrile is an amygdalin, a simple chemical compound consisting of two molecules of sugar, one molecule of benzaldehyde, and one molecule of cyanide. Nitrilosides are known as "laetrile" when used in medical dosage form.

Laetrile is a natural substance made from apricot pits and is claimed by its developers to have a specific cancer preventive and controlling effect. Dr. Ernest Krebs, Sr., who was the first to use laetrile therapeutically in this country, considered laetrile to be an essential vitamin and called it B_{17}.

However, laetrile has not been accepted as a cancer treatment in the United States because the Food and Drug Administration rejects its use in human cancer patients on the grounds that it may be poisonous due to the cyanide in the chemistry of the vitamin. This view is not held by Dr. Dean Burk, chief cytologist of the National Cancer Institute, who has conducted extensive tests including the use of laetrile and states that, "Laetrile is remarkably non-toxic . . . compared with virtually all cancer chemotherapeutic agents currently studied."[46] Other scientists claim that cyanide occurring naturally in food is not dangerous. Laetrile is manufactured and used legally in over 17 countries throughout the world, including Mexico, Germany, Italy, Belgium, and the Philippines.

Natural cyanide is locked in a sugar molecule. It is normally found in over 2,000 known unrefined foods and grasses. A concentration of about 2 or 3 percent laetrile is found in the whole kernels of most fruits, including apricots, apples, cherries, peaches, plums, and nectarines, and in some 70 plants commonly fed to animals for fodder. A sprouting seed produces from 10 to 30 times as much B_{17} as does the mature plant. Few citrus fruits contain laetrile, and it is one B vitamin that does not occur naturally in brewer's yeast. Shelled and unshelled apricot kernels contain 2 to 3 percent amygdalin and are also excellent sources of protein, unsaturated fatty acids, and minerals.

According to its advocates, laetrile is a highly selective substance that attacks only the cancerous cells. When laetrile is eaten and absorbed by normal cells, an enzyme called rhodanese detoxifies the cyanide, which is then excreted through the urine. But because cancer cells are completely deficient in rhodanese and are instead surrounded by another enzyme, beta-glucosidase, which releases the bound cyanide from the laetrile at the site of malignancy, laetrile is believed to attack only the malignant areas.

Absorption and Storage

Oral doses of B_{17} are not affected by the action of the acid medium of the stomach but pass directly into the intestine, where the substance is acted upon by bacterial enzymes. The bacterial enzymes in the intestine decompose the amygdalin into four components, which are then absorbed into the lymph and portal systems and circulated throughout the body.

Dosage and Toxicity

Although much research on B_{17} is still needed, the usual dosage is 0.25 to 1.0 gram taken with meals. Cumulative amounts of more than 3.0 grams are sometimes taken, but *more than 1.0 gram is never taken at any one time*. Dosages as high as 20 grams daily of combined oral intravenous administration have been used on patients whose detoxification and elimination levels of the vitamin were adequate.

Five to thirty apricot kernels eaten through the day may be a sufficient preventive amount, but they should never be taken all at one time. It is not considered desirable to prepare a slurry of ground up kernels (as in a solution of water, milk, or orange juice) and then let it stand for long periods of time before consumption.

Toxicity levels have not been established, and one should exercise extreme caution in order to avoid ingesting excessive amounts all at one time.

Deficiency Effects and Symptoms

Prolonged deficiency may lead to diminished resistance to malignancies.

Beneficial Effect on Ailments

Amygdalin may reduce the size of cancer tumors, ease accompanying pain, and inhibit the growth of cancer

---

[46]"Laetrile—An Answer to Cancer?" *Prevention*, December 1971, p. 162.

cells. In addition, it favorably regulates blood pressure and may have an antirheumatic and esthesizing effect.

NIACIN (NICOTINIC ACID, NIACINAMIDE, NICOTINAMIDE)

Description

Niacin, a member of the vitamin B complex, is water-soluble. It is more stable than thiamine or riboflavin and is remarkably resistant to heat, light, air, acids, and alkalies. There are also three synthetic forms of niacin: niacinamide, nicotinic acid, and nicotinamide. As a co-enzyme, niacin assists enzymes in the breakdown and utilization of proteins, fats, and carbohydrates. Niacin is effective in improving circulation and reducing the cholesterol level in the blood. It is vital to the proper activity of the nervous system and for formation and maintenance of healthy skin, tongue, and digestive-system tissues. Niacin is necessary for the synthesis of sex hormones.

Relatively small amounts of pure niacin are present in most foods. The niacin "equivalent" listed in dietary tables means either pure niacin or adequate supply of tryptophan, an amino acid that can be converted into niacin by the body. Lean meats, poultry, fish, and peanuts are rich daily sources of both niacin and tryptophan, as are such dietary supplements as brewer's yeast, wheat germ, and desiccated liver. Niacin is difficult to obtain except from these foods.

Absorption and Storage

Niacin is absorbed in the intestine and is stored primarily in the liver. Any excess is eliminated through the urine. Excessive consumption of sugar and starches will deplete the body's supply of niacin, as will certain antibiotics.

Dosage and Toxicity

The National Research Council suggests that daily allowances of niacin be based on caloric intake; 6.6 milligrams of niacin per 1000 calories is recommended. Tryptophan may provide part or all of the daily niacin requirements; 60 milligrams of tryptophan yield 1 milligram of niacin. The Recommended Dietary Allowance is 18 milligrams for men, 13 milligrams for women, and 9 to 16 milligrams for children. During pregnancy, lactation, illness, tissue trauma, and growth periods and after physical exercise, daily requirements are increased.

No real toxic effects are known, but large doses, usually 100 or more milligrams, may cause passing side effects such as tingling and itching sensations, intense flushing of the skin, and throbbing in the head due to a dilation of the lumen in the blood vessels. The flush is not considered dangerous. It lasts for approximately fifteen minutes and then disappears. By taking a synthetic form of niacin, niacinamide, a person gets all the benefits of niacin but avoids the above side effects. Acne and migraine headaches are two disturbances that do not respond as well to the synthetic forms as they do to the natural form.

Deficiency Effects and Symptoms

The symptoms of niacin deficiency are many. In the early stages, muscular weakness, general fatigue, loss of appetite, indigestion, and various skin eruptions occur. A niacin deficiency may also cause bad breath, small ulcers, canker sores, insomnia, irritability, nausea, vomiting, recurring headaches, tender gums, strain, tension, and deep depression. Severe niacin deficiency results in pellagra, which is characterized by dermatitis; dementia; diarrhea; rough, inflamed skin; tremors; and nervous disorders. Many digestive abnormalities causing irritation and inflammation of mucous membranes in the mouth and gastrointestinal tract develop from a niacin deficiency.

Beneficial Effect on Ailments

The amazing thing about niacin is the speed with which it can reverse disorders. Diarrhea has been cleared up in two days. Atherosclerosis, attacks of Ménière's syndrome (vertigo), and some cases of progressive deafness have improved or even disappeared. Niacin is often used to reduce high blood pressure and increase circulation in cramped, painful legs of the elderly. It also helps to stimulate the production of hydrochloric acid to aid impaired digestion. Acne has been successfully treated with niacin.

Lewis J. Silvers, M.D., writes: "Many a migraine headache can be prevented from developing into the excruciating painful stage by taking niacin at the first sign of attack."[47]   Large doses of niacin have effectively cured schizophrenia and have helped elderly patients who are mentally confused.

Drs. Richard M. Halpern and Robert A. Smith have reported research indicating that the flushless nicotinamide may be a factor in preventing cancer, due to enzyme regulation that protects normal cells and prevents them from becoming malignant.   Investigators have found niacin able to cure pellagra, a disease that affects the skin, intestinal tract, and nervous system.   When given in high doses, niacin may bring complete relief from delirium within 24 to 48 hours.

Human Tests

1. Niacin and Acne. 20 cases of acne were treated with 100 milligrams three times daily. This treatment continued for two or three weeks or until the patients experienced regular flushing.

Results.   The niacin treatment provided definite relief in all 20 cases. (Lewis J. Silvers, M.D., as reported in Clark, *Know Your Nutrition*, pp. 83-84.)

2. Niacin and Cancer. Drs. Richard M. Halpern and Robert A. Smith reported that malignancy is, in some way, associated with a deficiency of niacin. To prove that niacin could help prevent cancer, they exposed isolated malignant cells in their laboratory to nicotinamide and watched the vitamin suppress the malignancy. The doctors did not state dosages since individual needs vary so greatly. (Drs. Richard M. Halpern and Robert A. Smith, Molecular Biology Institute, as reported in Clark, *Know Your Nutrition*, p. 84.)

NIACIN MAY BE BENEFICIAL FOR THE FOLLOWING AILMENTS:

Body Member	Ailment
Blood/Circulatory system	Arteriosclerosis
	Atherosclerosis
	Cholesterol level, high
	Diabetes
	Hemophilia
	Hypertension
	Phlebitis
Bowel	Diarrhea
Brain/Nervous system	Dizziness
	Epilepsy
	Headache
	Insomnia
	Mental illness
	Multiple sclerosis
	Neuritis
	Parkinson's disease
Ear	Ménière's syndrome
Eye	Conjunctivitis
	Night blindness
Hair/Scalp	Baldness
Heart	Arteriosclerosis
	Atherosclerosis
	Hypertension
Intestine	Constipation
Joints	Arthritis
Leg	Phlebitis
Lungs/Respiratory system	Tuberculosis
Mouth	Canker sore
	Halitosis
Skin	Acne
	Bedsores
	Dermatitis
Stomach	Indigestion (dyspepsia)
Teeth/Gums	Pyorrhea
General	Alcoholism
	Cancer
	Stress

PARA-AMINOBENZOIC ACID (PABA)

Description

Para-aminobenzoic acid, an integral part of the vitamin B complex, is water-soluble and is considered unique in that it is a "vitamin within a vitamin," occurring in combination with folic acid.[48] PABA is found in liver, yeast, wheat germ, and molasses.

PABA stimulates the intestinal bacteria, enabling them to produce folic acid, which in turn aids in the production of pantothenic acid. As a coenzyme, PABA functions in the breakdown and utilization of proteins and in the formation of blood cells, especially red blood cells. PABA plays an important role in determining skin

[47]Clark, *Know Your Nutrition*, pp. 83-84.

[48]Krause and Hunscher, *Food, Nutrition and Diet Therapy*, p. 140.

health, hair pigmentation, and health of the intestines.[49] PABA acts as a sunscreen and is incorporated into some sunscreen ointments.[50]

Absorption and Storage

PABA is stored in the tissues but is synthesized by friendly bacteria in the intestines. This means that the body will manufacture its own PABA if conditions in the intestines are favorable.

Dosage and Toxicity

The need for PABA in human nutrition has not yet been established. PABA is available in supplements in potencies higher than 30 milligrams, but these higher doses (up to 100 milligrams) are used for therapeutic purposes. Continued ingestion of high doses of PABA is not recommended and can be toxic to the liver, heart, and kidneys.

Symptoms of toxicity are nausea and vomiting. Careful study must be done before any serious recommendations can be made for the use of PABA in dermatological conditions.[51]

Deficiency Effects and Symptoms

A deficiency of PABA may result from the use of sulfa drugs, which reduce the capacity of PABA to function properly in the intestines. Deficiency symptoms include fatigue, irritability, depression, nervousness, headache, constipation, and other digestive disorders.

Beneficial Effect on Ailments

PABA is used in treating vitiligo, a condition characterized by depigmentation or darkening of some areas of the skin, and in treating some parasitic diseases, including Rocky Mountain spotted fever. In certain laboratory animals, PABA, when combined with pantothenic acid, has helped restore color to hair that was turning gray and has prevented further graying. Research continues as to whether PABA has this effect on human hair.

According to Adelle Davis, the administration of PABA and folic acid has restored graying or white hair to its natural color. A daily intake of folic acid and PABA should be continued so that the restored hair is prevented from returning to its previous color.

PABA often soothes the pain of burns even more effectively than vitamin E.[52] PABA ointment has been effective in preventing and treating sunburn. Persons normally susceptible to sunburn have been able to remain many hours in the sun after applying PABA ointment. PABA alleviates the pain of sunburn and other burns immediately.[53] Adelle Davis has stated that PABA ointment may delay old-age skin changes such as wrinkles, dry skin, and dark spots.

Human Tests

1. PABA and Lupus Erythematosus (a Severe Skin Disorder). 33 patients with lupus erythematosus were given one to four grams of para-aminobenzoic acid at two- to three-hour intervals.

Results. Two of ten with chronic discord lupus showed no improvement, one patient had a poor response, and seven showed good to excellent responses. Improvement occurred in all of seven patients with scleroderma, a skin disorder; the sclerodermatous areas gradually softened and became thinner and more pliable. (*Zarafonetis: Ann. Intern. Med.*, vol. 30, p. 1188, 1949.)

PABA MAY BE BENEFICIAL FOR THE FOLLOWING AILMENTS:

Body Member	Ailment
Blood/Circulatory system	Anemia
Bowel	Constipation
Hair/Scalp	Baldness
Head	Headache
Skin	Burns
	Sunburn
	Vitiligo

PANGAMIC ACID (VITAMIN B$_{15}$)

Description

Pangamic acid is a water-soluble nutrient that was originally isolated in extracted apricot kernels and later was obtained in crystalline form from rice bran, rice polish, whole-grain cereals, brewer's yeast, steer blood,

---

[49] *The Vitamins Explained Simply*, p. 28.
[50] Hoover (ed.), *Remington's Pharmaceutical Sciences*, p. 1041.
[51] Goodhart and Shils, *Modern Nutrition in Health and Disease*, pp. 946-947.
[52] Davis, *Let's Get Well*, p. 37.
[53] Davis, *Let's Get Well*, p. 154.

and horse liver.[54] Pangamic acid promotes oxidation processes and cell respiration and stimulates glucose oxidation.[55] The chief merit of pangamic acid is its ability to eliminate the phenomena of hypoxia, an insufficient supply of oxygen in living tissue.[56] This is especially true in the cardiac and other muscles.

Pangamic acid is essential in promoting protein metabolism, particularly in the muscles of the heart. It regulates fat and sugar metabolism, which partly accounts for its effects on atherosclerosis and diabetes.[57] In some treatments, the action of B_{15} is improved by the addition of vitamins A and E.

Pangamic acid is helpful in stimulating the glandular and nervous system and is helpful in treating high blood cholesterol levels, impaired circulation, and premature aging.[58] It can help protect against the damaging effect of carbon monoxide poisoning.

Little is actually known about B_{15}, and only small quantities are used in the United States although it is used widely in Russia and other European countries. Pharmaceutical pangamic acid is derived from ground apricot pits. Good natural sources of pangamic acid are brewer's yeast, whole brown rice, whole grains, pumpkin seeds, and sesame seeds.

Absorption and Storage

Little is known about the absorption and storage of B_{15}, but excessive amounts are excreted through the kidneys and bowels and in perspiration.[59]

Dosage and Toxicity

The Recommended Dietary Allowance has not been established. According to Dr. Ernest T. Krebs, Jr., vitamin B_{15} has no undesirable effects and its toxic level for man is 100,000 times the therapeutic dose.[60] Clinical tests in which intramuscular injections of pangamic acid were given in doses of 2.5 to 10 milligrams daily proved completely nontoxic. After injections, some patients experienced a flushing of the skin. Similar effects were noted with niacin, but no laboratory changes were reported.[61] The valuable quality of the substance is its nontoxicity.

Deficiency Effects and Symptoms

A deficiency of vitamin B_{15} may cause diminished oxygenation of cells, hypoxia, heart disease, and glandular and nervous disorders.[62]

Beneficial Effect on Ailments

Many claims have been made concerning the therapeutic value of pangamic acid. In widespread Soviet clinical tests, over one-half of hospitalized sclerosis patients responded to vitamin B_{15} therapy.[63] Even patients who have had serious heart attacks have been restored to good health with treatments of B_{15}.[64] Most tests on B_{15} have been conducted in the USSR.

People complaining of headaches, chest pains, shortness of breath, tension, insomnia, and other common symptoms of advancing atherosclerosis have benefited from additional B_{15}. Pangamic acid has been found to alleviate hypoxia and has been used in cases of coronary artery insufficiency. It has been shown to relieve symptoms of angina, cyanosis (a discoloration of skin due to poor oxidation), and asthma.[65]

Good results have been obtained in the treatment of rheumatism, rheumatic heart disease, and acute and chronic cases of alcoholism.[66] Some alcoholics have lost their craving for alcohol when treated with vitamin B_{15}.[67] B_{15} has been helpful in treating chronic hepatitis and early stages of liver cirrhosis.[68]

Betty Lee Morales, a pangamic acid researcher, has had success using B_{15} in treating conditions such as circulatory problems, emphysema, and premature aging.[69] Dr. Ya. Yu. Shpirt, a Russian, developed a combination of vitamins A and E (AEVIT) which has proved to be

[54]Clark, *Know Your Nutrition*, p. 129.
[55]Ya. Yu. Shpirt, *Vitamin B15 (Pangamic Acid) Indications for Use and Efficacy in Internal Disease* (Moscow: V/O Medexport, 1968), p. 7.
[56]"The Life-Saving Banned Vitamin," Rodale (ed.), *Prevention*, May 1968.
[57]*Northern Neighbors*, November 1969, p. 6.
[58]Airola, *How to Get Well*, p. 268.
[59]"The Life-Saving Banned Vitamin," *Prevention*, May 1968.
[60]Shpirt, *Vitamin B15 (Pangamic Acid) Indications*, p. 7.
[61]"The Life-Saving Banned Vitamin," *Prevention*, May 1968.
[62]Airola, *How to Get Well*, p. 268.
[63]*Northern Neighbors*, November 1969, p. 6.
[64]*Northern Neighbors*, November 1969, p. 6.
[65]"The Life-Saving Banned Vitamin," *Prevention*, May 1968.
[66]"The Life-Saving Banned Vitamin," *Prevention*, May 1968.
[67]Clark, *Know Your Nutrition*, p. 128.
[68]Clark, *Know Your Nutrition*, p. 128.
[69]Clark, *Know Your Nutrition*, p. 127.

therapeutically successful in treating severe cases of atherosclerosis of the lower limbs.[70]

There are indications that pangamic acid may be a preventive substance in the treatment of cancer. Two-time Nobel prizewinner Dr. Felix Warburg states, "The primary cause of cancer is the replacement of the respiration of oxygen in normal body cells by a fermentation of sugar. All normal body cells meet their energy needs by respiration of oxygen, whereas cancer cells meet their energy needs in great part by fermentation, an oxidative decomposition of complex substances through the action of enzymes. All normal cells require oxygen and cancer cells can thrive without oxygen."[71] According to Warburg's theory, because of the lack of oxygen, the cell is faced with death. The cells without oxygen are able to change their metabolism and to derive their energy from glucose fermentation. These cells may become malignant. Thus a preventive treatment against deoxidation of cells is inclusion of sufficient B_{15} in the diet.

Human Tests

1. Pangamic Acid and Circulatory Disturbance. 42 patients suffering from circulatory problems were given B_{15} in the form of calcium pangamate. They were given 30 milligrams three times daily orally, for a total of 90 milligrams daily. The treatment lasted 20 days.

Results. All patients showed improvement in their clinical conditions. The pains in the heart subsided or disappeared. (Clark, *Know Your Nutrition*, pp. 127 and 128.)

2. Pangamic Acid and Cholesterol Level. A study was conducted on the general cholesterol levels of the same 42 cases mentioned in Test 1. They were measured before treatment, after 10 days of treatment, and at the end of 20 days of treatment.

Results. In most cases a drop of the cholesterol was noticed as early as 10 days after the treatment began and continued over the following period. Ten days after the end of treatment with B_{15}, the general level of

cholesterol was greatly reduced. (Clark, *Know Your Nutrition*, p. 128.)

3. Pangamic Acid and Coronary Sclerosis. 118 patients, all over fifty years of age, having coronary sclerosis, were observed after being treated with calcium pangamate. Both subjective symptoms and objective characteristics (EGG, biochemical analysis of the blood, and oscillation findings) were taken as criteria of the effectiveness of the treatment.

Results. Of all 118 cases, good results were obtained in 49 and satisfactory results in 55; in 11 cases the treatment had no effect; deterioration was noted in 3 cases. [Shpirt, *Vitamin B_{15} (Pangamic Acid) Indications*, p. 10.]

4. Pangamic Acid and Muscles of Injured Legs. Groups of athletes were given various amounts of substances to stimulate energy in muscular activity. Then they were given 300 milligrams of B_{15} on successive days.

Results. The B_{15} was effective in early healing of muscles of injured legs. (Clark, *Know Your Nutrition*, p. 129.)

5. Pangamic Acid and Cardiopulmonary Insufficiency. 16 patients suffering from cardiopulmonary insufficiency due to pneumosclerosis and bronchial asthma were treated with calcium pangamate. It was administered for 20 to 30 days orally in a dosage of 120 to 160 milligrams per day and as an aerosol in a dosage of 80 milligrams per day.

Results. 4 patients obtained good results, 10 obtained satisfactory results, and 2 showed no effects of the treatment. [Shpirt, *Vitamin B_{15} (Pangamic Acid) Indications*, pp. 24 and 25.]

6. Pangamic Acid and Atherosclerosis. 27 patients were receiving calcium pangamate for treatment of atherosclerosis. They were given 120 to 150 milligrams daily for 15 to 30 days.

Results. 15 patients showed good results, 8 showed satisfactory results, 2 showed no effects of treatment, and 2 showed relapse. [Shpirt, *Vitamin B_{15} (Pangamic Acid) Indications*, p. 25.]

---

[70]"The Life-Saving Banned Vitamin," *Prevention*, May 1968.
[71]"The Life-Saving Banned Vitamin," *Prevention*, May 1968.

PANGAMIC ACID MAY BE BENEFICIAL FOR THE
FOLLOWING AILMENTS:

Body Member	Ailment
Blood/Circulatory system	Angina pectoris
	Atherosclerosis
	Cholesterol level, high
	Hypertension
Brain/Nervous system	Hypertension
	Multiple sclerosis
Head	Headache
Heart	Angina pectoris
	Atherosclerosis
	Hypertension
Liver	Cirrhosis of liver
Lungs/Respiratory system	Asthma
	Emphysema
General	Alcoholism
	Cancer
	Hepatitis
	Hypoxia
	Rheumatic fever
	Rheumatism

PANTOTHENIC ACID

Description

Pantothenic acid, a part of the vitamin B complex, is water-soluble. It occurs in all living cells, being widely distributed in yeasts, molds, bacteria, and individual cells of all animals and plants. Organ meats, brewer's yeast, egg yolks, and whole-grain cereals are the richest sources. Pantothenic acid is synthesized in the body by the bacterial flora of the intestines.[72]

There is a close correlation between pantothenic acid tissue levels and functioning of the adrenal cortex. Pantothenic acid stimulates the adrenal glands and increases production of cortisone and other adrenal hormones important for healthy skin and nerves.

Pantothenic acid plays a vital role in cellular metabolism. As a coenzyme it participates in the release of energy from carbohydrates, fats, and proteins and in the utilization of other vitamins, especially riboflavin. Pantothenic acid is an essential constituent of the enzyme

COA, which forms active acetate and, as such, acts as an activating agent in metabolism. Pantothenic acid is essential for the synthesis of cholesterol, steroids (fat-soluble organic compounds), and fatty acids.[73] It is important in maintaining a healthy digestive tract.

Pantothenic acid can improve the body's ability to withstand stressful conditions. Adequate intake of pantothenic acid reduces the toxicity effects of many antibiotics. It aids in the prevention of premature aging and wrinkles. It also protects against cellular damage caused by excessive radiation.[74]

Absorption and Storage

Pantothenic acid is found in the blood, particularly in the plasma, which is the liquid part of the lymph. Pantothenic acid is excreted daily in the urine.

Approximately thirty-three percent of the pantothenic acid content of meat is lost during cooking and about fifty percent is lost by the milling of flour.[75] It is easily destroyed by acid, such as vinegar, or alkali, such as baking soda.

Dosage and Toxicity

Individual needs for pantothenic acid vary according to periods of stress, daily food intake, and urinary excretion levels. Several sources, including the National Research Council, suggest 5 to 10 milligrams daily for adults and children, respectively.[76] The Heinz Handbook of Nutrition suggests daily requirements to be 10 to 15 milligrams. Dr. Paavo Airola has estimated the optimum daily intake to be between 30 and 50 milligrams per day.

Therapeutic dosages usually range from 50 to 200 milligrams per day. In some studies, 1,000 and more milligrams were given daily for six months without side effects.[77] It is presumed that folic acid aids in the assimilation of pantothenic acid. There are no known toxic effects with pantothenic acid.

---

[72]Hoover (ed.), *Remington's Pharmaceutical Sciences*, p. 1030.

[73]Chaney and Ross, *Nutrition*, p. 304.

[74]Airola, *How to Get Well*, p. 265.

[75]Krause and Hunscher, *Food, Nutrition and Diet Therapy*, p. 138.

[76]Goodhart and Shils, *Modern Nutrition in Health and Disease*, p. 207.

[77]Airola, *How to Get Well*, p. 265.

Deficiency Effects and Symptoms

Pantothenic acid is so widely distributed in foods that an occurrence of deficiency is rare. The means of detecting deficiencies are limited, although low intakes may slow down many metabolic processes.[78]

Symptoms of a deficiency may include vomiting, restlessness, abdominal pains, burning feet, muscle cramps, sensitivity to insulin, decreased antibody formation, gastrointestinal disturbances, and upper respiratory infections. A deficiency may lead to skin disorders, adrenal exhaustion, and low blood sugar (hypoglycemia).[79] The list of deficiency symptoms reflects impaired health of cells in many tissues. A lack of pantothenic acid may result in duodenal ulcers. Deficiencies may occur when the body lacks the intestinal flora needed to synthesize pantothenic acid. The function of the adrenal gland is diminished, which may lead to physical and mental depression, insufficient secretions of hydrochloric acid in the stomach, and disturbances of the motor nerves.

Beneficial Effect on Ailments

Pantothenic acid has been used successfully to treat paralysis of the gastrointestinal tract after surgery.[80] It appears to stimulate gastrointestinal movement and aids in the prevention of nerve degeneration due to a deficiency. Nerve degeneration includes peripheral neuritis, nerve disorders, and epilepsy.

Blood pantothenic acid levels decrease during rheumatoid arthritis; the more severe the symptoms, the lower the acid level. Daily injections of pantothenic acid may lead to a rise in blood pantothenic acid levels. Pantothenic acid is important in the prevention of arthritis.[81] It is probably the greatest defense against stress and fatigue, and it also helps build antibodies for fighting infection.

Animal Tests

1. Pantothenic Acid and Duodenal Ulcers. Rats were kept on a diet deficient in pantothenic acid.

Results. Increased hormonal activity was shown to cause ulcers in 11 to 14 weeks. The same hormonal activity in rats that had been fed pantothenic acid did not pro-

[78]Guthrie, *Introductory Nutrition*, p. 261.
[79]Airola, *How to Get Well*, p. 265.
[80]Guthrie, *Introductory Nutrition*, p. 262.
[81]Williams, *Nutrition against Disease*, p. 126.

duce any ulcers. (*Drug Trade News*, March 11, 1957, as reported in J. I. Rodale, ed., *Best Health Articles from Prevention Magazine*, pp. 231 and 232.)

2. Pantothenic Acid and Infection. Rats were divided into two groups: one with a diet containing pantothenic acid and one without any. They were then exposed to an infection source.

Results. Spontaneous infections were widespread in the rats whose diet did not contain pantothenic acid. No infections were seen in the rats whose diet was complete. In the rats (deficient in pantothenic acid) that were inoculated with the infection source, 100 percent infection was noted. The rats whose diet included this vitamin showed an infection incidence of only 1 in 45 when given the same inoculation. (*Nutrition Review*, February 1957, as reported in Rodale, *Encyclopedia for Healthful Living*, p. 951.)

3. Pantothenic Acid and Life-Span. Mice were divided into two groups. They were treated alike except that each animal in the control group received 0.3 milligram of extra pantothenate per day in its drinking water. This amount was several times the amount that mice supposedly require.

Results. The 41 mice on the regular diet lived an average of 550 days. The 33 mice who received extra pantothenate lived an average of 653 days. (550 days is equivalent to 75 years for humans, and 653 days is equivalent to 89 years.) (Williams, *Nutrition against Disease*, pp. 141 and 142.)

PANTOTHENIC ACID MAY BE BENEFICIAL FOR THE FOLLOWING AILMENTS:

Body Member	Ailment
Blood/Circulatory system	Anemia
	Hypoglycemia
Bladder	Cystitis
Bones	Fracture
Bowel	Diarrhea
Brain/Nervous system	Epilepsy
	Fainting spells
	Insomnia
	Mental illness
	Multiple sclerosis

Body Member	Ailment
	Neuritis
Eye	Cataracts
Foot	Burning and tingling sensations
Glands	Adrenal exhaustion
Hair/Scalp	Baldness
Head	Headache
Intestine	Worms
Joints	Arthritis
	Gout
Leg	Leg cramp
	Phlebitis
Lungs/Respiratory system	Allergies
	Asthma
	Tuberculosis
Muscles	Muscular dystrophy
Skin	Acne
	Psoriasis
Stomach	Gastritis
	Indigestion (dyspepsia)
	Nausea
General	Alcoholism
	Cancer
	Depression
	Fatigue
	Infection
	Retarded growth
	Stress

VITAMIN C (ASCORBIC ACID)

Description

Vitamin C, also known as ascorbic acid, is a water-soluble nutrient. Although fairly stable in acid solution, it is normally the least stable of vitamins and is very sensitive to oxygen. Its potency can be lost through exposure to light, heat, and air, which stimulate the activity of oxidative enzymes.

A primary function of vitamin C is maintaining collagen, a protein necessary for the formation of connective tissue in skin, ligaments, and bones. Vitamin C plays a role in healing wounds and burns because it facilitates the formation of connective tissue in the scar. Vitamin C also aids in forming red blood cells and preventing hemorrhaging. In addition, vitamin C fights bacterial infections and reduces the effects on the body of some allergy-producing substances. For these reasons, vitamin C is frequently used in preventing and treating the common cold.

Vitamin C has significant relationships with other nutrients. It aids in the metabolism of the amino acids phenylalanine and tyrosine. Vitamin C converts the inactive form of folic acid to the active form, folinic acid, and may have a role in calcium metabolism.[82] In addition, vitamin C protects thiamine, riboflavin, folic acid, pantothenic acid, and vitamins A and E against oxidation.

Vitamin C is present in most fresh fruits and vegetables. Natural vitamin C dietary supplements are prepared from rose hips, acerola cherries, green peppers, and citrus fruits.

Absorption and Storage

The level of ascorbic acid in the blood reaches a maximum in two or three hours after ingestion of a moderate quantity, then decreases as it is eliminated in the urine and through perspiration.[83] Most vitamin C is out of the body in three or four hours. Because vitamin C is a "stress vitamin," it is used up even more rapidly under stressful conditions. Man, apes, and guinea pigs are the only animals that need vitamin C in their foodstuffs because they are unable to meet body needs by synthesis and must rely upon a dietary source. Ascorbic acid is readily absorbed from the gastrointestinal tract into the bloodstream. Two factors influencing absorption are the manner in which the vitamin is administered and the presence of other substances in the intestinal tract. The normal human body when fully saturated contains about 5,000 milligrams of vitamin C, of which 30 milligrams are found in the adrenal glands, 200 milligrams in the extracellular fluids, and the rest distributed in varying concentrations throughout the cells of the body. The body's ability to absorb vitamin C is reduced by smoking, stress, high fever, prolonged administration of antibiotics or cortisone, inhalation of DDT or fumes of petroleum, and ingestion of aspirin or other pain killers. Sulfa drugs increase urinary excretion of vitamin C by two or three times the normal amount. Baking soda creates an alkaline medium that destroys vitamin C. In

[82]Henrietta Fleck, *Introduction to Nutrition* (London: The Macmillan Co., 1971), p. 147.

[83]Linus C. Pauling, *Vitamin C and the Common Cold* (New York: Bantam Books, 1971), pp. 63 and 64.

addition, drinking excessive amounts of water will deplete the body's vitamin C. Cooking in copper utensils will destroy the vitamin C content of foods.

Dosage and Toxicity

The National Research Council recommends 45 milligrams of vitamin C for adults. According to Dr. Linus C. Pauling, Nobel Laureate Professor of Chemistry, University of California, Stanford, the optimum daily intake of vitamin C for most human adults is from 2,300 to 9,000 milligrams. The variation is caused by differences in weight, amount of activity, rate of metabolism, ailments, and age. Periods of stress, such as anxiety, infection, injury, surgery, burns, or fatigue, increase the body's need for this vitamin. It is better to take frequent small doses of the vitamin instead of a single large dose, because the body can absorb only a certain amount during a given period of time. For example, it is preferable to take one 250-milligram tablet of vitamin C six times daily rather than one or two gram tablets during the day. When megavitamin doses of vitamin C are given for colds, it is important that calcium intake be increased.

Toxicity symptoms usually do not occur with high intakes of vitamin C, because the body simply discharges whatever it cannot use. However, daily intake of between 5,000 and 15,000 milligrams may have side effects in some persons. Toxicity symptoms can be a slight burning sensation during urination, loose bowels, and/or skin rashes. When any symptom occurs, dosage should be reduced.

Deficiency Effects and Symptoms

Signs of deficiency are shortness of breath, impaired digestion, poor lactation, bleeding gums, weakened enamel or dentine, tendency to bruising, swollen or painful joints, nosebleeds, anemia, lowered resistance to infections, and slow healing of wounds and fractures. Severe deficiency results in scurvy. Breaks in the capillary walls are signs of vitamin C deficiency, and clots usually form at the point of the break. Therefore a lack of vitamin C is a probable cause of heart attacks and strokes initiated by clots. The blood level of ascorbic acid is known to be lowered by smoking. Nicotine added to a sample of human blood of known ascorbic acid content decreased the ascorbic acid content of the blood by 24 to 31 percent.[84]

[84] Rodale, *The Encyclopedia for Healthful Living*, p. 953.

Beneficial Effect on Ailments

Vitamin C plays an important role in preventing and relieving scurvy. Vitamin C promotes fine bone and tooth formation while protecting the dentine and pulp. Some types of viral and bacterial infections are prevented or cured by vitamin C, and it reduces the effects on the body of some allergy-producing substances. Vitamin C is frequently used in the prevention and treatment of the common cold.

The lubricating fluid of joints (synovial fluid) becomes thinner (allowing freer movement) when the serum levels of ascorbic acid are high. Therefore arthritic patients given vitamin C may find some relief of pain. It is an important nutrient in treating wounds because it speeds up the healing process. Ascorbic acid may lower blood cholesterol content of patients with artereosclerosis.

The need for vitamin C increases with age due to a greater need to regenerate collagen. With age, the sex glands develop a greater need for vitamin C and will draw it from other tissues, leaving these tissues vulnerable to disease. Therefore proper supplementation will help reduce depletion. Vitamin C is important in all stressful conditions. The tissue requirements for ascorbic acid are increased under conditions of increased metabolism.

Human Tests

1. Vitamin C and Whooping Cough. 90 children with whooping cough were given vitamin C orally or were injected with 5,000 milligrams daily for seven days, with the dosage being gradually reduced until a daily level of 100 milligrams was reached. A control group was given whooping cough vaccine.

Results. The duration of the disease in the children receiving ascorbic acid was 15 to 20 days, while the average duration for the children receiving vaccine was 34 days. When ascorbic acid therapy was started during the catarrhal stage, the spasmodic stage was prevented in 75 percent of the cases. (*Journal of the American Medical Association*, November 4, 1950, as reported in Rodale, *The Encyclopedia for Healthful Living*, p. 956.)

2. Vitamin C and Prickly Heat. 30 children were divided into two groups of 15. One group was given vitamin C in proportion to body weight; the other group was given placebos, in this case, sugar pills. Only the pharmacist knew who had which. After two weeks, Dr. Hindson and the pharmacist compared their notes:

Vitamin C Group	Placebo Group
1 same	9 same
4 improved	4 improved
10 free from lesions	2 worse

The 15 patients given the placebos were then given vitamin C following the first comparison. Within two months, no lesions were seen on any of the 30 children. (Dosage: Child of 38 pounds = 250 milligrams a day.) (Dr. C. Hindson, as reported in Rodale, ed., *Prevention*, July 1972.)

3. Vitamin C and Iron Deficiency. 30 females ages fourteen to forty-two were suffering from iron deficiency. They were given one tablet of 200 milligrams of ascorbic acid daily.

Results. After 60 days of treatment, the iron deficiency was alleviated. A chronic deficiency of iron is often complicated by the side effect of scurvy. In order to influence absorption of iron, a vitamin C intake of at least 200 to 500 milligrams per day is needed. (Enil Margo Schleicher, Director of Hematology at St. Barnabas Hospital, Minneapolis, as reported in Rodale, ed., *Prevention*, August 1970.)

4. Vitamin C and Nicotine. 14 smokers and 14 nonsmokers having similar characteristics and dietary habits were placed on vitamin C-deficient diets. Blood samples of all were taken. Then the subjects were given 1.1 grams of vitamin C and high doses of water-soluble vitamins to facilitate absorption. This process continued for five days, until the subjects' bodies were saturated with vitamin C. For three days vitamin C intakes were carefully limited, and the urine was closely examined.

Results. Blood tests showed that the smokers had about 30 percent less vitamin C in their blood than the nonsmokers. (Omar Pelletier of the Nutrition Research Division of the Food and Drug Directorate in Ottawa, Canada, as reported in Rodale, ed., *Prevention*, July 1969.)

5. Vitamin C and Inflammation of the Urethra. 12 men were suffering from painful inflammation of the urethra. The patients were examined, and each was given 3 grams of vitamin C daily for four days. The irritation was caused by phosphatic crystals formed in the urine due to insufficient acidity.

Results. The large doses of vitamin C proved to be a safe way of introducing enough acidity to force the crystals back into solution. What cured the patients was the "wasted" vitamin C, the part not stored in the body and spilled into the urine. The excess vitamin C in the urine proved to be 100 percent effective in relieving the symptoms. (Rodale, ed., *Prevention*, July 1973.)

Animal Tests

1. Vitamin C and Tooth Formation. In vitamin C-deficient guinea pigs, the dentine near the developing teeth ceased to form and the pulp was separated from the dentine by liquid. Either dentine ceased being manufactured, or it was of inferior quality. The pulp itself shrunk and once free from the dentine, was apparently floating in a liquid.

Results. Rapid repair followed the administration of vitamin C. (*Journal of Dentistry for Children*, Third Quarter, 1943, as reported in Rodale, *The Encyclopedia for Healthful Living*, pp. 953 and 954.)

2. Vitamin C and Mercury Poisoning. 20 guinea pigs were given 200 milligrams of vitamin C daily for six days (equivalent to 14 grams per day for humans). On the sixth day, each pig was given what should have been a fatal dosage of mercury. After the poisoning, they were put back on their regular diet, which included 200 milligrams of vitamin C daily.

Results. After two days, they lost weight but ate and behaved normally. The experiment was finally terminated. After 20 days the animals were considered saved. (Momcilo Mokranjae and Ceda Petrovic in the *C. R. Acad. Sc. Paris*, 1964, as reported in Rodale, ed., *Prevention*, July 1972, p. 82.)

3. Storage of Ascorbic Acid. Experimental guinea pigs supplied with natural sources of vitamin C had better storage in their tissues than when supplied with synthetic ascorbic acid. (Estelle E. Hawley, "The Effect of the Administration of Acid Content of Guinea Pigs Tissues," *Journal of Nutrition*, 1937, as reported in Rodale, ed., *Prevention*, July 1972.)

4. Vitamin C and Oxygen Starvation. 42 rats were placed in a decompression chamber until the atmospheric pressure equaled that at an altitude of 33,000 feet. All died within 13 minutes. A second group of rats were injected with vitamin C before being placed in the decompression chamber. The dosage given was equivalent to a human dosage of 7 grams.

Results. Three rats did not die; the others stayed alive for an average of 23.7 minutes. A third group of 44 rats were injected with double the vitamin C dosage of the second group (equivalent to a human dosage of 14 grams) and then were put in the decompression chamber.

Results. 21 rats did not die, and the others stayed alive for nearly an hour. The investigators admitted that they did not know why the vitamin C had this effect. (Kazuo Asahina and Katsumi Asano, Toho University School of Medicine, Tokyo, as reported in Rodale, ed., *Prevention*, July 1972.)

VITAMIN C MAY BE BENEFICIAL FOR THE FOLLOWING AILMENTS:

Body Member	Ailment
Bladder	Cystitis
Blood/Circulatory system	Alcoholism
	Anemia
	Angina pectoris
	Arteriosclerosis
	Bruising
	Cholesterol level, high
	Diabetes
	Hemophilia
	Hypertension
	Hypoglycemia
	Jaundice
	Leukemia
	Mononucleosis
	Pernicious anemia
	Phlebitis
	Stroke (cerebrovascular accident)
	Varicose veins
Bones	Fracture
	Osteomalacia
	Osteoporosis
	Rickets
Bowel	Celiac disease
	Colitis
	Cystic fibrosis
	Diarrhea
	Worms
Brain/Nervous system	Dizziness
	Epilepsy
	Fatigue
	Hypertension
	Hypoxia
	Insomnia
	Meningitis
	Mental illness
	Multiple sclerosis
	Parkinson's disease
	Shingles (herpes zoster)
	Stroke (cerebrovascular accident)
Ear	Ear infection
Eye	Amblyopia
	Cataracts
	Conjunctivitis
	Eyestrain
	Glaucoma
	Vision and focus disorders
Gallbladder	Gallstones
Glands	Adrenal exhaustion
	Cystic fibrosis
	Goiter
	Prostatitis
	Swollen glands
Hair/Scalp	Baldness
	Hair problems
Head	Headache
Heart	Angina pectoris
	Arteriosclerosis
	Hypertension
Intestine	Celiac disease
	Constipation
	Hemorrhoids
Joints	Arthritis
	Bursitis
	Gout
Kidney	Kidney stones (renal calculi)
	Nephritis
Leg	Leg cramp

Body Member	Ailment
	Phlebitis
	Varicose veins
Liver	Cirrhosis of liver
	Hepatitis
	Jaundice
Lungs/Respiratory system	Allergies
	Bronchitis
	Common cold
	Croup
	Emphysema
	Hay fever (allergic rhinitis)
	Influenza
	Pneumonia
	Tuberculosis
Mouth	Canker sore
	Halitosis
Muscles	Muscular dystrophy
	Rheumatism
Reproductive system	Prostatitis
Skin	Abscess
	Acne
	Athlete's foot
	Bedsores
	Boil (furuncle)
	Bruises
	Burns
	Carbuncle
	Eczema
	Impetigo
	Psoriasis
	Scurvy
	Shingles (herpes zoster)
Stomach	Gastritis
	Gastroenteritis
	Stomach ulcer (peptic)
Teeth/Gums	Pyorrhea
	Tooth and gum disorders
General	Alcoholism
	Arthritis
	Backache
	Beriberi
	Cancer
	Chicken pox

Body Member	Ailment
	Fever
	Infection
	Influenza
	Kwashiorkor
	Overweight and obesity
	Pregnancy
	Rheumatic fever
	Stress
	Stroke (cerebrovascular accident)

VITAMIN D

Description

Vitamin D is a fat-soluble vitamin, and it can be acquired either by ingestion or by exposure to sunlight. It is known as the "sunshine" vitamin because the action of the sun's ultraviolet rays activates a form of cholesterol, which is present in the skin, converting it to vitamin D.

The provitamins D are found in both plant and animal tissue. Vitamin D_2 is known as calciferol, a synthetic; vitamin D_3 is the natural form as it occurs in fish-liver oils. D_3 can be made synthetically by ultraviolet irradiation of 7-dehydrocholesterol, a derivative of cholesterol.

Vitamin D aids in the absorption of calcium from the intestinal tract and the breakdown and assimilation of phosphorus, which is required for bone formation.[85] It helps synthesize those enzymes in the mucous membranes which are involved in the active transport of available calcium. Vitamin D is necessary for normal growth in children, for without it bones and teeth do not calcify properly.

Adults also benefit from vitamin D. It is valuable in maintaining a stable nervous system, normal heart action, and normal blood clotting because all these functions are related to the body's supply and utilization of calcium and phosphorus. Vitamin D is best utilized when taken with vitamin A. Fish-liver oils are the best natural source of vitamins A and D.

Absorption and Storage

Ingested vitamin D is absorbed with the fats through the intestinal walls with the aid of bile. Vitamin D from

[85] Hoover (ed.), *Remington's Pharmaceutical Sciences* (Emmaus: Mack Pub. Co., 1970), p. 1017.

dehydrocholesterol by sun radiation is formed in the skin and absorbed into the circulatory system. Pigmentation is a factor in the absorption of ultraviolet rays. The more pigment there is in the skin, the less vitamin D is produced in the body by irradiation.

After absorption from the intestine or formation in the skin, vitamin D is transported to the liver for storage; other deposits are found in the skin, brain, spleen, and bones. The body can store sizable reserves of vitamin D. Mineral oil can destroy the vitamin D already stored in the intestinal tract.

Dosage and Toxicity

Most of the body's needs for vitamin D can be met by sufficient exposure to sunlight and from the ingestion of small amounts of food, but the sun's action on the skin can be inhibited by such factors as air pollution, clouds, window glass, or clothing. The National Research Council sets the dietary allowance of vitamin D at 400 IU per day to meet the requirements of practically all healthy individuals who have little or no exposure to ultraviolet light. This same dosage is recommended for infants, provided the calcium consumption at the same time is adequate. During pregnancy and lactation women need to include extra vitamin D in their diets. According to the National Research Council, there are no vitamin D recommendations for adults over twenty-two years of age since there is no data available upon which to base such a recommendation.

The adult rate of calcium and phosphorus loss from the skeletal system is thought to be less rapid than that of the growing organism.

It must be emphasized that good will result from the provision of adequate vitamin D *only* when the calcium and phosphorus requirements are met. No extra benefit is obtained from taking more than 400 IU daily except for therapeutic reasons; then dosages may range from 1,500 to 2,800 IU daily for several months. Increased heart activity requires increased calcium, which is not supplied unless there is enough vitamin D in the system.

It is known that "hypervitaminosis D" can occur and can cause pathological changes in the body. Excessive amounts may cause high levels of calcium and phosphorus in the blood and excessive excretion of calcium in the urine; this leads to calcification of soft tissues and of the walls of the blood vessels and kidney tubules, which is hypercalcemia.[86] Adelle Davis stated, "a toxic dose of vitamin D for adults appears to be 300,000 to 800,000 IU daily for many months. 30,000 IU daily or more over a period of time can easily produce toxic symptoms in babies and 50,000 IU are dangerous for children."[87]

Symptoms of acute overdosage are increased frequency of urination, loss of appetite, nausea, vomiting, diarrhea, muscular weakness, dizziness, weariness, and calcification of the soft tissues of the heart, blood vessels, and lungs. These symptoms will disappear within a few days when the overdosage is terminated.

Deficiency Effects and Symptoms

A deficiency of vitamin D leads to inadequate absorption of calcium from the intestinal tract and retention of phosphorus in the kidney, leading to faulty mineralization of bone structures. The inability of the soft bones to withstand the stress of weight results in skeletal malformations. Rickets, a bone disorder in children, is a direct result of vitamin D deficiency. Signs of rickets are softening of the skull; softening of the fragile bones with bowing of the legs and spinal curvature; enlargement of the wrist, knee, and ankle joints; poorly developed muscles; and nervous irritability.[88] "Adult rickets" called osteomalacia may also occur.

It is believed that vitamin D and parathyroid hormones work together to regulate the transport of calcium. A deficiency may cause tetany, a condition characterized by muscular numbness, tingling, and spasm. Thyroid glands need vitamin D to manufacture their hormones, so a vitamin D deficiency may cause flabbiness, poor metabolism, and diabetic distress.

Dr. Arthur A. Knapp, an ophthamologist, reported tests indicating that a vitamin D deficiency may cause myopia, or nearsightedness. An imbalance in calcium is the root of this disorder (see Animal and Human Tests). A vitamin D deficiency may also lead to faulty development of tooth structure.

Beneficial Effect on Ailments

Vitamin D helps prevent and cure rickets, a disease resulting from insufficient calcium, phosphorus, or vitamin D. It also aids in repairing osteomalacia in adults.

Vitamin D plays an important role in dentition. Besides being necessary for proper tooth eruption and linear growth, it continually strengthens the teeth. According to Adelle Davis, vitamin D helps in preventing

---

[86]Chaney and Ross, *Nutrition*, pp. 223-224.

[87]Rodale and Staff, *The Complete Book of Vitamins*, p. 340.
[88]Hoover (ed.), *Remington's Pharmaceutical Sciences*, p. 1017.

tooth decay and pyorrhea, an inflammation of the sockets of the teeth.

Vitamins D and A have been beneficial in reducing incidences of colds. The two vitamins taken along with vitamin C act as a preventive measure. Researchers have reported that the acidity of gastric juices is affected by the amount of vitamin D in the diet. These juices are named as a cause of stomach ulcers. Therefore an ulcer patient should be checked to see whether his diet has a sufficient supply of vitamin D.

Human Tests

1. Vitamin D and Myopia. 50,000 USP units of vitamin D in capsule and 1 gram of calcium, in the form of milk or dicalcium phosphate tables, were given daily to selected patients.

Results. In one group, 18 of 52 vitamin-fed patients showed a reduction in myopia, and 8 remained unchanged. (Rodale, ed., *Prevention*, May 1973, p. 95.)

2. Vitamin D and Conjunctivitis. 41 patients suffering from allergic conjunctivitis were given 50,000 units of vitamin D daily for seven weeks.

Results. 29 patients experienced complete relief with vitamin D therapy, 11 showed marked improvement, and 1 remained unchanged. (Dr. Arthur A. Knapp, Columbia College of Physicians and Surgeons, as reported in Rodale, ed., *Prevention*, September 1969, pp. 80-82.)

3. Vitamins D and A and Colds. 54 patients suffering from frequent colds, accompanied by high fever, were put into three groups. Group 1 received only vitamin A; Group 2 received only vitamin D; Group 3 received both vitamins D and A. Children under twelve were given half the adult dosage.

Results. None of the patients who received either vitamin D or A alone benefited by the treatment. In the group that received both vitamins, 80 percent showed a significant reduction in both the number and severity of common colds.

Animal Tests

1. Vitamin D and Myopia. Animals fed diets deficient in vitamin D and calcium developed axial myopia, keratoconus (a conical protrusion of the cornea), cataracts, and even arteriosclerosis comparable to the senile type observed clinically in human beings. (Dr. Arthur A. Knapp, Columbia College of Physicians and Surgeons, as reported in Rodale, ed., *Prevention*, September 1969, pp. 80-82.)

2. Vitamin D and Bone Growth. Experiments in which the calcium intake varied in rats showed that vitamin D was responsible for suppressing growth when dietary calcium was high and for stimulating growth when dietary calcium intake was low. (H. Steenback and D.C. Herting, *Nutrition Reviews*, vol. 14, p. 191, 1956.)

VITAMIN D MAY BE BENEFICIAL FOR THE FOLLOWING AILMENTS:

Body Member	Ailment
Bladder	Cystitis
Blood/Circulatory system	Cholesterol level, high
	Diabetes
Bones	Fracture
	Osteomalacia
	Osteoporosis
	Rickets
Brain/Nervous system	Epilepsy
	Meningitis
Eye	Bitot spots
	Cataracts
	Eyestrain
	Glaucoma
	Vision and focus disorders
Glands	Cystic fibrosis
Gallbladder	Gallstones
Head	Fever
Intestine	Celiac disease
	Constipation
	Worms
Joints	Arthritis
Leg	Leg cramp
	Sciatica
Liver	Cirrhosis of liver
	Jaundice
Lungs/Respiratory system	Allergies
	Bronchitis
	Common cold
	Emphysema
	Tuberculosis
Mouth	Canker sores

Body Member	Ailment
Muscles	Tetany
Reproductive system	Vaginitis
Skin	Acne
	Bedsores
	Burns
	Carbuncles
	Eczema
	Psoriasis
	Shingles (herpes zoster)
Teeth/Gums	Pyorrhea
General	Aging
	Alcoholism
	Backache
	Cancer
	Fatigue
	Insomnia
	Kwashiorkor
	Pregnancy
	Rheumatic fever
	Stress

VITAMIN E (TOCOPHEROL)

Description

Vitamin E, a fat-soluble vitamin, is composed of a group of compounds called tocopherols. Seven forms of tocopherol exist in nature: alpha, beta, delta, epsilon, eta, gamma, and zeta. Of these, alpha tocopherol is the most potent form of vitamin E and has the greatest nutritional and biological value. Tocopherols occur in highest concentrations in cold-pressed vegetable oils, all whole raw seeds and nuts, and soybeans. Wheat-germ oil is the source from which vitamin E was first obtained.

Vitamin E is an antioxidant, which means it opposes oxidation of substances in the body. It prevents saturated fatty acids and vitamin A from breaking down and combining with other substances that may become harmful to the body. The vitamin B complex and ascorbic acid are also protected against oxidation when vitamin E is present in the digestive tract.[89] Fats and oils containing vitamin E are less susceptible to rancidity than those devoid of vitamin E. Vitamin E has the ability to unite

[89] Guthrie, *Introductory Nutrition*, pp. 210-211.

with oxygen and prevent it from being converted into toxic peroxides; this leaves the red blood cells more fully supplied with the pure oxygen that the blood carries to the heart and other organs.

Vitamin E plays an essential role in cellular respiration of all muscles, especially cardiac and skeletal. Vitamin E makes it possible for these muscles and their nerves to function with less oxygen, thereby increasing their endurance and stamina. It also causes dilation of the blood vessels, permitting a fuller flow of blood to the heart. Vitamin E is a highly effective antithrombin in the bloodstream, inhibiting coagulation of blood by preventing clots from forming. It also aids in bringing nourishment to the cells, strengthening the capillary walls, and protecting the red blood cells from destruction by poisons, such as hydrogen peroxide, in the blood.

Vitamin E prevents both the pituitary and adrenal hormones from being oxidized and promotes proper functioning of linoleic acid, an unsaturated fatty acid. Because aging in the cells is due primarily to oxidation, vitamin E is useful in retarding this process. It is also necessary for proper focusing of the eyes in middle-aged persons.

Vitamin E is effective in the prevention of elevated scar formation on the body surface and within the body. In ointment form it is used on burns to promote healing and lessen the formation of scars. It stimulates urine excretion, which helps heart patients whose body tissues contain an excessive amount of tissue fluid (edema). As a diuretic, vitamin E helps lower elevated blood pressure. It protects against the damaging effects of many environmental poisons in the air, water, and food.[90] It protects the lungs and other tissues from damage by polluted air. Vitamin E has a dramatic effect on the reproductive organs; it helps prevent miscarriages, increases male and female fertility, and helps restore male potency.

Absorption and Storage

Vitamin E, as other fat-soluble vitamins, is absorbed in the presence of bile salts and fat. From the intestines, it is absorbed into the lymph and is transported in the bloodstream as tocopherol to the liver, where high concentrations of it are stored. It is also stored in the fatty tissues, heart, muscles, testes, uterus, blood, and adrenal and pituitary glands. Vitamin E in ointment form can

[90] Airola, *How to Get Well*, p. 206.

be absorbed through the skin and mucous membranes. Excessive amounts of vitamin E are excreted in the urine, and all effects of vitamin E disappear within three days.

There are several substances that interfere with, or even cause a depletion of, vitamin E in the body. For example, when iron, especially the inorganic form, and vitamin E are administered together, the absorption of both substances is impaired. Dr. Wilfred Shute, in *Vitamin E for Ailing and Healthy Hearts*, suggests that vitamin E should be taken in one dose and all iron taken 8 to 12 hours later for proper absorption. The best time to take vitamin E is before mealtime or bedtime. Chlorine in drinking water, ferric chloride, rancid oil or fat, and inorganic iron compounds destroy vitamin E in the body. Mineral oil used as a laxative depletes vitamin E. Vegetable oils dissolve alpha tocopherol and readily release it in the body, whereas mineral oil dissolves it but does not readily release it.

Large amounts of polyunsaturated fats or oils in the diet increase the rate of oxidation of vitamin E; the more unsaturated fats or oils consumed, the more vitamin E is necessary.[91] The female hormone estrogen is a vitamin E antagonist. Intake of this hormone makes it very difficult to estimate the amount of alpha tocopherol the individual is lacking.

Improper absorption may be partly responsible for muscular problems, such as muscular dystrophy and poor performance in athletes, and digestive problems, such as peptic ulcers and cancer of the colon.[92] Poor absorption can impair the survival of red blood cells.

Dosage and Toxicity

The daily intake of vitamin E recommended by the National Research Council is based upon the metabolic body size and the level of polyunsaturated fatty acids in the diet rather than upon weight or calorie intake. The requirements increase with gains in polyunsaturated fatty acids in the diet. Air pollution also increases the need for vitamin E. The RDA for infants is 4 to 5 IU daily; for children and adolescents the range is 7 to 12 IU; for adult males, 15 IU; for adult females, 12 IU; in pregnancy and lactation, needs increase to 15 IU daily. Many nutritionists consider these daily allowances exceedingly low. Adelle Davis recommends 30 IU daily for infants and children and 100 IU for adolescents and adults.[93] In cases of illness, doctors recommend 300 to 600 IU daily, although 2,000 IU have been used therapeutically with excellent results.[94]

Vitamin E has a tendency to raise blood pressure when it is given in large doses to someone whose body is not accustomed to it; therefore initial intake should be small, and as tolerance rises, the dosage should be gradually increased. It has been suggested that men start with 100 IU and gradually increase to 600 IU when used for preventive purposes. Women should begin with 100 IU and gradually increase to 400 IU.[95] The best way to determine the correct dosage is with the help of a doctor who is learned in vitamin E therapy.

Vitamin E is considered nontoxic except in two conditions: in high blood pressure patients, it elevates the pressure; starting a chronic rheumatic heart disease patient on high doses can lead to rapid deterioration or death. It is best to begin with small doses, gradually increasing the amount. When using vitamin E externally, Shute states that it is a good idea to take it orally while simultaneously applying it to the body. These methods complement each other.[96]

Deficiency Effects and Symptoms

The first clinical sign of a vitamin E deficiency is the rupture of red blood cells which results from their increased fragility. A deficiency could result in a reduction of membrane stability and a shrinkage in collagen, connective tissue. A vitamin E deficiency may result in a tendency toward muscular wasting or abnormal fat deposits in the muscles and an increased demand for oxygen. Without sufficient amounts of vitamin E in the body, the essential fatty acids are altered so that blood cells break down and hemoglobin formation is impaired. In addition, several amino acids cannot be utilized, and pituitary and adrenal glands reduce their level of functioning. Iron absorption and hemoglobin formation also are impaired. A severe deficiency can cause damage to the kidneys and liver.

[91] Clark, *Know Your Nutrition*, p. 49.

[92] Ruth Winter, *Vitamin E the Miracle Worker* (New York: Arco Publ. Co., 1972), p. 84.

[93] Davis, *Let's Get Well*, p. 398.

[94] Davis, *Let's Get Well*, p. 398.

[95] Carlson Wade, *The Rejuvenated Vitamin* (New York: Award Books, 1970), p. 21.

[96] Wilfred E. Shute and Harold J. Taub, *Vitamin E for Ailing and Healthy Hearts* (New York: Pyramid House, 1969), pp. 75-77.

Perhaps the widest incidence of vitamin E deficiency among adults in the United States is in gastrointestinal disease, where prolonged deficiency can cause faulty absorption of fat and of fat-soluble vitamins, possibly resulting in cystic fibrosis, blockage of the bile ducts, and chronic inflammation of the pancreas.[97] Poor utilization of the vitamin or an increased vitamin E demand peculiar to the individual can cause anemia and edema in premature and malnourished infants. Serious deficiencies of vitamin E in men may lead to degeneration of tissues in the testes. No amount of vitamin E therapy can repair the permanent damage, and such men may become sterile.[98] Women who are severely deficient in vitamin E cannot carry a pregnancy term successfully and often have miscarriages. Premature births frequently result from insufficient intake of vitamin E during pregnancy, leaving the infants more susceptible to anemia.[99] Hemorrhaging can occur in newborn infants who lack vitamin E. The blood cells of vitamin E–deficient babies are prone to weakness (hemolysis).

Vitamin E deficiencies can result in nephritis. This occurs when kidney tubules plug up with dead cells so that urine is unable to pass; dropsy and progressive degeneration then occur. Vitamin E deficiency appears to make red blood cells more susceptible to damage from medication and from environmental stresses.

A deficiency of vitamin E can produce heart disease.[100] Approximately 25,000 children are born with heart defects every year in the United States, where 50 percent of all deaths result from heart-related ailments. Evidence is accumulating to indicate that a lack of sufficient vitamin E may be a contributing factor in atherosclerosis and cancer.

According to Dr. Wilfred Shute, the lack of vitamin E in the American diet is partially due to the milling process which eliminates the highly perishable wheat germ, a significant source of vitamin E. About 90 percent of the vitamin E is lost in the milling process.

Beneficial Effect on Ailments

Vitamin E works to treat and prevent heart diseases such as coronary thrombosis, a heart attack in which the vessels are blocked by blood clots and part of the heart is deprived of its blood supply. Vitamin E causes arterial blood clots to disintegrate. Angina pectoris, a chest pain resulting from an insufficient supply of blood to the heart tissues, is successfully treated with alpha tocopherol.

According to Shute, rheumatic heart disease is responsible for 90 percent of defective hearts among children. Vitamin E aids rheumatic heart disease and early stages of cardiac complications by returning abnormal capillaries to normal and reducing fluid accumulation within and between cells. This promotes normal gas interchange across the cell membranes, which seems to arrest the disease.[101] Congenital heart disease results in structural defects of the heart. Vitamin E cannot alter the defective structure, but its oxygen-saving effects and its antithrombin activity are vital for patients who are not treated surgically. Many congenital heart disease patients have cyanosis, insufficient supply of oxygen in the blood, and with adequate dosage of vitamin E the cyanosis has disappeared.

Vitamin E is able to bring relief to intermittent claudication, a severe pain in calf muscles which results from inadequate blood supply caused by arterial spasm, atherosclerosis, or arteriosclerosis. Vitamin E is beneficial to persons with atherosclerosis if vitamin E therapy is used before irrepairable damage has occurred. It relieves pain in the extremities, speeds up blood flow, and reduces clotting tendencies.[102]

Vitamin E can aid in the healing of burned tissue, skin ulcers, and abrasions. It prevents or dissolves scar tissues. Vitamin E helps remove old acne scars, particularly if x-ray treatments have been given.[103] It is needed also to help dissolve scars in the arterial walls caused by toxic substances.

Vitamin E is helpful in counteracting premature aging of the skin.[104] It is useful to apply vitamin E to the skin in ointment form while taking it orally, because it affects the cell formation by replacing the cells on the outer layer of the skin. Vitamin E also helps counter the gradual decline in metabolic processes during aging. Dry, itchy skin is often part of the aging process; vitamin E ointment is able to relieve the itching.

Under normal conditions vitamin E reduces the formation of thrombin, a clotting agent; this tends to reduce the likelihood of thrombosis, the formation of a

[97] Martin Ebon, *The Truth about Vitamin E* (New York: Bantam Books, 1972), p. 7.

[98] Ebon, *The Truth about Vitamin E*, p. 30.

[99] Davis, *Let's Get Well*, p. 281.

[100] J.I. Rodale, *Complete Book of Minerals for Health* (Emmaus, Pa.: Rodale Books, 1972), p. 439.

[101] Shute and Taub, *Vitamin E for Ailing and Healthy Hearts*, pp. 61-64.

[102] Shute and Taub, *Vitamin E for Ailing and Healthy Hearts*, pp. 70-73.

[103] Davis, *Let's Get Well*, pp. 375-376.

[104] Ebon, *The Truth about Vitamin E*, p. 75.

blood clot. The intake of estrogen, found in contraceptive pills, may neutralize the effect of vitamin E. Intake of estrogen causes the collection of fibrin, an insoluble protein that promotes blood clotting by forming a fibrous network, to become greater. The greater amount of fibrin increases the chances of thromboembolism, the blocking of blood vessels.[105]

Vitamin E has been successful in regulating excessive or scanty flows during menstruation.[106] When vitamin E is added to the diet, it can correct menstrual rhythm. Vitamin E is recognized as a treatment for hot flashes and headaches during menopause. It has helped relieve itching and inflammation of the vagina when applied in ointment form and simultaneously ingested.

Bursitis, wry-neck, gout, and arthritis have improved with vitamin E therapy. Ingestion of large amounts has improved conditions of nearsightedness and crossed eyes. Vitamin E has also been used to prevent calcification of the kidneys caused by excessive vitamin D or other toxic substances.

Vitamin E has been used to help treat varicose veins, as an alternative to surgery. It also can relieve the pain of varicose veins by decreasing the amount of oxygen needed by the tissues involved.

Vitamin E has been successful in treating thrombosis and phlebitis, which are clots in the veins. In large doses it prevents clots from spreading, dissolves existing clots, and provides indirect circulation around obstructed veins. It should be used to prevent initial attacks of clotting after operations or childbirth.[107]

Individuals suffering from muscular dystrophy have benefited from massive doses of vitamin E.[108] Vitamin E may be able to clear up or control many forms of kidney disease, including nephritis. It also aids in restoring the functions of damaged livers.[109]

Vitamin E helps promote body defenses against virus infections and in some cases may be utilized as a flu vaccine.[110] High doses may build both the serum and the cellular levels of the body to high levels of immunity against flu.

Vitamin E therapy has been able to help diabetics. After administration of the vitamin, some patients found that their blood sugar levels became normal or near normal, and the amount of insulin required was reduced. Vitamin E has also been used to prevent and treat gangrene in diabetics.

Vitamins A and E may be beneficial in lowering blood cholesterol by preventing fat deposits. The vitamins help offset the high cholesterol accumulations deposited on the arterial walls.

Vitamin E is used for easing headaches because it preserves the oxygen in the blood for an extended period. This results in more efficiency as the blood is pumped through the blood vessels of the head. Vitamin E has also relieved migraine attacks. Vitamins C and E work together to keep blood vessels flexible, healthy, and less subject to painful disturbances.[111]

Human Tests

1. Vitamin E and Menopause. A woman had undergone a complete hysterectomy due to cancer of an ovary. The patient suffered from hot flashes. She was given 75 IU of alpha tocopherol daily.

Results. Administration of the vitamin proved valuable in diminishing or entirely removing the hot flashes. (*Journal of the American Medical Association*, vol. 167, p. 1806, 1958, as reported in Rodale, *The Encyclopedia for Healthful Living*, p. 980.)

2. Vitamin E and Varicose Veins. 51 patients with varicose veins were given 300 to 500 milligrams of vitamin E daily. They were kept on this treatment from two months to three years, depending upon the severity of the ailment.

Results. 9 of the patients showed improvement within 30 days; 7 were completely healed; and the other 35 all showed some relief of congestion, pain, and edema. No side effects were noted. (*La Riforma Medical*, Vol. 69, pp. 853-856, 1955, as reported in Rodale, *The Encyclopedia for Healthful Living*, p. 978.)

3. Vitamin E and Menstrual Pain. 100 women between eighteen and twenty-one years of age were suffering from pain and discomfort during their menstrual periods. They were divided into two groups. Each woman in the first group was given 50 milligrams of vitamin E daily for ten days before menstruation and for the next four days. Each woman in the second group was given a placebo. Treatment lasted three months.

---

[105] Ebon, *The Truth about Vitamin E*, p. 77.
[106] Ebon, *The Truth about Vitamin E*, p. 80.
[107] Ebon, *The Truth about Vitamin E*, p. 80.
[108] Herbert Bailey, *Vitamin E, Your Key to a Healthy Heart* (New York: Arc Books 1971), pp. 97-98.
[109] Bailey, *Vitamin E, Your Key to a Healthy Heart*, p. 99.
[110] Wade, *The Rejuvenation Vitamin*, p. 85.

[111] Wade, *The Rejuvenation Vitamin*, p. 155.

Results. 76 percent of the women in the first group noted improvement; only 29 percent of the women in the second group noted any improvement in three months. The patients experienced a recurrence of their pain two to six months after treatment ceased. (*The Lancet*, vol. I, pp. 844-847, 1955, as reported in Rodale, *The Encyclopedia for Healthful Living*, p. 988.)

4. Vitamin E and Coronary Occlusion (Blood Clot in the Coronary Artery). A forty-year-old male suffering from a coronary occlusion was treated with 60 IU of alpha tocopherol daily.

Results. The symptoms of angina (sense of suffocation) disappeared completely in four weeks. (Shute, *Vitamin E for Ailing and Healthy Hearts*, p. 39.)

5. Vitamin E and Athletic Performance. In a controlled study athletes were given large doses of alpha tocopherol.

Results. Their muscle performance, endurance, and speed of recovery improved. The effect was transient but persisted as long as the treatment was maintained. ("Resolving the Vitamin E Controversy," *Percival*, Summary 3.55, 1951.)

Animal Test

1. Vitamin E and Muscular Stamina in Racehorses. Dr. Evan Shute and William Gutterson devised an experiment with vitamin E and its effect on racehorses.

Results. The percentage of wins for each horse given vitamin E was 2.7, compared to 2.3 the year before, when a smaller dose of vitamin E was given. Two years before, when no vitamin E was given, the percentage of wins per horse had been 1.8. Although there was an improvement in the first year, the horses hit their peak the following year, when the dosages were doubled or tripled. (*The Summary*, December 1956, published by the Shute Foundation for Medical Research, London, Canada, as reported in Rodale, *The Encyclopedia for Healthful Living*, p. 777.)

VITAMIN E MAY BE BENEFICIAL FOR THE FOLLOWING AILMENTS:

Body Member	Ailment
Bladder	Cystitis
Blood/Circulatory system	Anemia
	Angina pectoris
	Arteriosclerosis
	Atherosclerosis
	Bruising
	Coronary thrombosis
	Diabetes
	Hypertension
	Pernicious anemia
	Phlebitis
	Stroke (cerebrovascular accident)
	Thrombophlebitis
	Varicose veins
Bones	Osteoporosis
Bowel	Colitis
Brain/Nervous system	Epilepsy
	Mental illness
	Multiple sclerosis
	Parkinson's disease
	Stroke (cerebrovascular accident)
Ear	Ménière's syndrome
Eye	Amblyopia
	Cataracts
	Eyestrain
Gallbladder	Gallstones
Glands	Cystic fibrosis
	Hyperthyroidism
	Prostatitis
Hair/Scalp	Baldness
	Dandruff
Head	Headache
	Sinusitis
Heart	Angina pectoris
	Arteriosclerosis
	Atherosclerosis
	Congestive heart failure
	Coronary thrombosis
	Hypertension
	Myocardial infarction
Intestine	Celiac disease
	Constipation
	Hemorrhoids
Joints	Arthritis
	Bursitis
	Gout
Kidney	Kidney stones (renal calculi)

Body Member	Ailment
	Nephritis
Leg	Leg cramp
	Phlebitis
	Sciatica
	Varicose veins
Lungs/Respiratory system	Allergies
	Bronchitis
	Common cold
	Emphysema
	Hay fever (allergic rhinitis)
Muscles	Muscular dystrophy
	Rheumatism
Reproductive system	Miscarriage
	Prostatitis
	Vaginitis
Skin	Abscess
	Acne
	Athlete's foot
	Bedsores
	Boil (furuncle)
	Bruises
	Burns
	Carbuncle
	Impetigo
	Ulcers
	Warts
Stomach	Gastritis
	Stomach ulcer (peptic)
General	Backache
	Cancer
	Measles
	Overweight and obesity
	Pregnancy
	Sunburn
	Thrombophlebitis

VITAMIN F (UNSATURATED FATTY ACIDS)

Description

Vitamin F is a fat-soluble vitamin consisting of the unsaturated fatty acids. Unsaturated fatty acids usually come in the form of liquid vegetable oils, while satu-rated fatty acids are usually found in solid animal fat. The saturated fatty acids are more slowly metabolized by the body than are the unsaturated fatty acids.

The body cannot manufacture the essential unsatu-rated fatty acids, linoleic, linolenic, and arachidonic, and they must be obtained from foods. Wheat germ; seeds; natural golden vegetable oils, such as safflower, soy, and corn; and cod-liver oil contain lecithin and are the best sources of the unsaturated fatty acids.

Unsaturated fatty acids are important for respiration of vital organs and make it easier for oxygen to be trans-ported by the bloodstream to all cells, tissues, and organs. They also help maintain resilience and lubrica-tion of all cells and combine with protein and choles-terol to form living membranes that hold the body cells together.[112]

Vitamin F helps to regulate the rate of blood coagula-tion and performs a vital function in breaking up cho-lestrol deposited on arterial walls. It is essential for normal glandular activity, especially of the adrenal glands and the thyroid gland.[113] Vitamin F nourishes the skin cells and is essential for healthy mucous mem-branes and nerves.

The unsaturated fatty acids function in the body by cooperating with vitamin D in making calcium available to the tissues, assisting in the assimilation of phosphorus, and stimulating the conversion of carotene into vita-min A. Fatty acids are related to normal functioning of the reproductive system.

Absorption and Storage

The stomach, small intestine, and pancreas normally produce liberal amounts of fat-splitting digestive en-zymes necessary for conversion of fats into fatty acids and glycerols (broken-down fatty acids). These are absorbed through the walls of the intestinal tract and are then transported through the portal vein to the liver, where they are usually metabolized as a source of energy. These changes must take place before the nutrients can enter the blood without causing food allergies.[114]

The digested fat is taken from the gastrointestinal tract as fatty acids and gylcerol. These then enter fat-collecting ducts that finally carry the fat to the lym-phatic system, which is primarily concerned with col-

[112] Arthur W. Snyder, *Vitamins and Minerals* (Los Angeles: Hansens, 1969), p. 10.
[113] Airola, *How to Get Well*, p. 272.
[114] Davis, *Let's Get Well*, p. 171.

lecting body fluids and returning them to the general circulatory system.[115] The fatty acids are stored in the adipose (containing massive amounts of fat cells) tissues.

Absorption of fat is decreased when there is increased movement in the gastrointestinal tract and when there is an absence of bile to break down the fat. X-ray treatments and radiation destroy the essential fatty acids within the body, although destruction can be prevented if large doses of vitamin E are taken. Vitamin F is easily destroyed when exposed to air and may become rancid.

Dosage and Toxicity

The National Research Council states that the fat intake should include essential unsaturated fatty acids to the extent of at least 1 percent of the total calories.[116] The level of essential fatty acids needed by infants has been set at 3 percent of the total calories.[117] The need for essential fatty acids is usually met when 2 percent of the calories are produced by linoleic acid, which is found in food sources such as the vegetable oils of soy, corn, sunflower, and wheat germ.

Men usually need five times more saturated fatty acids than women do. A balance of twice as much unsaturated fatty acids as saturated fatty acids in the daily diet is beneficial for heart and arterial health. About four or five tablespoons of vegetable oils per day are needed to maintain this balance.

The need for linoleic acid increases in proportion to the amount of solids eaten. If the intake of saturated fats is high, a deficiency of linoleic acid can occur even though oils are included in the diet, and increased consumption of such foods as butter, cream, and saturated fat increases the need for vitamin F. Eating a great deal of carbohydrates also increases the need for unsaturated fatty acids. When there is sufficient linoleic acid in the diet, the other two essential fatty acids can be synthesized from it.

In order to get the full benefit of vitamin F, one should take vitamin E with it at mealtimes. This ensures the best absorption. In addition, it is important that as the amount of oils and fats is increased, the dosage of vitamin E is increased.

There are no known toxic effects of vitamin F; however, excessive amounts of saturated fats may cause metabolic disturbances and abnormal weight gain.

Deficiency Effects and Symptoms

A vitamin F deficiency causes changes to occur in the structure and enzyme function within the nucleus of the cells, resulting in a number of disorders. A deficiency may be responsible for brittle and lusterless hair, nail problems, dandruff, and allergic conditions.[118] In addition, diarrhea, varicose veins, underweight, and gallstones may be a result of vitamin F deficiency. Skin disorders such as eczema, acne, and dry skin[119] have been linked with vitamin F deficiency; also ailments, such as diseases of the heart, circulatory system, and kidneys, associated with faulty fat metabolism. Without vitamin F, growth is retarded, teeth do not form properly, and prostaglandins, a group of fatty acids found in tissues of the prostrate gland, brain, kidney, and seminal and menstrual fluid, cannot be made by the cells.

Beneficial Effects on Ailments

Unsaturated fatty acids have been used to treat external ulcers, especially leg ulcers, with good results. The unsaturated fat preparation causes rapid granulation and regeneration of the skin.[120] It can also be used orally and externally for treating infantile eczema and the nonallergenic eczema that occurs in adolescents and adults. Psoriasis can benefit from treatment with unsaturated fatty acids. Arachidonic acid is effective in curing dermatitis.

Linoleic acid is effective in restoring growth. Hay fever has been successfully treated with vitamin F. It is also essential for the prevention and treatment of bronchial asthma and rheumatoid arthritis.

Vitamin F has been used in preventing heart disease. Vitamin F keeps cholesterol soft and prevents it from forming any hard deposits in the lumen of the blood vessels or under the skin.[121] This is especially important for the atherosclerosis patient. Because vitamin F lowers blood cholesterol, it helps prevent high blood pressure and hardening of the arteries.

Unsaturated fatty acids have helped prevent diarrhea and underweight. They have been useful in preventing prostate trouble and arthritis.[122] Any person who has

[115]Guthrie, *Introductory Nutrition*, p. 40.
[116]Rodale, *The Complete Book of Vitamins*, p, 410.
[117]Guthrie, *Introductory Nutrition*, p. 44.

[118]Rodale, *The Complete Book of Vitamins*, p. 411.
[119]Airola, *How to Get Well*, p. 272.
[120]Rodale, *The Health Seeker*, p. 732.
[121]Rodale, *Best Health Articles from* Prevention *Magazine*, p. 821.
[122]Rodale, *Best Health Articles from* Prevention *Magazine*, p. 205.

gallbladder problems or has had one removed needs to take extra bile in the form of a food supplement so as to ensure proper breakdown of fats.

Human Tests

1. Unsaturated Fatty Acids and Prostate Glands. 19 cases of prostate gland disorders were treated with unsaturated fatty acids.

Results. All 19 cases had a lessening of residual urine, that is, the urine that cannot be released from the bladder due to pressure from the enlarged prostate gland. In 12 cases there was no residual urine at the end of treatment. There was also a decrease in leg pains, fatigue, kidney disorders, and excessive urination at night. (James P. Hart and William de Grande Cooper, *Lee Report*, No. 1, as reported in Rodale, *The Health Builder*, p. 352.)

2. Fatty Acids and Asthma. Two doctors observed the effects of a diet supplement plus fatty acids in patients suffering from asthma.

Results. 40 percent of the patients were either entirely relieved of asthmatic symptoms or noticed some improvement. The other 60 percent did not respond to treatment. (*The Journal of Applied Nutrition*, Spring 1955, as reported in Rodale, *The Health Builder*, p. 357.)

3. Unsaturated Fatty Acids and Eczema. 87 chronic eczema patients were treated daily with corn oil (rich in unsaturated fatty acids) for a period of over four and one-half years.

Results. Standard treatments had been used but not with the same success that corn oil had on the patients. All patients responded and showed improvement with the corn oil treatment. (Lee Foundation Report, February 1942, as reported in Rodale, *The Encyclopedia for Healthful Living*, p. 777.)

VITAMIN F MAY BE BENEFICIAL FOR THE FOLLOWING AILMENTS:

Body Member	Ailment
Blood/Circulatory system	Cholesterol level, high
	Diabetes
Bowel	Colitis
	Diarrhea
Brain/Nervous system	Mental illness
	Multiple sclerosis
Ear	Ménière's syndrome
Glands	Prostatitis
Heart	Coronary thrombosis
Intestine	Constipation
Joints	Arthritis
Legs	Leg cramp
Lungs/Respiratory system	Asthma
	Bronchitis
Skin	Acne
	Dermatitis
	Eczema
	Psoriasis
Teeth/Gums	Tooth and gum disorders
General	Allergies
	Common cold
	Overweight and obesity
	Underweight

VITAMIN K

Description

There are three main K vitamins: K_1 and K_2 are fat-soluble and can be manufactured in the intestinal tract in the presence of certain intestinal flora (bacteria); K_3 is produced synthetically for the treatment of patients who are unable to utilize naturally occurring vitamin K because they lack bile, an enzyme necessary for the absorption of all fat-soluble vitamins.

If yogurt, kefir (a preparation of curdled milk), or acidophilus milk (fermented milk used to change intestinal bacteria) is included in the diet, the body may be able to manufacture sufficient amounts of vitamin K. In addition, unsaturated fatty acids and a low-carbohydrate diet increase the amounts of vitamin K produced by intestinal flora.[123]

Vitamin K is necessary for the formation of prothrombin, a chemical required in blood clotting. Vitamin K is involved in a body process, phosphorylation, in which phosphate, when combined with glucose, is

[123]Clark, *Know Your Nutrition*, p. 62.

passed through the cell membranes and converted into glycogen, a form in which carbohydrates are stored in the body.[124] It is also vital for normal liver functioning and is an important vitality and longevity factor.

Some natural sources of vitamin K are kelp, alfalfa, green plants, and leafy green vegetables. Cow's milk, yogurt, egg yolks, blackstrap molasses, safflower oil, fish-liver oils, and other polyunsaturated oils are other good sources. The most dependable supply is the intestinal bacteria.

Vitamin K can be safely used as a preservative to control fermentation in foods. It has no bleaching effect, no unpleasant odor, and when added to naturally colored fruits, helps maintain a stable and effective condition of the food.

Absorption and Storage

Vitamin K is absorbed in the upper intestinal tract with the aid of bile or bile salts and is transported to the liver, where it is essential for synthesis of prothrombin and several related proteins involved in the clotting of blood. Vitamin K is stored in very small amounts, and considerable quantities are excreted after administration of therapeutic doses.

Factors interfering with absorption of vitamin K include any obstruction of the bile duct limiting the secretion of fat-emulsifying bile salts; failure of the liver to secrete bile;[125] and dicumarol, an anticoagulant that reduces the activity of prothrombin in the blood plasma.

Frozen foods, rancid fats, radiation, x-rays, aspirin, and industrial air pollution all destroy vitamin K. Excessive use of antibiotics can destroy the intestinal flora.[126] Ingestion of mineral oil will cause rapid excretion of vitamin K.

Dosage and Toxicity

The National Research Council states that the abundance of vitamin K in most diets, along with synthesis by the intestinal bacteria, provides adequate intake of vitamin K.[127] The newborn infant needs a daily intake of 1 to 5 milligrams to prevent hemorrhagic disease, which is abnormal bleeding.[128] It is estimated that the average daily intake is between 300 and 500 micrograms, which is considered an adequate supply of vitamin K.[129]

Therapeutic dosages of vitamin K are often given before and after operations to reduce blood losses. Vitamin K injections are sometimes given to women prior to labor to protect against hemorrhaging.

Excessive doses of synthetic vitamin K can cause toxic reactions because the supplements will build up in the blood. Toxicity brings about a form of anemia that results in an increased breakdown in the red blood cells. In infants, kernicterus, a condition in which yellow pigment infiltrates the spinal cord and brain areas, can result, usually developing during the second to eighth days of life. Heinz bodies, or granules in the red blood cells resulting from damage to the hemoglobin molecules, are seen in infants suffering from an overdose. Toxicity has occurred when large dosages of synthetic vitamin K were injected into pregnant women. Flushing, sweating, and chest constrictions are symptoms of synthetic vitamin K toxicity. Natural vitamin K is stored in the body and produces no toxicity signs.

Deficiency Effects and Symptoms

Deficiencies of vitamin K usually result from inadequate absorption or the body's inability to utilize vitamin K in the liver.[130] Vitamin K deficiency is common in diseases such as celiac disease (intestinal malabsorption), sprue (malabsorption in adulthood), and colitis, which affect the absorbing mucosa of the small intestine and cause a rapid loss of intestinal contents. In such cases, intravenous administration of vitamin K may be needed.

In a deficiency, a condition of hypoprothrombinemia can occur, causing blood-clotting time to be greatly or even indefinitely prolonged. A deficiency can cause hemorrhages in any part of the body, including brain, spinal cord, and intestinal tract. A vitamin K deficiency can cause miscarriages and nosebleeds and can also be a factor in cellular disease and diarrhea.

Beneficial Effect on Ailments

Vitamin K is necessary to promote blood clotting, especially when jaundice is present. It is administered to heart patients who are using anticoagulant drugs to thin the consistency of their blood. Carefully measured doses

[124]Guthrie, *Introductory Nutrition*, p. 216.
[125]Guthrie, *Introductory Nutrition*, p. 216.
[126]Clark, *Know Your Nutrition*, p. 61.
[127]Krause and Hunscher, *Food, Nutrition and Diet Therapy*, p. 129.
[128]Guthrie, *Introductory Nutrition*, p. 216.

[129]Goodhart and Shils, *Modern Nutrition in Health and Disease*, p. 172.
[130]Krause and Hunscher, *Food, Nutrition and Diet Therapy*, p. 129.

of vitamin K are given to these patients to raise the prothrombin level slightly while not allowing it to completely counteract the effect of the anticoagulant.[131]

Vitamin K has proved beneficial in reducing the blood flow during prolonged menstruation, clots either diminish or disappear. It has often lessened or relieved menstrual cramps.

Vitamin K is frequently used with vitamin C in the prevention and improvement of hemorrhages in various parts of the eye.[132] Vitamin K is also used to prevent hemorrhaging following gallbladder operations and to prevent cerebral palsy.[133]

VITAMIN K MAY BE BENEFICIAL FOR THE FOLLOWING AILMENTS:

Body Member	Ailment
Blood/Circulatory system	Bruising
	Hemorrhage
Gallbladder	Gallstones
Glands	Cystic fibrosis
Intestine	Celiac disease
	Worms
Liver	Cirrhosis of liver
	Jaundice
Skin	Ulcers
General	Aging
	Alcoholism
	Cancer
	Hepatitis
	Kwashiorkor

BIOFLAVONOIDS (VITAMIN P)

Description

Bioflavonoids, known as vitamin P, are water-soluble and are composed of a group of brightly colored substances that often appear in fruits and vegetables as companions to vitamin C. The components of the bioflavonoids are citrin, hesperidin, rutin, flavones, and flavonals.

Bioflavonoids were first discovered as a substance in the white segments, not in the juices, of citrus fruits. There is ten times the concentration of bioflavonoids in the edible part of the fruit that there is in the strained juice. Sources of bioflavonoids include lemons, grapes, plums, black currants, grapefruit, apricots, buckwheat, cherries, blackberries, and rose hips.

Bioflavonoids are essential for the proper absorption and use of vitamin C. They assist vitamin C in keeping collagen, the intercellular cement, in healthy condition. They are vital in their ability to increase the strength of the capillaries and to regulate their permeability.[134] These actions help prevent hemorrhages and ruptures in the capillaries and connective tissues and build a protective barrier against infections.[135]

Absorption and Storage

The absorption and storage properties of bioflavonoids are very similar to those of vitamin C. The bioflavonoids are readily absorbed from the gastrointestinal tract into the bloodstream. Excessive amounts are excreted through urination and perspiration.

Dosage and Toxicity

There is no Recommended Dietary Allowance for this vitamin. Since bioflavonoids occur with vitamin C in natural food sources, synthetic vitamin C does not contain the bioflavonoids. When ingested together, bioflavonoids and C are more helpful than vitamin C taken alone.[136] Rutin, which comes from buckwheat leaves, is a good food source of bioflavonoids. Bioflavonoids are completely nontoxic.

Deficiency Effects and Symptoms

Symptoms of a bioflavonoid deficiency are closely related to those of a vitamin C deficiency. Especially noted is the increased tendency to bleed or hemorrhage and bruise easily. A deficiency of vitamins C and P may contribute to rheumatism and rheumatic fever.[137]

Beneficial Effect on Ailments

The body's utilization of vitamin C is increased when bioflavonoids are present. They are helpful in strengthening the capillaries and may help prevent colds and influenza. Bioflavonoids have proved to be beneficial in

---

[131] Rodale, *The Complete Book of Vitamins*, p. 439.
[132] Rodale, *The Health Builder*, p. 341.
[133] Clark, *Know Your Nutrition*, p. 61.

[134] Rodale, *The Health Builder*, p. 982.
[135] Dr. Paavo Airola, *Are You Confused?* (Phoenix, Ariz.: Health Plus Pub., 1971), p. 164.
[136] Rodale, *The Health Builder*, p. 980.
[137] Rodale, *The Health Seeker*, p. 76.

treating various degrees of capillary injury and have been found to minimize bruising that occurs in contact sports.[138]

Rutin is especially helpful in the prevention of recurrent bleeding arising from weakened blood vessels. It is sometimes used in the treatment of hemorrhoids and helps prevent the walls of the blood vessels from becoming fragile.

Bioflavonoids have been used successfully to treat ulcer patients and those suffering from dizziness caused by labyrinthitis, a disease of the inner ear. Weakness of the capillaries was found to be a major causative factor in both of these ailments.[139] Asthma has been successfully treated by the administration of bioflavonoids. Bioflavonoids have also been used as a protective agent against the harmful effects of x-rays.[140]

Bioflavonoids and vitamin C when taken together may help prevent habitual miscarriages. They are helpful in the treatment of disorders such as bleeding gums, eczema, and susceptibility to hemorrhaging. Rheumatism and rheumatic fever seem to be helped by vitamins C and P. The blood-vessel disorder of the eye which affects diabetics seems to respond to bioflavonoid–vitamin C treatment.[141] Administered together, these vitamins have also been beneficial in the treatment of muscular dystrophy because they help lower blood pressure moderately.

Human Tests

1. Bioflavonoids and Rheumatoid Arthritis. A fifty-two-year-old woman with rheumatoid arthritis in both hands, wrists, and elbows and in the right shoulder, knees, and ankles was given 3,000 milligrams of bioflavonoid complex.

Results. In seven days she "felt better." Two weeks later the pain had practically disappeared, her digestion was improved, and bowel action was normal. Her blood pressure dropped from 190 to 176, and by the end of five weeks she had more action in her joints and a great deal more endurance. (Dr. James R. West, Morrell

[138]Rodale, *The Health Seeker*, p. 77.
[139]Rodale, *The Encyclopedia for Healthful Living*, p. 70.
[140]Airola, *Are You Confused?*, p. 161.
[141]Rodale, *The Health Seeker*, p. 76.

Memorial Hospital, Lakeland, Florida, as reported in Rodale, *The Encyclopedia for Healthful Living*, p. 30.)

2. Bioflavonoids and Duodenal Ulcers. 36 cases of bleeding duodenal ulcers were treated with bioflavonoids and a diet consisting of an orange juice-milk-gelatin mixture given in doses of 4 to 6 ounces every two hours with bioflavonoid capsules, until bleeding was arrested. The bioflavonoid capsules were administered orally at the rate of three to nine capsules daily.

Results. All bleeding ceased on the fourth day. Then the patients were put on a bland diet. Vitamin supplements and bioflavonoid rations were added to the diet. All 36 patients responded with a return of mucous membrane and duodenal contour to a normal state. Total treatment took from 12 to 22 days. No recurrence of bleeding in two years or more occurred in 23 of the 36 cases. Twelve cases remained ulcer-free for one year or more, and the remaining cases were successfully treated and ulcer-free for four months. (Drs. Samuel Weiss, Jerome Weiss, and Bernard Weiss, *American Journal of Gastroenterology*, July 1958, as reported in Rodale, *The Encyclopedia for Healthful Living*, pp. 70-71.)

3. Bioflavonoids and Labyrinthitis (Disease of the Inner Ear). Nine cases were treated with four to six capsules of bioflavonoids daily with decreased salt intake.

Results. Positive results occurred in three to six days. The symptoms of dizziness, loss of balance, and nausea were successfully treated with no recurrence. (Dr. Theodore R. Miller, *Eye, Ear, Nose and Throat Monthly*, September 1958, as reported in Rodale, *The Encyclopedia for Healthful Living*, pp. 72-73.)

BIOFLAVONOIDS MAY BE BENEFICIAL FOR THE FOLLOWING AILMENTS:

Body Member	Ailment
Blood/Circulatory system	Arteriosclerosis
	Atherosclerosis
	Bruising
	Cholesterol level, high
	Hemophilia
	Hypertension

Body Member	Ailment
	Leukemia
	Stroke (cerebrovascular accident)
	Varicose veins
Heart	Arteriosclerosis
	Atherosclerosis
	Hypertension
	Hypoxia
Intestine	Hemorrhoids
Joints	Arthritis
	Rheumatic fever
	Rheumatism
Lungs/Respiratory system	Pneumonia
Skin	Ulcers
Teeth/Gums	Pyorrhea
	Scurvy
General	Common cold

VITAMIN T

Description

Vitamin T is often referred to as the "sesame seed factor." It reestablishes blood coagulation and is useful in correcting nutritional anemia. Vitamin T promotes the formation of blood platelets (round disks in the blood) and combats anemia and hemophilia, a hereditary blood disease characterized by prolonged coagulation time. It can also be useful in improving a fading memory.[142] Some natural sources of vitamin T are sesame seeds, raw sesame butter, and egg yolks.

VITAMIN U

Description

Vitamin U is a vitaminlike factor found in some vegetables. It promotes healing activity in peptic ulcers[143] and is particularly vital in healing duodenal ulcers. Important natural sources of vitamin U are raw cabbage juice, fresh cabbage, and homemade sauerkraut.[144]

[142] Airola, *How to Get Well*, p. 273.
[143] Airola, *How to Get Well*, p. 273.
[144] Airola, *How to Get Well*, p. 273.

MINERALS

ALUMINUM

Description

Aluminum is a trace mineral, but it can be dangerous, even fatal, if consumed in excessive amounts. There is no established function of aluminum in human nutrition. It is found in many plant and animal foods. It is also an ingredient in the bases of false teeth, children's aspirin tablets, some baking powders, and some white flour.

Aluminum weakens the living tissue of the alimentary canal, the digestive tube from the mouth to the anus. Many of aluminum's harmful effects result from its destruction of vitamins. It binds with many other substances and is never found alone in nature.

Absorption and Storage

Aluminum is easily absorbed by the body and is accumulated in the arteries. Foods cooked in aluminum utensils may absorb minute quantities of the mineral.

Dosage and Toxicity

The total aluminum content of the adult body is from 50 to 150 milligrams. The daily amount ingested in the average diet ranges from 10 milligrams to more than 100 milligrams.

Excessive amounts of aluminum can result in symptoms of poisoning. These symptoms include constipation, colic, loss of appetite, nausea, skin ailments, twitching of leg muscles, excessive perspiration, and loss of energy. Patients with aluminum poisoning should discontinue the use of aluminum cookware. Doctors often recommend that the drinking of tap water be discontinued.

Small quantities of soluble salts of aluminum present in the blood cause a slow form of poisoning characterized by motor paralysis and areas of local numbness, with fatty degeneration of the kidney and liver.[145] There are also anatomical changes in the nerve centers and symptoms of gastrointestinal inflammation. These symptoms result from the body's effort to eliminate the poison.

[145] Rodale, *Complete Book of Minerals for Health*, p. 387.

Deficiency Effects and Symptoms

No available information.

Beneficial Effect on Ailments

No available information.

BERYLLIUM

Description

Beryllium is a mineral that has definite adverse effects on the human body. This mineral can deplete the body's store of magnesium, allowing disease to result. When beryllium is absorbed into the bloodstream, it often lodges in vital organs and keeps them from performing their functions. It interferes with a number of the body's enzyme systems.[146] It does not allow the enzyme system to carry on its function in the body.

Beryllium is used in neon signs, electronic devices, some alloys including steel, bicycle wheels, fishing rods, and many common household products.[147]

Beryllium is a dangerous substance in industrial toxicology. Beryllium dust makes breathing difficult. This condition may lead to injury of the lungs, causing scarring or fibrosis. Some victims of beryllium poisoning become completely disabled by serious lung destruction.

CADMIUM

Description

Cadmium is a toxic trace mineral that has many structural similarities to zinc. There is no biological function for this element in humans. Its toxic effects are kept under control in the body by the presence of zinc.

Refining processes disturb the important cadmium-zinc balance. In whole wheat, cadmium is present in proportion to zinc in a ratio of 1 to 120.

Cadmium is found primarily in refined foods such as flour, rice, and white sugar. It is present in the air as an industrial contaminant. In addition, soft water usually contains higher levels of cadmium than does hard water. Coffee and tea also contain high levels of cadmium;

drinking about five cups of either per day doubles the average daily intake of cadmium.

Absorption and Storage

The liver and kidneys are storage areas for both cadmium and zinc. The total body concentration of cadmium increases with age and varies in different areas of the world.

When a deficit of zinc occurs in the diet, the body may make it up by storing cadmium instead. If the daily intake of zinc is high, zinc will be stored and cadmium will be excreted.

Dosage and Toxicity

Daily intakes of cadmium have been estimated at 0.2 to 0.5 milligram, with considerable variation according to sources and types of food.[148] Cadmium's toxic effects may stem from its being stored for use in the body in place of zinc when the proportion between the two metals is unfavorably out of balance.[149] Zinc is a natural antagonist to cadmium.

Dr. Henry A. Shroeder, a trace mineral researcher, has developed a theory about cadmium being a major causative factor in hypertension and related heart ailments.[150] Testing his theories on rats because of their biological similarity to humans, Dr. Schroeder found that regular high doses of cadmium caused increased tension. When he stopped administering the cadmium to the rats, they returned to normotension.

In humans, the urine of hypertensive patients contains up to 40 percent more cadmium than does the urine of normotensive persons. These findings may lend credibility to the theory that excessive cadmium can directly lead to hypertension.[151]

Deficiency Effects and Symptoms

No available information.

Beneficial Effect on Ailments

No available information.

[146] Rodale, *Complete Book of Minerals for Health*, p. 405.
[147] Rodale, *Complete Book of Minerals for Health*, p. 408.
[148] National Academy of Sciences, *Toxicants Occurring Naturally in Foods*, p. 64.
[149] Rodale, *Complete Book of Minerals for Health*, p. 410.
[150] Rodale, *Complete Book of Minerals for Health*, p. 413.
[151] Rodale, *Complete Book of Minerals for Health*, p. 277.

CALCIUM

Description

Calcium is the most abundant mineral in the body. About 99 percent of the calcium in the body is deposited in the bones and teeth, and the remainder is in the soft tissues. The ratio of calcium to phosphorus in the bones is 2.5 to 1. To function properly, calcium must be accompanied by magnesium, phosphorus, and vitamins A, C, and D.

The major function of calcium is to act in cooperation with phosphorus to build and maintain bones and teeth. It is essential for healthy blood, eases insomnia, and helps regulate the heartbeat. An important calcium partner in cardiovascular health is magnesium.

In addition, calcium assists in the process of blood clotting and helps prevent the accumulation of too much acid or too much alkali in the blood. It also plays a part in muscle growth, muscle contraction, and nerve transmission. Calcium aids in the body's utilization of iron, helps activate several enzymes (catalysts important for metabolism), and helps regulate the passage of nutrients in and out of the cell walls.

Calcium is present in significant amounts in a very limited number of foods. Milk and dairy products are dependable sources. The most common supplemental source is bone meal; it is well absorbed and utilized by most people. Those who are unable to use bone meal may use calcium gluconate or calcium lactate, natural derivatives of calcium which are even easier to absorb than is bone meal.

Absorption and Storage

Calcium absorption is very inefficient, and usually only 20 to 30 percent of ingested calcium is absorbed. Unabsorbed calcium is excreted in the feces. Absorption takes place in the duodenum and ceases in the lower part of the intestinal tract when the food content becomes alkaline. The amount absorbed depends largely on the diet, for unless calcium is in a water-soluble form in the intestine, it will not be absorbed properly.

Many other factors influence the actual amount of calcium absorbed. When in need, the body absorbs calcium more effectively; therefore the greater the need and the smaller the dietary supply, the more efficient the absorption. Absorption is also increased during periods of rapid growth.[152]

Calcium needs acid for proper assimilation. If acid in some form is not present in the body, calcium is not dissolved and therefore cannot be used as needed by the body. Instead it can build up in tissues or joints as calcium deposits, leading to a variety of disturbances.

Calcium absorption also depends upon the presence of adequate amounts of vitamin D, which works with the parathyroid hormone to regulate the amount of calcium in the blood. Phosphorus is needed in at least the same amount as calcium. Vitamins A and C are necessary for calcium absorption. Fat content in moderate amounts, moving slowly through the digestive tract, helps facilitate absorption. A high intake of protein also aids in the absorption of calcium.

Certain substances interfere with the absorption of calcium. When excessive amounts of fat combine with calcium, an insoluble compound is formed which cannot be absorbed. Oxalic acid, found in chocolate, spinach, and rhubarb, when combined with calcium makes another insoluble compound and may form into stones in the kidney or gallbladder. Large amounts of phytic acid, present in cereals and grains, may inhibit the absorption of calcium by the body. Other interfering factors include lack of exercise, excessive stress, and too rapid a flow of food through the intestinal tract.

Dosage and Toxicity

The National Research Council recommends 800 milligrams as a daily calcium intake; since only 20 to 30 percent is absorbed, 800 milligrams would maintain the necessary balance.[153] During pregnancy and lactation, this amount increases to 1,200 milligrams. With age, it seems the requirement also increases because the rate of absorption is reduced. If the calcium intake is high, the magnesium levels also need to be high.

A high intake of calcium and vitamin D is a potential source of hypercalcemia. This condition may result in excessive calcification of the bones and some tissues, such as the kidney's.

[152] Krause and Hunscher, *Food, Nutrition and Diet Therapy*, p. 102.
[153] Krause and Hunscher, *Food, Nutrition and Diet Therapy*, p. 102.

Deficiency Effects and Symptoms

One of the first signs of a calcium deficiency is a nervous affliction, tetany, characterized by muscle cramps and numbness and tingling in the arms and legs. A calcium deficiency can result in bone malformation, causing rickets in children and osteomalacia in adults. Another calcium deficiency ailment is osteoporosis, in which the bones become porous and fragile because calcium is withdrawn from the bones and other body areas faster than it is deposited in them.

Moderate cases of calcium deficiency may lead to cramps, joint pains, heart palpitation, slow pulse rates, tooth decay, insomnia, impaired growth, and excessive irritability of nerves and muscles. In extreme cases of deficiency, brittle or porous bone and tooth formation, slow blood clotting, or hemorrhaging may result.

Beneficial Effect on Ailments

Calcium has been successfully used in the treatment of osteoporosis. The hormones involved are stimulated by the concentration of calcium ions in the blood. Calcium is a natural tranquilizer and tends to calm the nerves.

Calcium has been beneficial in the treatment of cardiovascular disorders. In addition, calcium is a recognized aid for cramps in the feet or legs. It also helps patients suffering from "growing pains."

Calcium has been used in the treatment and prevention of sunburn. In addition to giving protection against effects of sun damage such as redness and subsequent peeling, it also protects against sun-caused skin cancers.[154] Calcium helps the skin to remain healthy. Vitamin A and calcium are a good combination for protection of the skin. This combination can also be used as a neutralizing agent against the poison of a black widow spider or a bee sting.

Arthritis, structural rigidity often caused by depletion of bone calcium, can be helped with regular supplements of bone meal. Early consumption of bone meal may help prevent arthritis. Rheumatism can also be treated successfully with calcium therapy.

Problems of menopause, such as nervousness, irritability, insomnia, and headaches, have been overcome with administration of calcium, magnesium, and vitamin D.[155] When there is not enough calcium in the body to be absorbed, the output of estrogen decreases.

Calcium can help prevent premenstrual tension and menstrual cramps.

High intakes of calcium may relieve the symptoms commonly associated with aging. Some of the disorders include bone pain, backaches, insomnia, brittle teeth with cavities, and tremors of the fingers.[156]

The parathyroid glands located in the neck help adjust the body's storage of calcium. If these glands are not functioning properly, calcium accumulation may occur. The remedy for this situation is to renew the proper function of the parathyroid glands rather than to cut down on calcium intake.[157]

Calcium treatments have been used successfully in treating rickets in children and osteomalacia in adults. In addition, nephritis has been cleared up with administration of calcium and other nutrients. Tooth and gum disorders are also relieved by higher intakes of calcium in the diet. A high dietary intake of calcium may protect against the harmful effects of radioactive strontium 90.

CALCIUM MAY BE BENEFICIAL FOR THE FOLLOWING AILMENTS:

Body Member	Ailment
Blood/Circulatory system	Anemia
	Diabetes
	Hemophilia
	Pernicious anemia
Bones	Fracture
	Osteomalacia
	Osteoporosis
	Rickets
Bowel	Colitis
	Diarrhea
Brain/Nervous system	Dizziness
	Epilepsy
	Insomnia
	Mental illness
	Parkinson's disease
Ear	Ménière's syndrome
Eye	Cataracts
Head	Fever
Heart	Arteriosclerosis
	Atherosclerosis

[154] Rodale, *Complete Book of Minerals for Health*, p. 37.
[155] Rodale, *Complete Book of Minerals for Health*, p. 37.
[156] Davis, *Let's Get Well*, p. 309.
[157] Rodale, *Best Health Articles from* Prevention *Magazine*, p. 598.

Body Member	Ailment
	Hypertension
Intestine	Celiac disease
	Constipation
	Hemorrhoids
	Worms
Joints	Arthritis
Kidney	Nephritis
Leg	Leg cramp
Lungs/Respiratory system	Allergies
	Common cold
	Tuberculosis
Muscles	General muscle cramps
	Tetany
Nails	Nail problems
Skin	Acne
Stomach	Stomach ulcer (peptic)
Teeth/Gums	Pyorrhea
	Tooth and gum disorders
General	Aging
	Fever
	Overweight and Obesity
	Sunburn

CHLORINE

Description

Chlorine is an essential mineral, occurring in the body mainly in compound form with sodium or potassium. It is widely distributed throughout the body in the form of chloride in amounts less than 15 percent of the total body weight.[158] Chlorine compounds such as sodium chloride, or salt, are found primarily within the cells.

Chlorine helps regulate the correct balance of acid and alkali in the blood and maintains pressure that causes fluids to pass in and out of cell membranes until the concentration of dissolved particles is equalized on both sides. It stimulates production of hydrochloric acid, an enzymatic juice needed in the stomach for digestion of tough, fibrous foods.

Chlorine stimulates the liver to function as a filter for wastes and helps clean toxic waste products out of the system.[159] It aids in keeping joints and tendons in youthful shape, and it helps to distribute hormones. Chlorine is sometimes added to water for purification purposes because it destroys waterborne diseases such as typhoid and hepatitis.

Chlorine in the diet is provided almost exclusively by sodium chloride, or table salt. It is also found in kelp, dulse, rye flour, ripe olives, and sea greens.

Absorption and Storage

Chlorine is absorbed in the intestine and excreted through urination and perspiration. The highest body concentrations are stored in the cerebrospinal fluid and in the secretions of the gastrointestinal tract. Muscle and nerve tissues are relatively low in chloride.[160] Excess chlorine is excreted; additional loss may be caused by conditions such as vomiting, diarrhea, or sweating.

There has been much controversy over the relative merits of adding chlorine to drinking water supplies because it is a highly reactive chemical and may join with inorganic minerals and other chemicals to form possibly harmful substances. It is known that chlorine in the drinking water destroys vitamin E. It also destroys many of the intestinal flora that help in the digestion of food.

Dosage and Toxicity

There is no Recommended Dietary Allowance for chlorine because the average person's salt intake is high and usually provides between 3 and 9 grams daily. Diets sufficient in sodium and potassium provide adequate chlorine. Daily intake of 14 to 28 grams of salt is considered excessive.[161]

Deficiency Effects and Symptoms

A deficiency of chlorine can cause hair and tooth loss, poor muscular contraction, and impaired digestion.[162]

Beneficial Effect on Ailments

Chlorine is beneficial in treating diarrhea and vomiting.

[158]Guthrie, *Introductory Nutrition*, p. 132.

[159]Carlson Wade, *Magic Minerals: Key to Better Health* (West Nyack, N.Y.: Parker, 1967), p. 26.
[160]Guthrie, *Introductory Nutrition*, p. 132.
[161]National Academy of Sciences, *Toxicants Occurring Naturally in Foods*, p. 30.
[162]Wade, *Magic Minerals: Key to Better Health*, p. 26.

CHLORINE MAY BE BENEFICIAL FOR THE FOLLOWING AILMENTS:

Body Member	Ailment
Bowel	Diarrhea
Stomach	Vomiting

CHROMIUM

Description

Chromium is an essential mineral found in concentrations of 20 parts of chromium per 1 billion parts of blood.[163] It has functions in both animal and human nutrition.

Chromium stimulates the activity of enzymes involved in the metabolism of glucose for energy and the synthesis of fatty acids and cholesterol. Chromium also appears to increase the effectiveness of insulin, thereby facilitating the transport of glucose into the cell. In the blood it competes with iron in the transport of protein. Chromium may also be involved in the synthesis of protein through its binding action with RNA molecules.

Sources of chromium include corn oil, clams, whole-grain cereals, and meats. Fruits and vegetables contain trace amounts. Brewer's yeast provides a dependable supply without the problems of high carbohydrate intake and high cholesterol levels.

Absorption and Storage

Chromium is difficult to absorb. Only about three percent of dietary chromium is retained in the body.[164] The mineral is stored primarily in the spleen, kidneys, and testes; small amounts are also stored in the heart, pancreas, lungs, and brain. Chromium has been found in some enzymes and in RNA.[165] Excretion occurs mainly through urination, with minor amounts lost in the feces. The amount of chromium stored in the body decreases with age.

Dosage and Toxicity

There is no Recommended Dietary Allowance for chromium. The daily chromium intake of humans is estimated to range from 80 to 100 micrograms.[166]

[163] Rodale, *Complete Book of Minerals for Health*, p. 171.
[164] Guthrie, *Introductory Nutrition*, p. 166.
[165] Chaney and Ross, *Nutrition*, p. 172.
[166] Krause and Hunscher, *Food, Nutrition and Diet Therapy*, p. 118.

Deficiency Effects and Symptoms

Even a very slight chromium deficiency will have serious effects on the body.[167] Tests indicate systematic deficiency of chromium to be common in the United States, although it rarely occurs in other countries. Americans tend to be deficient because their soil does not contain an adequate supply and thus chromium cannot be absorbed by the crops or reach the water supply. The refining of natural carbohydrates is another probable cause of chromium loss.

A chromium deficiency may be a factor that will upset the function of insulin and result in depressed growth rates and severe glucose intolerance in diabetics. It is also believed that the interaction of chromium and insulin is not limited to glucose metabolism but also applies to amino acid metabolism.[168] Chromium may inhibit the formation of aortic plaques, and a deficiency may contribute to atherosclerosis.

Beneficial Effect on Ailments

Chromium helps to regulate sugar levels in the blood. Infants suffering from kwashiorkor have benefited from oral administration of chromium.

CHROMIUM MAY BE BENEFICIAL FOR THE FOLLOWING AILMENTS:

Body Member	Ailment
Blood/Circulatory system	Diabetes
General	Kwashiorkor

COBALT

Description

Cobalt is considered an essential mineral and is an integral part of vitamin B_{12}, or cobalamin. Vitamin B_{12} and cobalt are so closely connected that the two terms can be used interchangeably.

Cobalt activates a number of enzymes in the body. It is necessary for normal functioning and maintenance of red blood cells as well as all other body cells.

The body does not have the ability to synthesize cobalt and must depend on animal sources for an

[167] Rodale, *Complete Book of Minerals for Health*, p. 171.
[168] Chaney and Ross, *Nutrition*, p. 173.

adequate supply of this nutrient.[169] For this reason, strict vegetarians are more susceptible to cobalt deficiency than are meat eaters. The best food sources are meats, especially liver and kidney, oysters, clams, and milk. Cobalt is present in ocean and sea vegetation but is lacking in almost all land green foods, although cobalt-enriched soil can yield minute amounts.

Absorption and Storage

Cobalt is not easily assimilated, and most of it passes through the intestinal tract unabsorbed. Most of what is absorbed is excreted in the urine after being used by the body. Cobalt is stored in the red blood cells and plasma; some storage occurs also in the liver, kidneys, pancreas, and spleen.[170]

Dosage and Toxicity

There is no Recommended Dietary Allowance for cobalt because the dietary need for it is low and can be supplied in protein foods. The average daily intake of cobalt is 5 to 8 micrograms.

There is evidence that high intakes of cobalt may result in an enlarged thyroid gland. Reduction in the cobalt intake should allow an enlarged thyroid to return to normal size.

Deficiency Effects and Symptoms

A deficiency of cobalt may be responsible for the symptoms of pernicious anemia and a slow rate of growth. If cobalt deficiency is not treated, permanent nervous disorders may result.[171]

Beneficial Effect on Ailments

Therapeutic doses of cobalt have been beneficial in the treatment of pernicious anemia. This action is attributed to cobalt's importance as a builder of red blood cells.

COBALT MAY BE BENEFICIAL FOR THE FOLLOWING AILMENTS:

Body Member	Ailment
Blood/Circulatory system	Pernicious anemia

[169] Guthrie, *Introductory Nutrition*, p. 166.
[170] Chaney and Ross, *Nutrition*, p. 188.
[171] Rodale, *Complete Book of Minerals For Health*, p. 187.

COPPER

Description

Copper is a trace mineral found in all body tissues. Copper assists in the formation of hemoglobin and red blood cells by facilitating iron absorption.

Copper is present in many enzymes that break down or build up body tissue. It aids in the conversion of the amino acid tyrosine into a dark pigment that colors the hair and skin. It is also involved in protein metabolism and in healing processes. Copper is required for the synthesis of phospholipids, substances essential in the formation of the protective myelin sheaths surrounding nerve fibers. Copper helps the body to oxidize vitamin C and works with this vitamin in the formation of elastin, a chief component of the elastic muscle fibers throughout the body. Copper is necessary for proper bone formation and maintenance. It is also necessary for the production of RNA.

Among the best food sources of copper are liver, whole-grain products, almonds, green leafy vegetables, and dried legumes. The amounts vary in plant sources, according to the mineral content in the soil in which they were grown. Most seafoods are also good sources of copper.

Absorption and Storage

Approximately 30 percent of ingested copper is used by the body; absorption takes place in the stomach and upper intestine. The copper moves from the intestine into the bloodstream 15 minutes after ingestion. Most of the dietary copper is excreted in the feces and bile, with very little lost in the urine.

Copper is stored in the tissues; highest concentrations of copper are in the liver, kidneys, heart, and brain. Bones and muscles have lower concentrations of copper, but because of their mass, they contain over 50 percent of the total copper in the body.[172]

Dosage and Toxicity

The National Research Council recommends a daily dietary intake of 2 milligrams of copper for adults. The average person ingests 2.5 to 5.0 milligrams per day. Toxicity is rare, since only a small amount of copper is absorbed and stored while the greatest part is excreted. However, the possibility of copper toxicity occurs with

[172] Krause and Hunscher, *Food, Nutrition and Diet Therapy*, p. 114.

Wilson's disease, a rare genetic disorder that results from abnormal copper metabolism, bringing about excess copper retention in the liver, brain, kidney, and corneas of the eyes.[173]

Deficiency Effects and Symptoms

Although copper deficiencies are relatively unknown, low blood levels of copper have been noted in children with iron-deficiency anemia, edema, and kwashiorkor. Symptoms of deficiency include general weakness, impaired respiration, and skin sores.[174]

Beneficial Effect on Ailments

Copper works with iron to form hemoglobin, thereby helping in the treatment of anemia. Copper is beneficial in the prevention and treatment of edema and kwashiorkor in children.

COPPER MAY BE BENEFICIAL FOR THE FOLLOWING AILMENTS:

Body Member	Ailment
Blood/Circulatory system	Anemia
	Leukemia
Bones	Osteoporosis
Hair	Baldness
Skin	Bedsores
General	Edema

FLUORINE (FLUORIDES)

Description

Fluorine is an essential trace mineral that is present in minute amounts in nearly every human tissue but is found primarily in the skeleton and teeth. Fluorine occurs in the body in compounds called fluorides. There are two types of fluorides: sodium fluoride is added to drinking water and is not the same as calcium fluoride, which is found in nature.

Recent research indicates that fluorine increases the deposition of calcium, thereby strengthening the bones. Fluorine also helps to reduce the formation of acid in the mouth caused by carbohydrates, thereby reducing the likelihood of decayed tooth enamel.[175] Although traces of fluorine are beneficial to the body, excessive amounts are definitely harmful. Fluorine can destroy the enzyme phosphotase, which is vital to many body processes including the metabolism of vitamins. Fluorine inhibits the activities of other important enzymes and appears to be especially antagonistic towards brain tissues.

Fluoridated water supplies are by far the most common source of this mineral, although this form (sodium fluoride) may be toxic. Toxic levels occur when the content of fluorine in drinking water exceeds 2 parts per million. Calcium is an antidote for fluoride poisoning. Other rich sources of fluorine include seafoods and gelatin. The fluorine content in plant foods varies according to environmental conditions such as type of soil, intensity of prevailing winds, and use of fertilizers and sprays that contain fluorine.

Absorption and Storage

Fluorine is absorbed primarily in the intestine, although some may be taken up by the stomach. About 90 percent of ingested fluorine appears in the bloodstream.[176] Half of this is excreted in the urine, and the other half is readily absorbed by the teeth and bones.

Substances interfering with absorption include aluminum salts of fluorine and insoluble calcium.

Dosage and Toxicity

An average diet will provide 0.25 to 0.35 milligram of fluorine daily. In addition, the average adult may ingest 1.0 to 1.5 milligrams from drinking and cooking water containing 1 part per million (ppm) of fluorine. Dental fluorosis may occur at fluoride concentrations of 2 to 8 ppm; osteosclerosis, at 8 to 20 ppm.[177] Higher levels can depress growth, cause calcification of the ligaments and tendons, and bring about degenerative changes in the kidneys, liver, adrenal glands, heart, central nervous system, and finally the reproductive organs. Fatal poisoning can occur at 50 ppm, or 2,500 times the recommended level.[178] There are some areas in the United States where fluorine levels in the water are high

---

[173] Guthrie, *Introductory Nutrition*, p. 165.
[174] Wade, *Magic Minerals: Key to Health*, p. 24.
[175] Guthrie, *Introductory Nutrition*, p. 170.
[176] Guthrie, *Introductory Nutrition*, p. 170.
[177] Krause and Hunscher, *Food, Nutrition and Diet Therapy*, p. 115.
[178] Guthrie, *Introductory Nutrition*, p. 171.

and tooth mottling (enamel discoloration) is epidemic, and there are other areas where fluorine is not added to the water and dental decay is high.

Dr. Ionel Rapaport, a University of Wisconsin researcher, suggests that there is a direct relationship between the incidence of mongolism and fluoridated drinking water.[179] Higher than average incidences of mongolism have been noted in areas where mottled teeth indicate an excess concentration of fluorides in the water.[180]

Deficiency Effects and Symptoms

A diet deficient in fluorine may lead to poor tooth development and subsequent dental caries. Fluorine deficiencies are unusual in the American diet.

Beneficial Effect on Ailments

Fluorides have been used in the treatment and prevention of osteoporosis and dental caries.

FLUORINE MAY BE BENEFICIAL FOR THE FOLLOWING AILMENTS:

Body Member	Ailment
Bones	Osteoporosis
Teeth/Gums	Tooth decay
	Tooth and gum disorders

IODINE (IODIDE)

Description

Iodine is a trace mineral most of which is converted into iodide in the body. Iodine aids in the development and functioning of the thyroid gland and is an integral part of thyroxine, a principal hormone produced by the thyroid gland. It is estimated that the body contains 25 milligrams of iodine, about 0.0004 percent of the total weight.[181]

Iodine plays an important role in regulating the body's production of energy, promotes growth and development, and stimulates the rate of metabolism, helping the body burn excess fat. Mentality; speech; and the condition of hair, nails, skin, and teeth are depend-

ent upon a well-functioning thyroid gland.[182] The conversion of carotene to vitamin A, the synthesis of protein by ribosomes, and the absorption of carbohydrates from the intestine all work more efficiently when thyroxine production is normal.[183] The synthesis of cholesterol is stimulated by thyroxine levels.

Both types of sea life, plant and animal, absorb iodine from seawater and are excellent sources of this mineral. Mushrooms and Irish moss are good sources, too, but only if they are grown in soil rich in iodine.

Absorption and Storage

Iodine is readily absorbed from the gastrointestinal tract and is transported via the bloodstream to the thyroid gland, where it is oxidized and converted into thyroxine.[184] About 30 percent of the iodide in the blood is absorbed by the thyroid gland; the rest is absorbed by the kidneys and excreted in the urine.

Dosage and Toxicity

The National Research Council has suggested that an intake of 1 microgram of iodine per kilogram of body weight is adequate for most adults.[185] They recommend a daily intake of 130 micrograms for men and 100 micrograms for women, 125 micrograms during pregnancy, and 150 micrograms during lactation.

There have been no reported cases of toxicity resulting from too much iodine as it naturally occurs in food or water. However, iodine prepared as a drug or medicine must be carefully prescribed, because an overdose can be serious.[186] Sudden large doses of iodine administered to humans with a normal thyroid may impair the synthesis of thyroid hormones. For individuals on low-salt therapeutic diets, iodine supplements may be desirable.

Deficiency Effects and Symptoms

An iodine deficiency results in simple goiter characterized by thyroid enlargement and hypothyroidism (an abnormally low rate of secretion of thyroid hormones, including thyroxine).

[182] Rodale, *Complete Book of Minerals for Health*, p. 204.
[183] Gunthrie, *Introductory Nutrition*, p. 151.
[184] Krause and Hunscher, *Food, Nutrition and Diet Therapy*, p. 116.
[185] Guthrie, *Introductory Nutrition*, p. 152.
[186] Rodale, *Complete Book of Minerals for Health*, p. 215.

[179] Rodale, *Complete Book of Minerals for Health*, pp. 367-370.
[180] Rodale, *Complete Book of Minerals for Health*, pp. 367-370.
[181] Chaney and Ross, *Nutrition*, p. 158.

Iodine deficiency may lead to hardening of the arteries, obesity, sluggish metabolism, slowed mental reactions, dry hair, rapid pulse, heart palpitation, tremor, nervousness, restlessness, and irritability. An iodine deficiency may also result in cretinism, which is a congenital disease characterized by physical and mental retardation in children born to mothers who have had a limited iodine intake during adolescence and pregnancy. Polio has also been associated with iodine deficiency. The higher rate of occurrence of polio cases in the summer may be caused in part by higher losses of iodine through perspiration.[187]

An iodine deficiency may be caused by certain compounds present in some raw foods, such as cabbage and nuts, which may interfere with the utilization of iodine in thyroid-hormone production. This will not occur unless excessive amounts of these raw foods are eaten and the intake of iodine is low to begin with.

Beneficial Effect on Ailments

Iodine therapy has been used successfully in the treatment and prevention of simple goiter.

Hardening of the arteries occurs when a disturbance in normal fat metabolism allows cholesterol to collect in the arteries instead of being used or expelled. Iodine is needed to prevent this metabolic malfunction. Sufficient dietary iodine will also reduce the danger of radioactive iodine collecting in the thyroid gland.

Iodine is beneficial to children suffering from cretinism, if treatment is started soon after birth. Many of the symptoms are reversible, but if conditions persist beyond childbirth, the mental and physical retardation will be permanent.

IODINE MAY BE BENEFICIAL FOR THE FOLLOWING AILMENTS:

Body Member	Ailment
Blood/Circulatory system	Angina pectoris
Hair	Hair problems
Heart	Arteriosclerosis
	Atherosclerosis
Joints	Arthritis
Thyroid	Goiter
	Hyperthyroidism
	Hypothyroidism

[187]Rodale, *Complete Book of Minerals for Health*, p. 207.

Body Member	Ailment
General	Cretinism
	Loss of physical and mental vigor

IRON

Description

Iron is a mineral concentrate in the blood which is present in every living cell. All iron exists in the body combined with protein.

The major function of iron is to combine with protein and copper in making hemoglobin, the coloring matter of red blood cells. Hemoglobin transports oxygen in the blood from the lungs to the tissues, which need oxygen to maintain the basic life functions. Thus iron builds up the quality of the blood and increases resistance to stress and disease. Iron is also necessary for the formation of myoglobin, which is found only in muscle tissue. Myoglobin is also a transporter of oxygen; it supplies oxygen to the muscle cells for use in the chemical reaction that results in muscle contraction.

Iron is present in enzymes that promote protein metabolism, and it works with other nutrients to improve respiratory action. Calcium and copper must be present for iron to function properly.

The best source of dietary iron is liver, with oysters, heart, lean meat, and tongue as second choices. Leafy green vegetables are the best plant sources.

Absorption and Storage

The body can utilize either ferric or ferrous iron, but evidence indicates that naturally occurring ferrous iron is used more efficiently and that most iron is reduced to ferrous iron before being absorbed.[188] It is absorbed from food in regulated amounts into the blood and bone marrow. Absorption occurs in the upper part of the small intestines. Iron is usually absorbed within four hours after ingestion; from 2 to 4 percent of the iron found in the food is used by the body. It is primarily stored in the liver, spleen, bone marrow, and blood.

The iron in the body is normally used efficiently. It is neither used up nor destroyed, but it is conserved to be used repeatedly. Only very small amounts are normally

[188]Guthrie, *Introductory Nutrition*, p. 140.

excreted from the body. Virtually no iron is excreted in the urine, but unabsorbed iron is detected in the feces.

There are many factors that influence the absorption of iron. Ascorbic acid enhances absorption by helping reduce ferric to ferrous iron. Vitamin E also aids in the assimilation of iron. The iron found in animal protein is more readily absorbed than the iron in vegetables. The degree of gastric acidity regulates the solubility and availability of the iron in food.[189]

The balance of calcium, phosphorus, and iron is very important. Excess phosphorus hinders iron absorption, although if calcium is present in sufficient amounts, it will combine with the phosphates and free the iron for use. In addition, the lack of hydrochloric acid; the administration of alkalis; a high intake of cellulose, coffee, and tea; the presence of insoluble iron complexes (phytates, oxalates, and phosphates); and increased intestinal mobility all interfere with iron absorption.[190]

Dosage and Toxicity

The National Research Council suggests a daily iron intake of 18 milligrams for women and 10 milligrams for men. The need for iron increases during menstruation, hemorrhage, periods of rapid growth, or whenever there is a loss of blood. Additional iron is required during pregnancy, when the developing fetus builds up his own reserve supply of iron in the liver.

A toxic level of iron may occur in an individual due to a genetic error of metabolism, due to blood transfusion, or due to a prolonged oral intake of iron. Excessive deposits of iron in the liver and spleen, in certain individuals, may result from such conditions as cirrhosis of the liver, diabetes, and pancreas insufficiency.[191]

Deficiency Effects and Symptoms

The most common deficiency of iron is iron-deficiency anemia (hypochromic anemia), in which the amount of hemoglobin in the red blood cells is reduced and the cells consequently become smaller. As in other forms of anemia, iron-deficiency anemia reduces the oxygen-carrying capacity of the blood, resulting in pale skin and abnormal fatigue. Symptoms of anemia may include constipation, lusterless, brittle nails, and difficult breathing.

Hemorrhagic anemia, marked by internal hemorrhaging, may not be detected for some time, especially when associated with the bleeding that may occur in peptic ulcers.[192] Excessive donation of blood may cause this type of anemia.

Infections and peptic ulcers may also lead to anemia.

Beneficial Effect on Ailments

When iron-deficiency anemia, with its symptoms of pallor, easy fatigue and decreased resistance to disease, is diagnosed, a diet high in iron-rich foods with a concurrent intake of vitamin C will speed up the restoration of hemoglobin levels to normal. Pernicious anemia is successfully treated with therapeutic doses of organic and inorganic iron salts.

Iron is the most important mineral for the prevention of anemia during menstruation. Iron may also be beneficial in the treatment of leukemia and colitis.

IRON MAY BE BENEFICIAL FOR THE FOLLOWING AILMENTS:

Body Member	Ailment
Blood/Circulatory system	Anemia
	Diabetes
	Leukemia
	Menstruation
	Pernicious anemia
Bowel	Colitis
	Diarrhea
Brain/Nervous system	Alcoholism
Intestine	Celiac disease
	Colitis
	Worms
Joint	Gout
Kidney	Nephritis
Lungs/Respiratory system	Tuberculosis
Nails	Nail problems
Reproductive system	Menstruation
	Pregnancy
Skin	Scurvy
	Ulcers

[189]Krause and Hunscher, *Food, Nutrition and Diet Therapy*, p. 106.

[190]Krause and Hunscher, *Food, Nutrition and Diet Therapy*, p. 106.

[191]Goodhart and Shils, *Modern Nutrition in Health and Disease*, pp. 320-321.

[192]Chaney and Ross, *Nutrition*, p. 149.

Body Member	Ailment
Stomach	Gastritis
	Stomach ulcer (peptic)
Teeth/Gums	Tooth and gum disorders
General	Aging
	Alcoholism
	Bruises
	Cancer
	Pregnancy

LEAD

Description

Lead is a highly toxic trace mineral. In recent years human exposure to lead poisoning has changed in origin and probably has increased in magnitude.[193]

The human body can tolerate only 1 to 2 milligrams (about 0.00003 of an ounce) of lead without suffering toxic effects.[194] Two pounds of food contaminated by only one part per million of lead contain almost a milligram of lead, so there is not a very wide margin of safety.

The single most effective way to prevent lead poisoning is to include a small amount of algin in the daily diet. Algin is a nonnutritive substance found in Pacific kelp, which is sometimes used as a thickening agent in the preparation of various foods. It attaches itself to any lead that is present and carries it harmlessly out of the system.[195]

Absorption and Storage

Lead contained in food is poorly absorbed and is excreted mainly in the feces. Lead may enter the body via the skin and the gastrointestinal tract. The lead that is absorbed enters the blood and is stored in the bones and the soft tissues, including the liver. Up to certain levels of consumption, lead excretion keeps pace with ingestion so that retention is negligible.

Dosage and Toxicity

Critical levels of intake, above which significant lead retention occurs, cannot be quoted with any accu-

racy.[196] Toxic intake can come from consumption of moonshine whiskey and fruit juices stored in lead-glazed earthenware pottery. Sources of poisoning include drinking water, food from lead-lined containers, lead-based paint, lead in water pipes, cosmetics, cigarette smoking, and motor vehicle exhausts. The accumulation of lead in the body from motor vehicle exhausts is caused directly by inhalation and indirectly through deposition in the soil and plants along highways and in urban areas.

Acute lead toxicity is manifested in abdominal colic, encephalopathy (dysfunction of the brain), myelopathy (any pathological condition of the spinal cord), and anemia. The anemia is hypochromic and is rarely severe. Acute lead poisoning attacks the central nervous system and is a possible cause of hyperactivity in children.[197]

There is considerable difference of opinion as to the treatment for lead poisoning. The usual treatment during acute stages consists of a diet high in calcium plus injections of a calcium chloride solution and administration of vitamin D.[198] The additional calcium and vitamin D help prevent lead from being leeched out of the bones into the circulatory system. Calcium and vitamin D also appear to facilitate the return of lead from the blood to the bones.

Deficiency Effects and Symptoms

No available information.

Beneficial Effect on Ailments

No available information.

MAGNESIUM

Description

Magnesium is an essential mineral that accounts for about 0.05 percent of the body's total weight. Nearly 70 percent of the body's supply is located in the bones together with calcium and phosphorus, while 30 percent is found in the soft tissues and body fluids.

Magnesium is involved in many essential metabolic processes. Most magnesium is found inside the cell,

[193]National Academy of Sciences, *Toxicants Occurring Naturally in Foods,* p. 61.
[194]Rodale, *Complete Book of Minerals for Health,* p. 446.
[195]"Problem Children, Lead and What to Do about It," *Prevention,* October 1973, p. 87.

[196]National Academy of Sciences, *Toxicants Occurring Naturally in Foods,* pp. 61-62.
[197]"Problem Children, Lead and What to Do about It," pp. 81-88.
[198]Krause and Hunscher, *Food, Nutrition and Diet Therapy,* p. 519.

where it activates enzymes necessary for the metabolism of carbohydrates and amino acids. By countering the stimulative effect of calcium, magnesium plays an important role in neuromuscular contractions.[199] It also helps regulate the acid-alkaline balance in the body.

Magnesium helps promote absorption and metabolism of other minerals, such as calcium, phosphorus, sodium, and potassium. It also helps utilize the B complex and vitamins C and E in the body. It aids during bone growth and is necessary for proper functioning of the nerves and muscles, including those of the heart. Evidence suggests that magnesium is associated with the regulation of body temperature. Sufficient amounts of magnesium are needed in the conversion of blood sugar into energy.

Magnesium appears to be widely distributed in foods, being found chiefly in fresh green vegetables, where it is an essential element of chlorophyll. Other excellent sources include raw, unmilled wheat germ, soybeans, figs, corn, apples, and oil-rich seeds and nuts, especially almonds. Dolomite, a natural dietary supplement, is also rich in magnesium and is a good source of calcium and essential trace minerals as well.

Absorption and Storage

Nearly 50 percent of the average daily intake of magnesium is absorbed in the small intestine. The rate of absorption is influenced by the parathyroid hormones, the rate of water absorption, and the amounts of calcium, phosphate, and lactose (milk sugar) in the body.[200] When the intake of magnesium is low, the rate of absorption may be as high as 75 percent; when the intake is high, the rate of absorption may be as low as 25 percent.[201]

The adrenal gland secretes a hormone called aldosterone, which helps to regulate the rate of magnesium excretion through the kidneys. Losses tend to increase with the use of diuretics and with the consumption of alcohol.

Dosage and Toxicity

The National Research Council recommends a daily magnesium intake of 350 milligrams for the adult male and 300 milligrams for the adult female. The amount increases to 450 milligrams during pregnancy and lactation.[202] It is estimated that the typical American diet provides 120 milligrams per 1000 kilocalories, a level that will barely provide the recommended daily intake.

Evidence suggests that the balance between calcium and magnesium is especially important. If calcium consumption is high, magnesium intake needs to be high also. The amounts of protein, phosphorus, and vitamin D in the diet also influence the magnesium requirement. The need for magnesium is increased when blood cholesterol levels are high and when consumption of protein is high. Magnesium oxide is preferred over dolomite, but if dolomite is taken, additional supplementation of hydrochloric acid is needed to ensure that the dolomite is dissolved properly. Because magnesium acts as an alkali, it should not be taken after meals.

Large amounts of magnesium can be toxic, especially if the calcium intake is low and the phosphorus intake is high. Excessive magnesium is usually excreted adequately, but in the event of a kidney failure, there is greater danger of toxicity because the rate of excretion will be much lower.

Deficiency Effects and Symptoms

Magnesium deficiency can occur in patients with diabetes, pancreatitis, chronic alcoholism, kwashiorkor, kidney malfunction, a high-carbohydrate diet, or severe malabsorption as caused by chronic diarrhea or vomiting. Some hormones when used as drugs can upset metabolism and cause local deficiencies.[203]

Magnesium deficiency is thought to be closely related to coronary heart disease.[204] An inadequate supply of this mineral may result in the formation of clots in the heart and brain and may contribute to calcium deposits in the kidneys, blood vessels, and heart.

Symptoms of magnesium deficiency may include apprehensiveness, muscle twitch, tremors, confusion, and disorientation. The first step in treating the symptoms of a magnesium deficiency, especially among children, is to eliminate milk from the diet.[205] Calciferol (synthetic vitamin D), like fluorine, tends to bind with magnesium and carry it out of the body; since milk contains high amounts of this substance, it contributes

[199] Guthrie, *Introductory Nutrition*, p. 133.

[200] Ruth L. Pike and Myrtle L. Brown, *Nutrition: An Integrated Approach* (New York: Wiley, 1971), p. 444.

[201] Guthrie, *Introductory Nutrition*, p. 133.

[202] Krause and Hunscher, *Food, Nutrition and Diet Therapy*, p. 109.

[203] Rodale, *Complete Book of Minerals for Health*, p. 82.

[204] Williams, *Nutrition against Disease*, p. 80.

[205] Rodale, *Complete Book of Minerals for Health*, p. 99.

to the deficiency. Herein lies another good reason to supplement the diet with natural fish-liver oil instead of synthetic vitamin D, which is ten times more active as a magnesium-binding agent.

Beneficial Effect on Ailments

Magnesium is vital in helping prevent heart attacks and severe coronary thrombosis. Magnesium seems to be important in controlling the manner in which electrical charges are utilized by the body to induce the passage of nutrients in and out of cells. It has been successfully used to treat prostate troubles, polio, and depression. It has also proved beneficial in the treatment of neuromuscular disorders, nervousness, tantrums, sensitivity to noise, and hand tremor.[206]

In alcoholics, the magnesium levels in the blood and muscles are low. Magnesium treatment helps the body retain magnesium and often helps control delirium tremens.

Magnesium helps to protect the accumulation of calcium deposits in the urinary tract. It makes the calcium and phosphorus soluble in the urine and prevents them from turning into hard stones. Adequate amounts of magnesium can help reduce blood cholesterol and help keep the arteries healthy.

Magnesium, not calcium, helps form the kind of hard tooth enamel that resists decay.[207] No matter how much calcium is ingested, only a soft enamel will be formed unless magnesium is present. The magnesium supplement dolomite is beneficial in fighting tooth decay.

Magnesium therapy has been effective in treating diarrhea, vomiting, nervousness, and kwashiorkor. Since magnesium works to preserve the health of the nervous system, it has been successfully used in controlling convulsions in pregnant women and epileptic patients. Because magnesium is very alkaline, it acts as an antacid and can be used in place of over-the-counter antacid compounds.

Human Tests

1. Magnesium and Kidney Stones. A thirty three-year-old pregnant woman had passed at least 8 to 12 stones

[206] Linda Clark, *Get Well Naturally* (New York: Pyramid Communications, 1968), p. 122.
[207] Rodale, *Complete Book of Minerals for Health*, p. 105.

during previous pregnancies. She was given 500 to 1,500 milligrams of magnesium daily over a period of 6 weeks.

Results. The pregnancy during which she was given the oral dose of magnesium was the first one during which she did not pass a single kidney stone. (F. Peter Kohler and Charles A. W. Uhle, *Journal of Urology*, November 1966, as reported in Rodale, *Complete Book of Minerals for Health*, p. 78.)

MAGNESIUM MAY BE BENEFICIAL FOR THE FOLLOWING AILMENTS:

Body Member	Ailment
Blood/Circulatory system	Arteriosclerosis
	Atherosclerosis
	Cholesterol level, high
	Diabetes
	Hypertension
Bones	Fracture
	Osteoporosis
	Rickets
Bowel	Colitis
	Diarrhea
Brain/Nervous system	Alcoholism
	Epilepsy
	Mental illness
	Multiple sclerosis
	Nervousness
	Neuritis
	Parkinson's disease
Heart	Arteriosclerosis
	Atherosclerosis
	Hypertension
Intestine	Celiac disease
Joint	Arthritis
Kidney	Kidney stones (renal calculi)
	Nephritis
Leg	Leg cramp
Muscles	Muscular excitability
Skin	Psoriasis
Stomach	Vomiting
General	Alcoholism
	Backache

Body Member	Ailment
	Kwashiorkor
	Overweight and obesity

MANGANESE

Description

Manganese is a trace mineral and plays a role in activating numerous enzymes. Manganese aids in the utilization of choline and is an activator of enzymes that are necessary for utilization of biotin, thiamine, and ascorbic acid.[208] Manganese is a catalyst in the synthesis of fatty acids and cholesterol. It also plays a part in protein, carbohydrate, and fat production; is necessary for normal skeletal development; and may be important for the formation of blood.[209] Manganese is important for the production of milk and the formation of urea, a part of the urine. It helps maintain sex-hormone production. Manganese also helps nourish the nerves and brain.

Whole-grain cereals, egg yolks, and green vegetables are among the better sources of manganese, but the content will vary depending upon the amount present in the soil.

Absorption and Storage

Manganese is very poorly absorbed while in the intestinal tract. Large intakes of calcium and phosphorus in the diet will depress the rate of absorption. Excretion of manganese occurs via the feces, much of it in the form of choline complex in the bile.[210]

The adult body contains only 10 to 20 milligrams of manganese. The highest concentrations of it are in the bones, liver, pancreas, and pituitary gland.

Dosage and Toxicity

The National Research Council sets no Recommended Dietary Allowance for manganese. The average daily diet contains approximately four milligrams, which is within the amount (3 to 9 milligrams) estimated to be required for an adult.[211]

A high calcium and phosphorus intake will increase the need for manganese. Very high dosages of manganese result in reduced storage and utilization of iron.

Industrial workers frequently exposed to manganese dust may absorb enough of the metal in the respiratory tract to develop toxic symptoms.[212] Weakness and psychological and motor difficulties can result from high tissue levels of manganese.

Deficiency Effects and Symptoms

A deficiency of manganese can affect glucose tolerance, resulting in the inability to remove excess sugar from the blood by oxidation and/or storage.[213] Ataxia, the failure of muscular coordination, has been linked with the inadequate intake of manganese. Deficiencies may also lead to paralysis, convulsion, blindness, and deafness in infants. Dizziness, ear noises, and loss of hearing may occur in adults.

Beneficial Effect on Ailments

Manganese has been beneficial in the treatment of diabetes. When combined with the B vitamins, manganese has helped children and adults who are suffering from devastating weakness by stimulating the transmission of impulses between nerve and muscle. Manganese also helps treat myasthenia gravis (failure of muscular coordination and loss of muscle strength).[214] Research suggests that manganese may play a role in the treatment of multiple sclerosis.[215]

MANGANESE MAY BE BENEFICIAL FOR THE FOLLOWING AILMENTS:

Body Member	Ailment
Blood/Circulatory system	Diabetes
Brain/Nervous system	Multiple sclerosis
Lungs/Respiratory system	Allergies
	Asthma
General	Fatigue

---

[208] Rodale, *Complete Book of Minerals for Health*, pp. 228-229.

[209] Linnea Anderson, Marjorie V. Dibble, Helen S. Mitchell, and Hendrika J. Rynbergen, *Cooper's Nutrition in Health and Disease* (Philadelphia: J.B. Lippincott Co., 1968), p. 73.

[210] Chaney and Ross, *Nutrition*, p. 182.

[211] Krause and Hunscher, *Food, Nutrition and Diet Therapy*, p. 116.

[212] Rodale, *Complete Book of Minerals for Health*, p. 223.

[213] Rodale, *Complete Book of Minerals for Health*, p. 224.

[214] Clark, *Know Your Nutrition*, pp. 166-167.

[215] Clark, *Know Your Nutrition*, pp. 166-167.

MERCURY

Description

Mercury occurs widely in the biosphere and is a toxic element presenting occupational hazards associated with both ingestion and inhalation. Mercury has no essential function in the human body.

Dr. Henry A. Shroeder, a prominent trace mineral researcher, has stated that the only fish that need to be avoided for fear of mercury poisoning are fish from inland waters known to be polluted by toxic-mercury dumping. People eating well-balanced meals, not exclusively fish, have not reported any mercury poisoning.

Mercury's danger to the body lies in exposure to specific compounds, rather than inorganic forms, of this trace mineral. Methyl mercury and ethyl mercury are two highly toxic forms.[216] Methyl mercury can be found throughout agriculture and industry in pesticides, in fungicides, in the chemical by-product of chlorine, and in a form of mercury vapor from smokestacks. All of these chemicals can threaten the environment and the human body because they are retained in the tissues for long periods and adversely effect the central nervous system.

Symptoms of subacute mercury poisoning may be salivation, stomatitis, and diarrhea; or they may be neurological, such as Parkinsonian tremors, vertigo, irritability, moodiness, and depression.[217] Methyl mercury attacks the central nervous system and can cause brain damage. It usually takes the body 70 days to flush out half of the amount that originally was ingested. Symptoms of methyl mercury poisoning include loss of coordination, intellectual ability, vision, and hearing.

The average intake of mercury from food is estimated to be only 0.5 milligram daily. Oral ingestion of as little as 100 milligrams of mercury chloride produces toxic symptoms, and 500 milligrams is usually always fatal unless immediate treatment is given.

MOLYBDENUM

Description

Molybdenum is a trace mineral found in practically all plant and animal tissues. It is an essential part of two enzymes: xanthine oxidase, which aids in the mobiliza-

tion of iron from the liver reserves; and aldehyde oxidase, which is necessary for the oxidation of fats.

Food sources of molybdenum include legumes, cereal grains, and some of the dark-green leafy vegetables. The food's mineral content is completely dependent upon the soil content.

Absorption and Storage

Molybdenum is found in minute amounts in the body, being readily absorbed from the gastrointestinal tract and excreted in the urine. Molybdenum is stored in the liver, kidneys, and bones.[218]

Dosage and Toxicity

There is no Recommended Dietary Allowance for molybdenum because it is so widely distributed in commonly used foods. Toxicity symptoms include diarrhea, anemia, and depressed growth rate.[219] High intake may also result in a copper deficiency.[220]

Deficiency Effects and Symptoms

There are no known molybdenum deficiency effects.

Beneficial Effect on Ailments

Molybdenum may play a part in the prevention of anemia.

MOLYBDENUM MAY BE BENEFICIAL FOR THE FOLLOWING AILMENTS:

Body Member	Ailment
Liver	Anemia

NICKEL

Description

Nickel is a trace mineral found in large amounts in the body. Nickel catalysts are involved in the hydrogenation of edible vegetable oils such as corn, peanut, and cottonseed oil. This is one reason for large amounts of nickel being present in the human body tissue. Nickel is an essential mineral, but its application in human nutrition is unknown.[221]

---

[216] Rodale, *Complete Book of Minerals for Health*, p. 419.
[217] National Academy of Sciences, *Toxicants Occurring Naturally in Foods*, p. 67.
[218] Guthrie, *Introductory Nutrition*, p. 165.
[219] Chaney and Ross, *Nutrition*, p. 183.
[220] Chaney and Ross, *Nutrition*, p. 183.
[221] National Academy of Sciences, *Recommended Dietary Allowances*, Washington, p. 102.

PHOSPHORUS

Description

Phosphorus is the second most abundant mineral in the body and is found in every cell. It often functions along with calcium, and the healthy body maintains a specific calcium-phosphorus balance in the bones of 2.5 parts calcium to 1 part phosphorus, although phosphorus is in higher ratio in the soft tissues. This balance of calcium and phosphorus is needed for these minerals to be effectively used by the body.

Phosphorus plays a part in almost every chemical reaction within the body because it is present in every cell. It is important in the utilization of carbohydrates, fats, and protein for the growth, maintenance, and repair of cells and for the production of energy. It stimulates muscle contractions, including the regular contractions of the heart muscle. Niacin and riboflavin cannot be digested unless phosphorus is present. Phosphorus is an essential part of nucleoproteins, which are responsible for cell division and reproduction and the transference of hereditary traits from parents to offspring. It is also necessary for proper skeletal growth, tooth development, kidney functioning, and transference of nerve impulses.

Phospholipids, such as lecithin, help break up and transport fats and fatty acids. They help prevent the accumulation of too much acid or too much alkali in the blood, assist in the passage of substances through the cell walls, and promote the secretion of glandular hormones. They are also needed for healthy nerves and efficient mental activity.

Foods rich in protein are also rich in phosphorus. Meat, fish, poultry, eggs, whole grains, seeds, and nuts are primary sources of phosphorus.

Absorption and Storage

Unlike calcium, which is poorly absorbed, most dietary phosphorus is absorbed from the intestine into the bloodstream. About 70 percent of the phosphorus ingested in foods is absorbed. About 88 percent of the absorbed phosphorus is stored in the bones and teeth, along with calcium, although antacids can deplete the storage. There is relatively little control over the rate of absorption, so the body content is regulated by urinary excretion.

Phosphorus absorption depends on the presence of vitamin D and calcium. Absorption can be interfered with by excessive amounts of iron, aluminum, and magnesium, which tend to form insoluble phosphates.[222] The calcium-phosphorus balance is disturbed in the presence of white sugar. High fat diets or digestive conditions that prevent the absorption of fat increase the absorption of phosphorus in the intestine, but such conditions are not healthful because they also decrease the amount of calcium absorbed and upset the calcium-phosphorus balance.[223]

Dosage and Toxicity

The National Research Council recommends a daily dietary intake of 800 milligrams of phosphorus for men and women. During pregnancy and lactation the amount increases to 1,200 milligrams. This is equal to the daily requirement for calcium. If the phosphorus content of the body is high, additional calcium should be taken to maintain a proper balance. There is no known toxicity of phosphorus.

Deficiency Effects and Symptoms

An insufficient supply of phosphorus, calcium, or vitamin D may result in stunted growth, poor quality of bones and teeth, or other bone disorders. A deficiency in the calcium-phosphorus balance may result in diseases such as arthritis, pyorrhea, rickets, and tooth decay.[224]

A phosphorus deficiency can cause lack of appetite and weight loss or, conversely, overweight. Irregular breathing, mental and physical fatigue, and nervous disorders may occur.

Beneficial Effect on Ailments

Dietary phosphate has speeded up the healing process in bone fractures and has reduced the expected loss of calcium in such patients. It has been used successfully in the treatment of osteomalacia and osteoporosis. It also helps to prevent or cure rickets and to prevent stunted growth in children.

Mental stress can cause an upset in the body chemistry and bring on strong arthritic symptoms such as aching joints. The calcium-phosphorus balance can help treat the stressful condition and can also help alleviate the arthritis.

Recent research has shown that phosphorus may be important in cancer prevention. Investigators have discovered that phosphorus is more easily lost from

[222] Guthrie, *Introductory Nutrition* p. 126.
[223] Rodale, *Complete Book of Minerals for Health*, p. 65.
[224] Rodale, *Complete Book of Minerals for Health*, p. 65.

cancerous cells than from normal cells.[225] Phosphorus is essential in treating disorders of the teeth and gums.

PHOSPHORUS MAY BE BENEFICIAL FOR THE FOLLOWING AILMENTS:

Body Member	Ailment
Bones	Fracture
	Osteomalacia
	Osteoporosis
	Rickets
	Stunted growth
Bowel	Colitis
Brain/Nervous system	Mental illness
Heart	Arteriosclerosis
	Atherosclerosis
Joints	Arthritis
Leg	Leg cramp
Teeth/Gums	Tooth and gum disorders
General	Backache
	Cancer
	Pregnancy
	Stress

POTASSIUM

Description

Potassium is an essential mineral found mainly in the intracellular fluid; a small amount occurs in the extracellular fluid. Potassium constitutes 5 percent of the total mineral content of the body.[226] Potassium and sodium help regulate water balance within the body; that is, they help regulate the distribution of fluids on either side of the cell walls.

Potassium is necessary for normal growth, to stimulate nerve impulses for muscle contraction, and to preserve proper alkalinity of the body fluids. It aids in keeping the skin healthy. Potassium assists in the conversion of glucose to glycogen, the form in which glucose can be stored in the liver. It functions in cell metabolism, enzyme reactions, and the synthesis of muscle protein from amino acids in the blood. It

stimulates the kidneys to eliminate poisonous body wastes.

Potassium works with sodium to help normalize the heartbeat and nourish the muscular system.[227] It unites with phosphorus to send oxygen to the brain and also functions with calcium in the regulation of neuromuscular activity.[228]

Food sources of potassium include all vegetables, especially green leafy vegetables, oranges, whole grains, sunflower seeds, and mint leaves. Large amounts of potassium are found in potatoes, especially in the peelings, and in bananas.

Absorption and Storage

Potassium is rapidly absorbed from the small intestine. It is excreted mainly through urination and perspiration, with very little lost in the feces. The kidneys are able to maintain normal serum levels through their ability to filter, secrete, and excrete potassium. Aldosterone, an adrenal hormone, stimulates potassium excretion.

Excessive potassium buildup may result from kidney failure or from severe lack of fluid.

Because sodium and potassium must be in balance, the excessive use of salt depletes the body's conservation of its often scarce potassium supplies. In addition, potassium can be depleted by prolonged diarrhea, excessive sweating, vomiting, and the use of diuretics.

Alcohol and coffee increase the urinary excretion of potassium. Alcohol is a double antagonist since it also depletes the magnesium reserve.[229] Excessive intake of sugar is also antagonistic towards potassium.

A low blood sugar level is a stressful condition that strains the adrenal glands, causing additional potassium to be lost in the urine while water and salt are held in the tissues. An adequate supply of magnesium is needed to retain the storage of potassium in the cells.

Dosage and Toxicity

A Recommended Dietary Allowance for potassium has not been established, but many authorities suggest that between 2,000 and 2,500 milligrams be included in the diet daily. The amount of potassium in the average American's daily diet has been estimated at 2,000 to

[225] Rodale, *The Health Builder*, p. 664.
[226] Krause and Hunscher, *Food, Nutrition and Diet Therapy*, p. 110.

[227] Wade, *Magic Minerals: Key to Health*, p. 22.
[228] Krause and Hunscher, *Food, Nutrition and Diet Therapy*, p. 110.
[229] Lisa Cosman, "Potassium: The Neglected Mineral," *Bestways*, October 1973, p. 19.

6,000 milligrams per day, since it is distributed in many different foods.[230] There is no known toxicity of potassium.

Deficiency Effects and Symptoms

Excessive urinary losses induced by high salt intake have caused potassium deficiencies to be commonplace. A potassium deficiency can result from an excessive intake of sodium chloride or from an inadequate intake of fruits and vegetables. Refined sugar can cause the urine to become alkaline so that minerals cannot be held in solution. Deficiency can be caused by prolonged intravenous administration of saline, which induces potassium excretion.[231] Vomiting, severe malnutrition, and stress, both mental and physical, may also lead to potassium deficiency.

A potassium deficiency may cause nervous disorders, insomnia, constipation, slow and irregular heartbeat, and muscle damage. When a deficiency of potassium impairs glucose metabolism, energy is no longer available to the muscles and they become more or less paralyzed.

When the body is lacking potassium, the sodium content of the heart and muscles increases. Infants suffering from diarrhea may have a potassium deficiency because the passage of the intestinal contents is so rapid that there is decreased absorption of potassium.[232] Diabetic patients are often deficient in potassium.[233] Persons suffering from diseases of the digestive tract are frequently found to be potassium-deficient. A person loses potassium when taking hormone products such as cortisone and aldosterone. Sodium is retained and potassium is excreted when these drugs are administered.

Early symptoms of potassium deficiency include general weakness and impairment of neuromuscular function, poor reflexes, and soft, sagging muscles. In adolescents, acne can result; in older persons, dry skin may occur.

Beneficial Effect on Ailments

Potassium has been used to treat cases of high blood pressure which were directly caused by excessive salt intake. Colic in infants has disappeared after injections of potassium chloride. Potassium chloride has also proven effective in treating allergies.

Giving potassium to patients with mild diabetes can reduce blood pressure and blood sugar levels.[234] Since potassium is essential for the transmission of nerve impulses to the brain, it has been effective in the treatment of headache-causing allergies.[235]

Potassium has also been used in the treatment of diarrhea in infants and adults. Therapeutic doses of potassium are sometimes used to slow the heartbeat in cases of severe injury, such as burns.

POTASSIUM MAY BE BENEFICIAL FOR THE FOLLOWING AILMENTS:

Body Member	Ailment
Blood/Circulatory system	Angina pectoris
	Diabetes
	Hypertension
	Mononucleosis
	Stroke (cerebrovascular accident)
Bones	Fracture
Bowel	Colitis
	Diarrhea
Brain/Nervous system	Alcoholism
	Hypertension
	Insomnia
	Polio
Glands	Mononucleosis
Head	Fever
	Headache
Intestine	Constipation
	Worms
Heart	Angina pectoris
	Congestive heart failure
	Hypertension
	Myocardial infarction
Joints	Arthritis
	Gout
Lungs/Respiratory system	Allergies
Muscles	Impaired muscle activity
	Muscular dystrophy

[230] Guthrie, *Introductory Nutrition*, p. 128.
[231] Williams, *Nutrition against Disease*, pp. 156-157.
[232] Guthrie, *Introductory Nutrition*, p. 128.
[233] Davis, *Let's Get Well*, p. 115.
[234] Rodale, *The Health Builder*, p. 695.
[235] Rodale, *The Best Health Articles from* Prevention *Magazine*, p. 578.

Body Member	Ailment
	Rheumatism
Skin	Acne
	Burns
	Dermatitis
Stomach	Gastroenteritis
Teeth/Gums	Tooth and gum disorders
General	Alcoholism
	Cancer
	Fever
	Stress

SELENIUM

Description

Selenium is an essential mineral found in minute amounts in the body. It works closely with vitamin E in some of its metabolic actions and in the promotion of normal body growth and fertility. Selenium is a natural antioxidant and appears to preserve elasticity of tissue by delaying oxidation of polyunsaturated fatty acids that can cause solidification of tissue proteins.[236]

The selenium content of food is dependent upon the extent of its presence in the soil in which the food was grown. Selenium is found in the bran and germ of cereals; in vegetables such as broccoli, onions, and tomatoes; and in tuna.

Absorption and Storage

The liver and kidneys contain four to five times as much selenium as do the muscles and other tissues. Selenium is normally excreted in the urine; its presence in the feces is an indication of improper absorption.[237]

Dosage and Toxicity

The Recommended Dietary Allowance of selenium for adults is extremely minute; 5 to 10 parts per million is considered toxic. This is due to the tendency of selenium to replace sulfur in biological compounds and inhibit the action of some enzymes.[238] Selenium can be toxic in its pure form and should be obtained from natural foods only.[239] Reported instances of toxicity

have occurred in areas where the selenium content of the soil was high.

Deficiency Effects and Symptoms

A deficiency of selenium may lead to premature aging. This is because selenium preserves tissue elasticity.

Beneficial Effect on Ailments

Selenium when combined with protein is beneficial in treating kwashiorkor, a protein-deficiency disease.

SELENIUM MAY BE BENEFICIAL FOR THE FOLLOWING AILMENT:

Body Member	Ailment
General	Kwashiorkor

SODIUM

Description

Sodium is an essential mineral found predominantly in the extracellular fluids; the vascular fluids within the blood vessels, arteries, veins, and capillaries; and the intestinal fluids surrounding the cells.[240] About 50 percent of the body's sodium is found in these fluids and the remaining amount is found within the bones.[241]

Sodium functions with potassium to equalize the acid-alkali factor in the blood. Along with potassium, it helps regulate water balance within the body; that is, it helps regulate the distribution of fluids on either side of the cell walls. Sodium and potassium are also involved in muscle contraction and expansion and in nerve stimulation.

Another important function of sodium is keeping the other blood minerals soluble, so that they will not build up as deposits in the bloodstream.[242] It acts with chlorine to improve blood and lymph health, helps purge carbon dioxide from the body and aids digestion.[243] Sodium is also necessary for hydrochloric acid production in the stomach.

Sodium is found in virtually all foods, especially sodium chloride, or salt. High concentrations are contained in seafoods, carrots, beets, poultry, and meat. Kelp is an excellent supplemental source of sodium.

[236] Rodale, *Complete Book of Minerals for Health*, p. 235.
[237] Guthrie, *Introductory Nutrition*, p. 162.
[238] Guthrie, *Introductory Nutrition*, p. 162.
[239] Rodale, *Complete Book of Minerals for Health*, p. 236.

[240] Guthrie, *Introductory Nutrition*, p. 129.
[241] Guthrie, *Introductory Nutrition*, p. 129.
[242] Wade, *Magic Minerals: Key to Health*, p. 21.
[243] Rodale, *Complete Book of Minerals for Health*, p. 133.

Absorption and Storage

Sodium is readily absorbed in the small intestine and the stomach and is carried by the blood to the kidneys, where it is filtered out and returned to the blood in amounts needed to maintain blood levels required by the body.[244] The absorption of sodium requires energy. Any excess, which usually amounts to 90 to 95 percent of ingested sodium, is excreted in the urine.[245]

The adrenal hormone aldosterone is an important regulator of sodium metabolism. Excessive salt in food interferes with absorption and utilization, especially in the case of protein foods.[246] Vomiting, diarrhea, or excessive perspiration may result in a depletion of sodium. Sodium supplements to prevent sodium deficiency may be needed in such cases. The levels of sodium in the urine reflect the dietary intake; therefore when there is a high intake of sodium the rate of excretion is high, and if the intake is low the excretion rate is low.

Dosage and Toxicity

There is no established dietary requirement for sodium, but it is generally observed that the usual intake far exceeds the need. The average American ingests 3 to 7 grams of sodium and 6 to 18 grams of sodium chloride each day.[247] The National Research Council recommends a daily sodium chloride intake of 1 gram per kilogram of water consumed.[248]

An excess of sodium in the diet may cause potassium to be lost in the urine. Abnormal fluid retention accompanied by dizziness and swelling of such areas as legs and face can also occur. An intake of 14 to 28 grams of salt (sodium chloride) daily is considered excessive.[249]

Diets containing excessive amounts of sodium contribute to the increasing incidences of high blood pressure. The simplest way to reduce sodium intake is to eliminate the use of table salt.

[244]Guthrie, *Introductory Nutrition*, p. 129.
[245]Krause and Hunscher, *Food, Nutrition and Diet Therapy*, p. 110.
[246]Rodale, *The Health Builder*, pp. 841-842.
[247]Krause and Hunscher, *Food, Nutrition and Diet Therapy*, p. 110.
[248]Krause and Hunscher, *Food, Nutrition and Diet Therapy*, p. 110.
[249]National Academy of Sciences, *Toxicants Occurring Naturally in Foods*, p. 270.

Deficiency Effects and Symptoms

Deficiencies are very uncommon because nearly all foods contain some sodium, with meats containing especially high amounts. A sodium deficiency can cause intestinal gas, weight loss, vomiting, and muscle shrinkage. The conversion of carbohydrates into fat for digestion is impaired when sodium is absent. Arthritis, rheumatism, and neuralgia, a sharp pain along a nerve, may be caused by acids that accumulate in the absence of sodium.

Beneficial Effect on Ailments

An individual suffering from high blood pressure is advised to maintain a low-sodium diet, since sodium may aggravate this ailment. Resistance to heat cramps and heat strokes may be increased by moderate sodium intake. Sodium helps keep calcium in a solution that is necessary for nerve strength.[250] Clinical studies indicate that low-sodium diets are effective in preventing or relieving the symptoms of toxemia (bacterial poisoning), edema (swelling), proteinuria (albumin in the urine), and blurred vision.

SODIUM MAY BE BENEFICIAL FOR THE FOLLOWING AILMENTS:

Body Member	Ailment
Bowel	Diarrhea
Glands	Adrenal exhaustion
	Cystic Fibrosis
Leg	Leg cramp
Teeth/Gums	Tooth and gum disorders
General	Dehydration
	Fever
	Polio

SULFUR

Description

Sulfur is a nonmetallic element that occurs widely in nature, being present in every cell of animals and plants. Sulfur makes up 0.25 percent of the human body weight. It is called nature's "beauty mineral" because it keeps the hair glossy and smooth and keeps the complexion clear and youthful.

[250]Wade, *Magic Minerals: Key to Health*, p. 22.

Sulfur has an important relationship with protein. It is contained in the amino acids methionine, cystine, and cysteine, and it appears to be necessary for collagen synthesis.[251] Sulfur is prevalent in keratin, a tough protein substance necessary for health and maintenance of the skin, nails, and hair.[252] It is found in insulin, the hormone that regulates carbohydrate metabolism.[253] It also occurs in carbohydrates such as heparin, an anticoagulant found in the liver and other tissues.

Sulfur works with thiamine, pantothenic acid, biotin, and lipoic acid, which are needed for metabolism and strong nerve health. In addition, sulfur plays a part in tissue respiration, the process whereby oxygen and other substances are used to build cells and release energy. It works with the liver to secrete bile. Sulfur also helps to maintain overall body balance.

Sulfur is found in protein-containing foods such as meat, fish, legumes, and nuts. Other natural sources include eggs, cabbage, dried beans, and brussels sprouts.

Absorption and Storage

Sulfur is stored in every cell of the body. The highest concentrations are found in the hair, skin, and nails. Excess sulfur is excreted in the urine and the feces.

Dosage and Toxicity

There is no Recommended Dietary Allowance for sulfur because it is assumed that a person's sulfur requirement is met when the protein intake is adequate.[254] Sulfur can be used in various forms such as ointments, creams, lotions, and dusting powders. Excessive intake of inorganic sulfur may result in toxicity.

Deficiency Effects and Symptoms

There are no known deficiency effects or symptoms.

Beneficial Effect on Ailments

Sulfur is important in the treatment of arthritis. The level of cystine, a sulfur-containing amino acid, in arthritic patients is usually much lower than normal.

When used topically in the form of an ointment, sulfur is helpful in treating skin disorders, such as psoriasis, eczema, and dermatitis. It also may be beneficial in treating ringworm.

SULPHUR MAY BE BENEFICIAL FOR THE FOLLOWING AILMENTS:

Body Member	Ailment
Intestine	Worms
Joints	Arthritis
Skin	Dermatitis
	Eczema
	Psoriasis

VANADIUM

Description

Vanadium is a trace mineral found in varying quantities in vegetables. Marine life is the most reliable source.

Vanadium is part of the natural circulatory regulating system. The presence of it in the brain inhibits cholesterol formation in the blood vessels. In addition, the formation of cholesterol in the human central nervous system can be reduced by administering vanadium orally.[255]

It is difficult to measure vanadium levels in humans, although 90 percent of ingested vanadium is eliminated in the urine. An overdose of vanadium, even in synthetic form, is easily induced. Vanadium should be taken in the natural form, and fish is an excellent source.

ZINC

Description

Zinc is an essential trace mineral occurring in the body in larger amounts than any other trace element except iron. The human body contains approximately 1.8 grams of zinc compared to nearly 5 grams of iron.

Zinc has a variety of functions. It is related to the normal absorption and action of vitamins, especially the B complex. It is a constituent of at least 25 enzymes involved in digestion and metabolism, including carbonic anhydrase, which is necessary for tissue respiration. Zinc is a component of insulin, and it is part of the enzyme that is needed to break down alcohol. It also plays a part in carbohydrate digestion and phosphorus

[251] Guthrie, *Introductory Nutrition*, pp. 128-129.
[252] Wade, *Magic Minerals: Key to Health*, p. 24.
[253] Krause and Hunscher, *Food, Nutrition and Diet Therapy*, p. 108.
[254] Chaney and Ross, *Nutrition*, p. 187.
[255] Rodale, *Complete Book of Minerals for Health*, p. 251.

metabolism. In addition, it is essential in the synthesis of nucleic acid, which controls the formation of different proteins in the cell. Zinc is essential for general growth and proper development of the reproductive organs and for normal functioning of the prostate gland.

Recent medical findings indicate that zinc is important in healing wounds and burns. It may also be required in the synthesis of DNA, which is the master substance of life, carrying all inherited traits and directing the activity of each cell.[256]

The best sources of all trace elements in proper balance are natural unprocessed foods, preferably those grown in organically enriched soil. Diets high in protein, whole-grain products, brewer's yeast, wheat bran, wheat germ, and pumpkin seeds are usually high in zinc. The zinc content of most municipal drinking water is negligible.[257]

Absorption and Storage

Zinc is readily absorbed in the upper small intestine. The major route of excretion is through the gastrointestinal tract; little is lost in the urine. The largest storage of zinc occurs in the liver, pancreas, kidney, bones, and voluntary muscles. Zinc is also stored in parts of the eyes, prostate gland and spermatozoa, skin, hair, fingernails, and toenails as well as being present in the white blood cells.[258]

A high intake of calcium and phytic acid, found in certain grains, may prevent absorption of zinc. If the intake of calcium and phytic acid is higher, zinc consumption should be increased.

Dosage and Toxicity

The National Research Council recommends a daily dietary intake of 15 milligrams of zinc for adults. An additional 15 milligrams is recommended during pregnancy, and an additional 25 milligrams is recommended during lactation. The average zinc content of a mixed diet is between 10 and 15 milligrams.[259]

Zinc is relatively nontoxic, although poisoning may result from eating foods that have been stored in

galvanized containers. High intakes of zinc interfere with copper utilization, causing incomplete iron metabolism. Excessive intake of zinc may result in a loss of iron and copper from the liver. When zinc is added to the diet, vitamin A is also needed in larger amounts.

Deficiency Effects and Symptoms

The most common cause of zinc deficiency is an unbalanced diet, although other factors may also be responsible. For example, the consumption of alcohol may precipitate a deficiency by flushing stored zinc out of the liver and into the urine.[260] Zinc deficiency is also a factor in increased fatigue, susceptibility to infection, injury, and decreased alertness.[261]

Zinc deficiency can cause retarded growth, delayed sexual maturity, and prolonged healing of wounds. A deficiency of zinc, copper, and vanadium may result in atherosclerosis.

Cadmium, a toxic mineral, also plays an important role in zinc deficiencies. High intakes of cadmium will accentuate the signs of a zinc deficiency, and the cadmium will be stored in the body in the absence of zinc. This creates a detrimental situation that can be reversed by increasing the consumption of zinc.

Recent studies demonstrate conclusively that zinc deficiency causes sterility and dwarfism in humans. The deficiency leads to unhealthy changes in the size and structure of the prostate gland, which contains more zinc than any other part of the human anatomy. In prostate problems, particularly prostate cancer, the levels of zinc in the prostate gland decline.

James A. Halstead and J. Cecil Smith, Jr., of the Trace Element Research Laboratory, Washington, D.C., have made interesting studies on zinc. They found low zinc levels in the blood plasma of people suffering from alcoholic cirrhosis, other types of liver disease, ulcers, heart attacks, mongolism, and cystic fibrosis. Pregnant women and women taking oral contraceptives also had low levels of zinc in their blood plasma.

Excessive zinc excretion occurs in leukemia and Hodgkin's disease, but the causes of this are unknown. A zinc deficiency is characterized by abnormal fatigue and may cause a loss of normal taste sensitivity, poor appetite, and suboptimal growth.

[256] Rodale, *Complete Book of Minerals for Health*, p. 259.
[257] National Academy of Sciences, *Recommended Dietary Allowances*, p. 101.
[258] Krause and Hunscher, *Food, Nutrition and Diet Therapy*, p. 117.
[259] National Academy of Sciences, *Recommended Dietary Allowances*, p. 100.

[260] Rodale, *Complete Book of Minerals for Health*, p. 226.
[261] Clark, *Know Your Nutrition*, p. 168.

Beneficial Effect on Ailments

Zinc helps eliminate cholesterol deposits and has been successfully used in the treatment of atherosclerosis. Zinc may contribute to the rapid healing of internal wounds or any injury to the arteries. Zinc supplements given in therapeutic doses will speed up the rate at which the body heals certain external wounds and injuries.

Zinc is beneficial in the prevention and treatment of infertility. It also helps in the proper growth and maturity of the sex organs.

The administration of zinc may benefit patients suffering from Hodgkin's disease and leukemia. It also is used in treatment of cirrhosis of the liver and alcoholism.

Zinc is beneficial to the diabetic because of its regulatory affect on insulin in the blood. It has been found that the addition of zinc to insulin prolongs its effect on blood sugar.[262] A diabetic pancreas contains only about half as much zinc as does a healthy one.

ZINC MAY BE BENEFICIAL FOR THE FOLLOWING AILMENTS:

Body Member	Ailment
Blood/Circulatory system	Arteriosclerosis
	Atherosclerosis
	Cholesterol level, high
	Diabetes
	Hodgkin's disease
Brain/Nervous system	Alcoholism
Glands	Prostatitis
Heart	Arteriosclerosis
	Atherosclerosis
Reproductive system	Prostatitis
	Retarded sexual activity
Skin	Burns
	Wounds
General	Alcoholism
	Retarded growth

BORON, LITHIUM, SILICON, STRONTIUM, TIN, AND TRITIUM

These are essential trace minerals, but their role in human nutrition is unknown.

[262] Rodale, *The Encyclopedia of Common Disease*, p. 273.

WATER

Water is not only the most abundant nutrient found in the body (accounting for roughly two-thirds of body weight), it also is by far the most important nutrient. Responsible for and involved in nearly every body process, including digestion, absorption, circulation, and excretion, water is the primary transporter of nutrients throughout the body and is necessary for all building functions in the body. Water helps maintain a normal body temperature and is essential for carrying waste material out of the body.

Nearly all foods contain water that is absorbed by the body during digestion. Fruits and vegetables are especially good sources of chemically pure water, which is 100 percent pure hydrogen and oxygen.

The average adult body contains approximately 45 quarts of water and loses about 3 quarts daily through excretion and perspiration.[263] Rate of water loss depends almost entirely upon level of activity and environmental conditions and may range from less than 1 quart per day for a sedentary person in a temperate climate to more than 10 quarts per day in a desert.[264] If severe deficiencies are not corrected as soon as possible, salt depletion and dehydration will occur, eventually resulting in death.

There are nearly as many types of water as there are uses for it. Most *tap water* comes from streams, rivers, and lakes. This surface water may contain pollutants and agricultural wastes, such as fertilizer and insecticide residue that is carried by rainwater runoff into nearby waterways. Air pollutants, such as lead from automobile and factory exhausts, also end up in our rivers and streams. Chemicals, including chlorine, fluorine, phosphates, alum, sodium aluminates, soda ash, carbon, and lime, are frequently added to drinking water for purification. These substances are needed to kill bacteria, but questions have been raised regarding potential cancer-causing effects of some of these chemicals. Poisonous substances such as arsenic, cadmium, cyanides, asbestos, etc.—common industrial wastes—can combine with other chemicals in water and form carcinogenic substances. Boiling water, whether hot or cold tap water or bottled

[263] Paul C. Bragg, *The Shocking Truth about Water* (Burbank, Calif.: Health Science, 1972).
[264] National Academy of Sciences, *Recommended Dietary Allowances*, p. 22.

water, for long periods of time for purification is *not* recommended because, although the bacteria will be destroyed, the purest water will be lost in the form of steam and any heavy metals or nitrates in the water will be more concentrated in the final amount.

Another source of tap water is *well water*. Unlike most surface water, which has relatively uniform mineral content, well water varies so drastically in mineral content from one location to the next that the hardness and total dissolved solids in the water can range from nearly nothing to excessive extremes. Water should not be relied upon as a healthy source of minerals because it may contain *inorganic* minerals, including calcium, copper, magnesium, mercury, iron, and silicon, some of which cannot be assimilated by the body. Instead they are deposited in the joints, arteries, and internal organs in the forms of arthritis, calcium-hardened arteries, and stones. However, *organic* minerals, those of or derived from living organisms, are more readily utilized by the body than are *inorganic* minerals. Plants "distill" the water they consume and convert the inorganic minerals into organic minerals, which can then be assimilated by the body.

Distilled water is the only "pure" water there is, being found in nature in the form of rainwater and in all fruits and vegetables. Even rainwater may be contaminated by atmospheric pollutants it picks up on the way to the ground. Distilling water for human consumption is a relatively simple process: water is heated to boiling, which kills any bacteria; steam vapors, which cannot hold any chemical, bacterial or mineral impurities, are released from the boiling water; the vapors are then collected and condensed back into water which is free of all contaminants. Distilling removes *all* minerals, whether beneficial or harmful, from the water. It has been suggested that a person switching to distilled water should make an effort to provide an adequate mineral intake by eating mineral-rich foods or supplementing the diet. This diet allows the consumption of minerals in manageable quantities that will fill individual needs. This is the only way to ensure a proper mineral balance without taking the risk of pollutants, chemicals, bacteria, and inorganic minerals.

SUMMARY CHART OF NUTRIENTS

Nutrients	Importance	Deficiency Symptoms	RDA*	Toxicity Level
Carbohydrate	Provides energy for body functions and muscular exertions. Assists in digestion and assimilation of foods.	Loss of energy. Fatigue. Excessive protein breakdown. Disturbed balance of water, sodium, potassium, and chloride.	See "Nutrient Allowance Chart," p. 235.	Intake should not exceed what is needed to maintain desirable weight.
Fat	Provides energy. Acts as a carrier for fat-soluble vitamins A, D, E, and K. Supplies essential fatty acids needed for growth, health, and smooth skin.	Eczema or skin disorders. Retarded growth.	See "Nutrient Allowance Chart," p. 235.	Intake should not exceed what is needed to maintain desirable weight.
Protein	Is necessary for growth and development. Acts in formation of hormones, enzymes, and antibodies. Maintains acid-alkali balance. Is source of heat and energy.	Fatigue. Loss of appetite. Diarrhea and vomiting. Stunted growth. Edema.	See "Nutrient Allowance Chart," p. 235.	Intake should not exceed what is needed to maintain desirable weight.
VITAMINS				
Vitamin A (Carotene)	Is necessary for growth and repair of body tissues. Is important to health of the eyes. Fights bacteria and infection. Maintains healthy epithelial tissue. Aids in bone and teeth formation.	Night blindness. Rough, dry, scaly skin. Increased susceptibility to infections. Frequent fatigue. Loss of smell and appetite.	5,000 IU.	50,000 or more IU may be toxic if there is no deficiency. 10,000 IU is the maximum single dose that can be bought without a prescription.
Vitamin B Complex	Is necessary for carbohydrate, fat, and protein metabolism. Helps functioning of the nervous system. Helps maintain muscle tone in the gastrointestinal tract.	Dry, rough, cracked skin. Acne. Dull, dry, or gray hair. Fatigue. Poor appetite. Gastrointestinal tract disorders.	See individual B vitamins.	See individual B vitamins; relatively nontoxic.

*Recommended Dietary Allowances.

Nutrients	Importance	Deficiency Symptoms	RDA*	Toxicity Level
	Maintains health of skin, hair, eyes, mouth, and liver.			
Vitamin B$_1$ (Thiamine)	Is necessary for carbohydrate metabolism. Helps maintain healthy nervous system. Stabilizes the appetite. Stimulates growth and good muscle tone.	Gastrointestinal problems. Fatigue. Loss of appetite. Nerve disorders. Heart disorders.	0.5 mg per 1000 calories consumed. 1.4 mg for men, 1.0 mg for women.	No known oral toxicity. Single doses of up to 500 mg are available without prescription.
Vitamin B$_2$ (Riboflavin)	Is necessary for carbohydrate, fat, and protein metabolism. Aids in formation of antibodies and red blood cells. Maintains cell respiration.	Eye problems. Cracks and sores in mouth. Dermatitis. Retarded growth. Digestive disturbances.	0.55 mg per 1000 calories consumed. 1.6 mg for adults.	No known oral toxicity. Single doses of 100 mg are available without prescription.
Vitamin B$_6$ (Pyridoxine)	Is necessary for carbohydrate, fat, and protein metabolism. Aids in formation of antibodies. Helps maintain balance of sodium and phosphorus.	Anemia. Mouth disorders. Nervousness. Muscular weakness. Dermatitis. Sensitivity to insulin.	0.2 mg for each 100 mg of protein. 1.8 mg men, 1.5 mg women.	No known oral toxicity. Single doses up to 100 mg are available without prescription.
Vitamin B$_{12}$ (Cyanocobalamin)	Is essential for normal formation of blood cells. Is necessary for carbohydrate, fat, and protein metabolism. Maintains healthy nervous system.	Pernicious anemia. Brain damage. Nervousness. Neuritis.	3 mcg for adults.	No known oral toxicity even with intake as high as 600-1,200 mcg.
Vitamin B$_{13}$ (Orotic acid)	Is needed for metabolism of some B vitamins.	Degenerative disorders.	No RDA.	No known toxicity.
Biotin	Necessary for carbohydrate, fat, and protein metabolism. Aids in utilization of other B vitamins.	Dermatitis. Grayish skin color. Depression. Muscle pain. Impairment of fat metabolism. Poor appetite.	150-300 mcg usually meets daily needs. No RDA.	No known oral toxicity. Single doses up to 50 mcg are available without prescription.

*Recommended Dietary Allowances.

Nutrients	Importance	Deficiency Symptoms	RDA*	Toxicity Level
Choline	Is important in normal nerve transmission. Aids metabolism and transport of fats. Helps regulate liver and gallbladder.	Fatty liver. Hemorrhaging kidneys. High blood pressure.	No RDA, but the average diet yields 500-900 mg per day.	No known oral toxicity, even with intake as high as 50,000 mg daily for one week.
Folic acid (Folacin)	Is important in red blood cell formation. Aids metabolism of proteins. Is necessary for growth and division of body cells.	Poor growth. Gastrointestinal disorders. Anemia. B_{12} deficiency.	400 mcg for adults.	No toxic effects. Single doses up to 400 mcg are available without prescription.
Inositol	Is necessary for formation of lecithin. May be indirectly connected with metabolism of fats, including cholesterol. Is vital for hair growth.	Constipation. Eczema. Hair loss. High blood cholesterol.	No RDA.	No known toxicity. Single doses up to 500 mg are available without prescription.
Laetrile (Vitamin B_{17})	Has been linked to cancer prevention.	Diminished resistance to malignancies.	No RDA.	More than 1.0 g taken at one time may prove toxic. 0.25-1.0 g at a mealtime is usual dosage.
Niacin (Nicotinic acid, Niacinamide)	Is necessary for carbohydrate, fat, and protein metabolism. Helps maintain health of skin, tongue, and digestive system.	Dermatitis. Nervous disorders.	6.6 mg per 1000 calories. 1.8 mg men, 13 mg women.	100-300 mg nicotinic acid orally or 30 mg intraveneously may produce side effects for some individuals. No effects with niacinamide.
PABA	Aids bacteria in producing folic acid. Acts as a coenzyme in the breakdown and utilization of proteins. Aids in formation of red blood cells. Acts as a sunscreen.	Fatigue. Irritability. Depression. Nervousness. Constipation. Headache. Digestive disorders. Graying hair.	No RDA.	Single doses of 100 mg are available without prescription. Continued high ingestion may be toxic.
Pangamic acid (Vitamin B_{15})	Helps eliminate hypoxia. Helps promote protein metabolism. Stimulates nervous and glandular system.	Diminished oxygenation of cells.	No RDA.	500 mg tolerated daily with no toxic effect.

*Recommended Dietary Allowances.

Nutrients	Importance	Deficiency Symptoms	RDA*	Toxicity Level
Pantothenic acid	Aids in formation of some fats. Participates in the release of energy from carbohydrates, fats, and protein. Aids in the utilization of some vitamins. Improves body's resistance to stress.	Vomiting. Restlessness. Stomach stress. Increased susceptibility to infection. Sensitivity to insulin.	0.5-10.0 mg for both adults and children is considered adequate.	10,000-20,000 mg as a calcium salt may have side effects in some persons.
Vitamin C	Maintains collagen. Helps heal wounds, scar tissue, and fractures. Gives strength to blood vessels. May provide resistance to infections. Aids in absorption of iron.	Bleeding gums. Swollen or painful joints. Slow-healing wounds and fractures. Bruising. Nosebleeds. Impaired digestion.	45 mg for adults.	Essentially nontoxic. 5,000-15,000 mg daily over a prolonged period may have side effects in some persons.
Vitamin D	Improves absorption and utilization of calcium and phosphorus required for bone formation. Maintains stable nervous system and normal heart action.	Poor bone and tooth formation. Softening of bones and teeth. Inadequate absorption of calcium. Retention of phosphorus in kidney.	400 IU for adults.	25,000 IU may be toxic in some individuals over extended period of time. 400 IU is the maximum single dose that can be purchased without a prescription.
Vitamin E	Protects fat-soluble vitamins. Protects red blood cells. Is essential in cellular respiration. Inhibits coagulation of blood by preventing blood clots.	Rupture of red blood cells. Muscular wasting. Abnormal fat deposits in muscles.	15 IU men, 12 IU women.	Essentially nontoxic. 4.0-12.0 g (4,000-30,000 IU) of tocopherol for prolonged periods produces side effects in some persons.
Vitamin F	Is important for respiration of vital organs. Helps maintain resilience and lubrication of cells. Helps regulate blood coagulation. Is essential for normal glandular activity.	Brittle, lusterless hair. Brittle nails. Dandruff. Diarrhea. Varicose veins.	No RDA, 10% of total calories. Men need five times more than women.	Intake should not exceed what is needed to maintain desirable weight.

*Recommended Dietary Allowances.

Nutrients	Importance	Deficiency Symptoms	RDA*	Toxicity Level
Vitamin K	Is necessary for formation of prothrombin; is needed for blood coagulation.	Lack of prothrombin, increasing the tendency to hemorrhage.	No RDA; 300-500 mcg daily is considered adequate.	The menadione (synthetic vitamin K) may have side effects in newborn infants. Available in alfalfa tablet form.
Bioflavonoids	Help increase strength of capillaries.	Tendency to bleed and bruise easily.	No RDA.	No known toxicity.
MINERALS				
Calcium	Sustains development and maintenance of strong bones and teeth. Assists normal blood clotting, muscle action, nerve function, and heart function.	Tetany. Softening bones. Back and leg pains. Brittle bones.	800-1,400 mg, depending upon age.	Excessive intakes of calcium may have side effects in certain persons. No known oral toxicity.
Chlorine	Regulates acid-base balance. Maintains osmotic pressure. Stimulates production of hydrochloric acid. Helps maintain joints and tendons.	Loss of hair and teeth. Poor muscular contractibility. Impaired digestion.	No RDA.	Daily intake of 14-28 g of salt (sodium chloride) is considered excessive. Excess intake of chlorine may have adverse effects.
Chromium	Stimulates enzymes in metabolism of energy and synthesis of fatty acids, cholesterol, and protein. Increases effectiveness of insulin.	Depressed growth rate. Glucose intolerance in diabetics. Atherosclerosis.	No RDA; average daily intake is 80-100 mcg for adults.	No known toxicity.
Cobalt	Functions as part of vitamin B_{12}. Maintains red blood cells. Activates a number of enzymes in the body.	Pernicious anemia. Slow rate of growth.	No RDA; average daily intake is 5.0-8.0 mcg.	Excessive intakes of cobalt may have side effects in certain persons. Available by prescription only.
Copper	Aids in formation of red blood cells. Is part of many enzymes. Works with vitamin C to form elastin.	General weakness. Impaired respiration. Skin sores.	0.08 mg per kilogram of body weight. 2 mg for adults.	20 times RDA over prolonged period may cause toxicity.

*Recommended Dietary Allowances.

Nutrients	Importance	Deficiency Symptoms	RDA*	Toxicity Level
Fluorine	May reduce tooth decay by discouraging the growth of acid-forming bacteria.	Tooth decay.	No RDA.	Excessive intake of fluorine may have side effects in some persons.
Iodine	Is essential part of the hormone thyroxine. Is necessary for the prevention of goiter. Regulates production of energy and rate of metabolism. Promotes growth.	Enlarged thyroid gland. Dry skin and hair. Loss of physical and mental vigor. Cretinism in children born to iodine-deficient mothers.	100 mcg women, 130 mcg men.	Up to 1,000 mcg daily produced no toxic effects in persons with a normal thyroid.[†]
Iron	Is necessary for hemoglobin and myoglobin formation. Helps in protein metabolism. Promotes growth.	Weakness. Paleness of skin. Constipation. Anemia.	10 mg men, 18 mg women.	100 mg daily over prolonged period of time may be toxic in some individuals.
Magnesium	Acts as a catalyst in the utilization of carbohydrates, fats, protein, calcium, phosphorus, and possibly potassium.	Nervousness. Muscular excitability. Tremors.	350 mg men, 300 mg women.	30,000 mg daily may be toxic in certain individuals with kidney malfunctions.
Manganese	Is enzyme activator. Plays a part in carbohydrate and fat production. Is necessary for normal skeletal development. Maintains sex-hormone production.	Paralysis. Convulsions. Dizziness. Ataxia. Blindness and deafness in infants.	No RDA. Average diet supplies 3.0-9.0 mg.	Excessive intake may have side effects in certain persons. Single doses of up to 60 mg are available without prescription.
Molybdenum	Acts in oxidation of fats and aldehydes. Aids in mobilization of iron from liver reserves.	Premature aging.	No RDA. Minute amounts found in body.	5.0-10 ppm is considered toxic.
Phosphorus	Works with calcium to build bones and teeth. Utilizes carbohydrates, fats, and proteins.	Loss of weight and appetite. Irregular breathing. Pyorrhea.	800 mg for adults.	No known toxicity.

*Recommended Dietary Allowances.
[†]Goodhart and Shils, *Modern Nutrition in Health and Disease*, p. 365.

Nutrients	Importance	Deficiency Symptoms	RDA*	Toxicity Level
	Stimulates muscular contraction.			
Potassium	Works to control activity of heart muscles, nervous system, and kidneys.	Poor reflexes. Respiratory failure. Cardiac arrest.	No RDA. Average daily intake is 2,000-2,500 mg.	No known toxicity.
Selenium	Works with vitamin E. Preserves tissue elasticity.	Premature aging.	No RDA.	5.0-10 ppm is considered toxic.
Sodium	Maintains normal fluid levels in cells. Maintains health of the nervous, muscular, blood, and lymph systems.	Muscle weakness. Muscle shrinkage. Nausea. Loss of appetite. Intestinal gas.	3.0-7.0 g sodium. 6.0-18 g sodium chloride.	Excessive sodium intake may have adverse effects. Intake of 14-28 g of sodium chloride (salt) is considered excessive.
Sulfur	Is part of amino acids. Is essential for formation of body tissues. Is part of the B vitamins. Plays a part in tissue respiration. Is necessary for collagen synthesis.	—	The RDA of protein supplies sufficient amounts of sulfur.	Not available for over-the-counter sales.
Vanadium	Inhibits cholesterol formation.	—	No RDA.	No known toxicity.
Zinc	Is component of insulin and male reproductive fluid. Aids in digestion and metabolism of phosphorus. Aids in healing process.	Retarded growth. Delayed sexual maturity. Prolonged healing of wounds.	15 mg for adults.	Relatively nontoxic. 50 mg available without prescription.
Water	Part of blood, lymph, and body secretions. Aids in digestion. Regulates body temperature. Transports nutrients and body wastes.	Dehydration.	—	—

*Recommended Dietary Allowances.

NUTRIENTS THAT FUNCTION TOGETHER

When nutrients are taken in supplemental form, they function best when taken together in particular combinations. Some nutrients are so closely interrelated that their effectiveness in the body is markedly improved when they are taken together with other nutrients. Minerals are especially important in aiding the effectiveness of specific vitamins.

For example, if one is suffering from athlete's foot (see p. 114), vitamin A is recommended for treatment. Vitamin A can be utilized more effectively within the body when taken with the B-complex vitamins, choline, and vitamins C, D, E, and F. Calcium, phosphorus, and zinc are also recommended to increase the effectiveness of vitamin A.

The following chart provides a basic guide to nutrients that function best when taken together.

A. VITAMINS

1. VITAMIN A IS MORE EFFECTIVE WHEN TAKEN WITH

Vitamin B complex	Helps preserve stored vitamin A.
Choline	
Vitamin C	Helps protect against toxic effects of vitamin A.
	Helps prevent oxidation.
Vitamin D	1 part vitamin D to 10 parts vitamin A.
Vitamin E	Acts as an antioxidant.
Vitamin F	When vitamin E dosage is increased, increase supply of vitamin A.
Calcium	When vitamin A dosage is increased, increase supply of calcium and phosphorus.
Phosphorus	When vitamin A dosage is increased, increase supply of calcium and phosphorus.
Zinc	Helps in the absorption of vitamin A.

VITAMIN A EFFECTIVENESS IS DIMINISHED BY

Mineral oil

Lack of vitamin D in the body

2. VITAMIN B COMPLEX IS MORE EFFECTIVE WHEN TAKEN WITH

Vitamin C

Vitamin E

Calcium

Phosphorus

3. VITAMIN B_1 (THIAMINE) IS MORE EFFECTIVE WHEN TAKEN WITH

Vitamin B complex	
Vitamin B_2 (riboflavin)	
Folic acid	
Niacin	
Vitamin C	Helps protect against oxidation.
Vitamin E	
Manganese	
Sulfur	

4. VITAMIN B_2 (RIBOFLAVIN) IS MORE EFFECTIVE WHEN TAKEN WITH

Vitamin B complex	
Vitamin B_6	Vitamin B_2 and vitamin B_6 doses should always be the same.
Niacin	
Vitamin C	Helps protect against oxidation.

5. VITAMIN B_6 (PYRIDOXINE) IS MORE EFFECTIVE WHEN TAKEN WITH

Vitamin B complex	
Vitamin B_1 (thiamine)	Vitamin B_1 and vitamin B_6 doses should always be the same.
Vitamin B_2 (riboflavin)	Vitamin B_2 and vitamin B_6 doses should always be the same.
Pantothenic acid	
Vitamin C	
Magnesium	
Potassium	
Linoleic acid	
Sodium	

6. VITAMIN B_{12} (CYANOCOBALAMIN) IS MORE EFFECTIVE WHEN TAKEN WITH

Vitamin B complex

Vitamin B_6 (pyridoxine)   Helps increase absorption of vitamin B_{12}.

Choline

Folic acid

Inositol

Vitamin C   Helps increase absorption of vitamin B_{12}.

Potassium

Sodium

7. BIOTIN IS MORE EFFECTIVE WHEN TAKEN WITH

Vitamin B complex

Vitamin B_{12} (cyanocobalamin)

Folic acid

Pantothenic acid

Vitamin C

Sulfur

8. CHOLINE IS MORE EFFECTIVE WHEN TAKEN WITH

Vitamin A

Vitamin B complex

Vitamin B_{12} Helps synthesize choline.

Folic acid   Helps synthesize choline.

Inositol

Linoleic acid

9. FOLIC ACID IS MORE EFFECTIVE WHEN TAKEN WITH

Vitamin B complex

Vitamin B_{12}

Biotin

Pantothenic acid

Vitamin C   Helps protect against oxidation.

10. INOSITOL IS MORE EFFECTIVE WHEN TAKEN WITH

Vitamin B complex

Vitamin B_{12}

Choline

Linoleic acid

11. LAETRILE (B_{17}) IS MORE EFFECTIVE WHEN TAKEN WITH

Vitamin A

Vitamin B complex

Pangamic acid

Vitamin C

Vitamin E

12. NIACIN IS MORE EFFECTIVE WHEN TAKEN WITH

Vitamin B complex

Vitamin B_1 (thiamine)

Vitamin B_2 (riboflavin)

Vitamin C   Helps protect against oxidation.

13. PARA-AMINOBENZOIC ACID (PABA) IS MORE EFFECTIVE WHEN TAKEN WITH
    Vitamin B complex
    Folic acid
    Vitamin C

14. PANGAMIC ACID (VITAMIN B_{15}) IS MORE EFFECTIVE WHEN TAKEN WITH
    Vitamin B complex
    Vitamin C
    Vitamin E

15. PANTOTHENIC ACID IS MORE EFFECTIVE WHEN TAKEN WITH
    Vitamin B complex
    Vitamin B_6 (pyridoxine)
    Vitamin B_{12} (cyanocobalamin)
    Biotin   Aids in the absorption of pantothenic acid.
    Folic acid   Aids in the absorption of pantothenic acid.
    Vitamin C   Helps protect against oxidation.
    Sulfur

16. VITAMIN C IS MORE EFFECTIVE WHEN TAKEN WITH
    All vitamins and minerals
    Bioflavonoids
    Calcium   Helps body utilize vitamin C.
    Magnesium   Helps body utilize vitamin C.

17. VITAMIN D IS MORE EFFECTIVE WHEN TAKEN WITH
    Vitamin A   10 parts vitamin A to 1 part vitamin D.
    Choline   Helps to prevent toxicity.
    Vitamin C   Helps to prevent toxicity.
    Vitamin F
    Calcium
    Phosphorus

18. VITAMIN E IS MORE EFFECTIVE WHEN TAKEN WITH
    Vitamin A
    Vitamin B complex
    Vitamin B_1 (thiamine)
    Inositol   Helps body utilize vitamin E.
    Vitamin C   Helps protect against oxidation.
    Vitamin F
    Manganese   Helps body utilize vitamin E.
    Selenium

    VITAMIN E EFFECTIVENESS IS DIMINISHED BY
    Choline   Destructive towards vitamin E.
    Iron   Taking synthetic iron simultaneously with vitamin E.

19. VITAMIN F IS MORE EFFECTIVE WHEN TAKEN WITH
    Vitamin A
    Vitamin C
    Vitamin D

Vitamin E   Helps prevent oxidation and depletion.

Phosphorus

20. VITAMIN K IS MORE EFFECTIVE WHEN TAKEN WITH

No information is available at this time.

21. BIOFLAVONOIDS (VITAMIN P) ARE MORE EFFECTIVE WHEN TAKEN WITH

Vitamin C

B. MINERALS

1. CALCIUM IS MORE EFFECTIVE WHEN TAKEN WITH

Vitamin A	Aids in absorption.
Vitamin C	Aids in absorption.
Vitamin D	Helps in the reabsorption of calcium in kidney tubules and in the retention and utilization of calcium.
Vitamin F	Helps make calcium available to tissues.
Iron	Aids in absorption.
Magnesium	2 parts calcium to 1 part magnesium.
Manganese	
Phosphorus	2.5 parts calcium to 1 part phosphorus.
Hydrochloric acid	

CALCIUM EFFECTIVENESS IS DIMINISHED BY

Lack of hydrochloric acid

Lack of vitamin D

Lack of magnesium

2. CHLORINE IS MORE EFFECTIVE WHEN TAKEN WITH

No information is available at this time.

3. CHROMIUM IS MORE EFFECTIVE WHEN TAKEN WITH*

No information is available at this time.

4. COBALT IS MORE EFFECTIVE WHEN TAKEN WITH*

Copper

Iron

Zinc

5. COPPER IS MORE EFFECTIVE WHEN TAKEN WITH

Cobalt

Iron

Zinc

6. FLUORINE IS MORE EFFECTIVE WHEN TAKEN WITH*

No information is available at this time.

7. IODINE IS MORE EFFECTIVE WHEN TAKEN WITH*

No information is available at this time.

8. IRON IS MORE EFFECTIVE WHEN TAKEN WITH*

Vitamin B_{12} Helps iron function in the body.

Folic acid

*Denotes essential trace mineral.

Vitamin C   Aids in absorption
Calcium
Cobalt
Copper
Phosphorus
Hydrochloric acid   Needed for assimilation of iron.

9. MAGNESIUM IS MORE EFFECTIVE WHEN TAKEN WITH
Vitamin B_6
Vitamin C
Vitamin D
Calcium   1 part magnesium to 2 parts calcium.
Phosphorus
Protein

10. MANGANESE IS MORE EFFECTIVE WHEN TAKEN WITH*
Vitamin B_1 (thiamine)
Vitamin E
Calcium
Phosphorus

11. MOLYBDENUM IS MORE EFFECTIVE WHEN TAKEN WITH†
No information is available at this time.

12. PHOSPHORUS IS MORE EFFECTIVE WHEN TAKEN WITH
Vitamin A
Vitamin D
Vitamin F
Calcium   1 part phosphorus to 2.5 parts calcium.
Iron
Manganese
Protein

13. POTASSIUM IS MORE EFFECTIVE WHEN TAKEN WITH
Vitamin B_6
Sodium

14. SELENIUM IS MORE EFFECTIVE WHEN TAKEN WITH†
Vitamin E

15. SODIUM IS MORE EFFECTIVE WHEN TAKEN WITH
Vitamin D

SODIUM EFFECTIVENESS IS DIMINISHED BY
Lack of chlorine
Lack of potassium

16. SULFUR IS MORE EFFECTIVE WHEN TAKEN WITH
Vitamin B complex

*Denotes essential trace mineral.
†Denotes trace element whose biological importance to man is unknown.

Vitamin B$_1$ (thiamine)

Biotin

Pantothenic acid

SULFUR EFFECTIVENESS IS DIMINISHED BY

Insufficient protein

17. VANADIUM IS MORE EFFECTIVE WHEN TAKEN WITH[†]

No information is available at this time.

18. ZINC IS MORE EFFECTIVE WHEN TAKEN WITH[*]

Vitamin A

Calcium

Copper

Phosphorus

ZINC EFFECTIVENESS IS DIMINISHED BY

Lack of phosphorus

[*]Denotes essential trace element.
[†]Denotes trace element whose biological importance to man is unknown.

AVAILABLE FORMS OF NUTRIENT SUPPLEMENTS

NATURAL AND SYNTHETIC

Because of individual differences such as sex, age, environment, stress, and state of health, many people do not receive the full benefit of the nutrients provided in their daily diet. For this reason vitamin and mineral supplements are used.

Vitamin supplements come in two forms, natural and synthetic. A natural vitamin exists in its original state in nature. It is not artificial, and its source is either a plant or an animal. A synthetic vitamin, in most instances, has the same chemical structure as the natural vitamin, but it is produced artificially by synthesis of simpler materials. There may be factors such as enzymes, synergists, catalysts, minerals, proteins, or even unidentified vitamins which are found in the natural nutrient but not in its synthetic counterpart. Compounds found in the natural vitamins contain nutrients in their natural ratios and do not contain potentially harmful ingredients such as artificial coloring or flavorings, as may be found in the synthetic product.

Labels do not always tell the full story. A natural vitamin should be a whole food product with nothing removed. Many so-called natural vitamins are not completely natural but rather are a combination of both natural and synthetic nutrients called "co-natural" vitamins. Synthetic nutrients are added to increase the potency or stability and to standardize the amount of nutrients per capsule or per batch.

Synthetic vitamins and minerals often contain a salt form that is used to increase stability of the nutrient. These salt forms are palmatate, sulfate, nitrate, hydrochloride, chloride, succinate, bitartrate, acetate, and gluconate. This information may aid in the determination of whether a nutrient is natural or synthetic. A label may read, "Vitamin A Palmitate," thus indicating that it is synthetic rather than natural.

ORGANIC AND INORGANIC

If a vitamin supplement is labeled "organic," it is composed of, or contains, matter of plant or animal origin. "Inorganic" means that the vitamin supplement is composed of something other than organic materials such as those found in water and soil. Foods and supplements derived from organic sources are probably better assimilated by the body than are inorganic supplements.

FORMS OF SUPPLEMENTAL NUTRIENTS

Nearly all the nutrient supplements are available in many forms: tablet, capsule, liquid, powder, drops, or ointment. This variety allows people to choose a supplement form that best suits their needs.

The *tablet* is a compressed block of material available in a variety of potencies, especially higher ones. If kept in a closed bottle, it can be stored indefinitely. However, once opened, all nutrients in this form should be stored in a cool, dark place because exposure to air will reduce potency.

The *capsule* is a small container made of gelatin or other soluble materials. The ingredients inside the container can either be powder or liquid. The advantage of the powder-filled capsule is that it can be opened and sprinkled on food or in beverages, a useful factor for those people who have difficulty swallowing. The liquid-filled capsule, as in vitamin E, has distinct advantages too. For example, a person suffering from a cold sore may pick up a capsule, insert a pin, gently squeeze, and apply the oil directly to the sore. The capsule will then seal itself, become airtight, and be ready for use again. The capsule is available in the same potencies as the tablet, and its storage properties are also the same.

Nutrients in liquid form are easily taken and are especially good for children or elderly persons who find swallowing a tablet or a capsule difficult. Vitamin C is available in liquid and may be the preferred form if one is suffering from a cold and finds swallowing a pill painful. The liquid is usually found in lower potencies and should be stored in the refrigerator. Once opened, a bottle of liquid nutrients rapidly loses potency.

Nutrients in powdered form can be sprinkled on foods and in beverages and are also easy for children or the elderly to consume. They are an excellent way to provide the essential amino acids. Vegetarians may find this form useful. Powder should be kept in a dark place away from high humidity.

In some cases it may be desirable to obtain the nutrients in drops or ointments. For example, vitamin E ointment is recommended for treatment of burns to promote healing and reduce scarring.

To avoid confusion and insure the best possible benefits from nutrient supplements, it is important to schedule their consumption. Schedules will vary with specific needs, ailments, eating habits, environment, etc. Vitamins and minerals should be taken with meals, and it is advantageous to take the most vitamins with the largest meal for best absorption. It is wise to take the fat-soluble vitamins with fat-containing foods to ensure adequate amounts of bile for absorption. The water-soluble vitamins need to be taken throughout the day because they are lost through excretion. It is also necessary to be aware of which nutrients function together and which are antagonists. For example, vitamin E and iron should be taken 8 to 12 hours apart. For further information, see individual nutrients and "Nutrients That Function Together," pp. 93-99.

The following table gives the various supplemental forms in which a nutrient may be found, together with its source. Supplemental forms are subject to change and may vary in different localities.

Nutrient	Form	Source	Explanation
VITAMINS			
Vitamin A	Fish-liver oils	Natural	Excellent natural sources; good source of oil in diet.
	Carrot (oil)	Natural	Cannot be tolerated by persons suffering from gall-bladder problems and other digestive problems. Not absorbed by the body as easily as fish-liver oils.
	Lemon grass	Natural	An herbal grass that is a good source of oil.
	Vitamin A palmatate	Synthetic	Recommended for pregnant women and persons with fish-liver-oil absorption problems.
	Vitamin A acetate	Synthetic	Recommended for pregnant women and persons with fish-liver-oil absorption problems.
Vitamin B complex	Brewer's yeast	Natural	Low-potency form; all B factors, protein, enzymes, and possibly some unidentified nutrients included.
	Nutritional yeast	Natural	Usually higher potency and better flavor than brewer's yeast.
Vitamin B_1 (thiamine)	Yeast or rice bran	Natural	Natural ingredient in capsule or tablet form.
	Thiamine hydrochloride	Synthetic	High-potency.
	Thiamine chloride	Synthetic	High-potency.
	Thiamine mononitrate	Synthetic	High-potency.
Vitamin B_2 (riboflavin)	Yeast or bran	Natural	Natural ingredient in capsule or tablet form.
	Riboflavin	Synthetic	High-potency.
Vitamin B_6 (pyridoxine)	Yeast or bran	Natural	Natural ingredient in capsule or tablet form.
	Pyridoxine hydrochloride	Synthetic	High potency.
Vitamin B_{12} (cobalamin)	Yeast or rice bran	Natural	Natural ingredient in capsule or tablet form.
	Fermentation concentrate	Natural	More easily absorbed than other forms of B_{12}.
	Cobalamin	Natural	High-potency natural fermentation product.
	Cyanocobalamin	Natural	Natural fermentation product.
Vitamin B_{13} (orotic acid)	Orotic acid	Natural	May not be available yet in health stores in U.S.
Biotin	Yeast	Natural	
	D-biotin	Synthetic	High-potency.
Choline	Soybeans	Natural	Other factors may be present which may not be in synthetic form; found in powder, tablet, and capsule forms.
	Yeast	Natural	Other factors may be present which may not be in synthetic form; found in powder, tablet, and capsule forms.
	Choline bitartrate	Synthetic	Obtained in high-potency dosage.
Folic acid	Yeast	Natural	Other factors may be present which may not be in synthetic form.
	Pleroylglutamic	Synthetic	High-potency.
Inositol	Soybeans	Natural	Other factors may be present which may not be in synthetic form; found in powder, tablet, and capsule forms.
	Corn or yeast	Natural	Other factors may be present which may not be in synthetic form; found in powder, tablet, and capsule forms.

Nutrient	Form	Source	Explanation
Laetrile (vitamin B_{17})	Apricot kernels	Natural	More inexpensive and more readily available than amygdalin.
	Amygdalin	Natural	More expensive than apricot kernels.
Niacin	Yeast or bran	Natural	Other factors may be present which may not be in synthetic form.
	Niacinamide	Synthetic	Will not cause flushing or tingling sensation (see "Niacin") when dosage is over 100 mg.
	Nicotinic acid	Synthetic	
	Niacin	Synthetic	Will cause flushing or tingling sensation (100 mg or more); more effective than niacinamide for migraine headaches.
Pantothenic acid	Yeast	—	Other factors may be present which may not be in synthetic forms.
	Calcium D-pantothenate	Synthetic	High-potency.
Para-aminobenzoic acid (PABA)	Yeast	—	Other factors may be present which may not be in synthetic forms.
	Para-aminobenzoic acid	Synthetic	High-potency.
Pangamic acid (vitamin B_{15})	Apricot kernels	Natural	More inexpensive and more readily absorbed than other forms.
	Pangamic acid	Synthetic	Russian formula for B_{15} has recently become available in the U.S.; high-potency.
	Calcium pangamate	—	High-potency.
Vitamin C	Rose hips	Natural	Available in all forms, capsule, tablet, etc.
	Acerola cherries	Natural	Available in all forms, capsule, tablet, etc.
	Citrus fruits	Natural	Available in all forms, capsule, tablet, etc.
	Green peppers	Natural	
	Ascorbic acid	Synthetic	Most economical source but without bioflavonoids; added to vitamin C to increase potency and stability.
Vitamin D	Cod-liver oil	Natural	An excellent natural source; cannot be tolerated by persons suffering from gallbladder or other digestive problems.
	Irradiated ergosterol	Synthetic	High-potency.
	Calciferol	Synthetic	High-potency.
Vitamin E	Vegetable oils	Natural	Good way to get essential oils.
	Wheat germ	Natural	Low-potency.
	Mixed tocopheryl	Natural	D-alpha and other tocopheryls that help alpha function better.
	d-alpha tocopheryl	Natural	Most active form of tocopheryl which helps alpha function better.
	d-alpha tocopheryl acetate	Co-natural	A natural derivative with synthetic products added.
	dl-alpha tocopheryl	Synthetic	Considered by some a more stable form.
	dl-alpha tocopheryl acetate	Synthetic	Considered by some a more stable form; Shute clinics recommend this form.
	dl-alpha tocopheryl succinate	Synthetic	Considered by some a more stable form.

Nutrient	Form	Source	Explanation
Vitamin F	Unsaturated fatty acids	Natural	Good way to provide oil for diet.
	Essential fatty acids	Natural	Good way to provide oil for diet.
Vitamin K	Alfalfa	Natural	Contains chlorophyll enzymes, and other factors; high mineral source.
	Menodoine	Synthetic	
Bioflavonoids	Rutin	Natural	Are factors that make vitamin C more effective.
	Hesperiden	Natural	Are factors that make vitamin C more effective.
	Flavons	Natural	Are factors that make vitamin C more effective.
	Bioflavonoids in combination with vitamin C	Natural	Are factors that make vitamin C more effective.
MINERALS			
Calcium	Calcium lactate	Natural	A salt of lactic acid from milk; easily absorbed; low-potency.
	Calcium gluconate	Natural	A salt of gluconic acid from glucose; easily absorbed; one needs to take more to get equivalent potencies.
	Calcium pantothenate	Natural	A salt of pantothenic acid (from B complex).
	Bone meal	Natural	Dried bones of cattle; type of calcium closest to calcium found in human bones and teeth; poorly absorbed; has high potency with other trace minerals.
	Dolomite	Natural	Calcium and magnesium also available with vitamin A and D; not to be used by the elderly or persons with poor hydrochloric acid secretions.
	Di-cal phosphate	Co-natural	Bone meal or bone ash with additional 22% phosphorus.
	Eggshell calcium	Natural	Dried eggshell.
	Oyster-shell calcium	Natural	Natural calcium form with minimal phosphorus interference but with natural trace minerals.
	Liquid calcium	Natural	Good for person who has calcium-absorption problems.
Chloride	—	—	Not available singly but in some complete-multimineral supplements.
Cobalt	—	—	Not available singly but in some complete-multimineral supplements.
Copper	Copper sulfate	Synthetic	Available in other salt forms.
Chromium	—	—	Not available singly but in some complete-multimineral supplements.
Fluorine	—	—	Not available singly but in some complete-multimineral supplements.
Iodine	Sea kelp	Natural	Includes trace minerals and other substances.
	Sea salt	Natural	Includes trace minerals and other substances.
	Seaweed	Natural	Includes trace minerals and other substances.
	Potassium oxide	Synthetic	Table salt.

Nutrient	Form	Source	Explanation
Iron	Desiccated liver	Natural	Dried liver of cattle; low-potency; good for women.
	Yeast	Natural	Low-potency; good for women.
	Molasses	Natural	Low-potency; good for women.
	Ferrous fumerate	Synthetic	High-potency.
	Ferrous gluconate	Synthetic	High-potency; more readily absorbed than ferrous fumerate.
	Ferrous sulfate	Synthetic	High-potency.
Magnesium	Dolomite	Natural	Calcium and magnesium in natural balance (2:1); not recommended for persons with poor hydrochloric acid secretions.
	Magnesium palmatate	Synthetic	Available in other salt forms; high-potency.
	Magnesium sulfate	Synthetic	Epsom salts; calcium-free.
Manganese	Manganese gluconate	Synthetic	Easily absorbed.
Molybdenum	—	—	
Phosphorus	Bone meal	Natural	Contains additional calcium and other nutrients.
	Calcium phosphate	Synthetic	High-potency.
Potassium	Potassium gluconate	Synthetic	Easily absorbed.
	Potassium chloride	Synthetic	
Selenium	—	—	
Sodium	Sodium chloride	Synthetic	Table salt.
Sulfur	—	—	Available in ointment form and in some complete-multimineral supplements.
Zinc	Zinc gluconate	Synthetic	More readily absorbed than zinc sulfate.
	Zinc sulfate	Synthetic	
Protein	Meat or fish	Natural	Available in powder and tablet forms.
	Eggs or milk	Natural	Available in powder and tablet forms.
	Soybeans	Natural	Good source for vegetarians.
	Amino acid compounds	Natural	Available in tablet, liquid, and powder form.

APPROXIMATE NUTRIENT COMPOSITION OF THE BODY

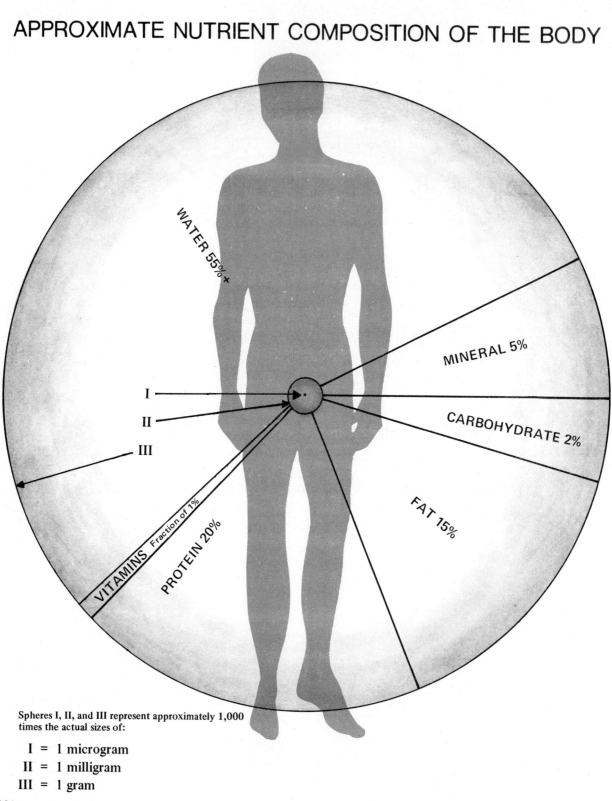

WATER 55%+

MINERAL 5%

CARBOHYDRATE 2%

FAT 15%

VITAMINS Fraction of 1%

PROTEIN 20%

I

II

III

Spheres I, II, and III represent approximately 1,000 times the actual sizes of:

I = 1 microgram
II = 1 milligram
III = 1 gram

Ailments and Other Stressful Conditions

Good health is a product of heredity, environment, and nutrition. Nutritional deficiency, resulting in malnutrition or disease, is one of the major problems in modern society despite adequate food supply, primarily because of ignorance of good nutrition. A well-balanced diet, rich in all essential nutrients, is necessary to maintain a healthy body and mind.

Authorities have found that a number of diseases can appear when there is a deficiency of one or more nutrients. Most diseases caused by such deficiencies can be corrected when all essential nutrients are supplied. However, in some instances of severe deficiency, irreparable damage may be done.

The following pages list common ailments and stressful conditions that many authorities believe are related to nutrition. Common ailments are listed alphabetically by ailment together with explanations, including pertinent nutritional information regarding the nature of most of the ailments. These explanations are designed to give an understanding of the specific ailments.

The body member affected by each ailment is also identified. Nutrient listings for each ailment are given. These include those nutrients found by nutrition researchers to be beneficial in the treatment of the given ailment.

Nutrient quantities are given for some nutrients. They represent amounts of these nutrients which have been found by some researchers to be effective in the treatment of the ailment. All amounts are daily unless otherwise stated. When no quantity is listed, available research did not indicate an amount.

Note: These and the following quantity-of-nutrient listings do not constitute prescriptive amounts. They only represent research findings.

Many of the seemingly high doses result from clinical tests on ailing persons. These amounts would not necessarily be required, or even recommended, for a healthy person. Most dosages used in research are greater than those cited as daily allowances. We repeat:

These amounts are not prescriptive.

Individual tolerances to the nutrients may differ significantly. Each individual must determine, according to his own tolerances, the quantity of each nutrient that will be beneficial in the treatment of disease.

Factors influencing individual tolerances include a person's normal eating habits, previous amounts of vitamins ingested, height, weight, metabolic rate, reaction to stress, and environmental variances. Build up the dosages slowly: it took a long time for your body to become ill, so take your time in trying to heal it. If you wish to take large amounts of a nutrient, it would be wise to consult a physician.

AILMENTS

ABSCESS

An abscess is a localized infection with a collection of pus in any part of the body. An abscess may be located externally or internally and may be initiated by lowered resistance to infection, bacterial contamination, or injury. Symptoms of abscess include tenderness and swelling in the infected area, fever, and chills.

Antibiotics may be used to treat the infection, although in the case of a severe abscess, surgery may be necessary. Because the antibiotics used in treatment may interfere with the absorption of the B vitamins, supplementary B complex may be required. Fever increases the body's need for calories; vitamins A, C, and E; and extra fluids.

NUTRIENTS THAT MAY BE BENEFICIAL IN TREATMENT OF ABSCESS

Body Member	Nutrients	Quantity*
Body/Skin	Vitamin A	100,000 IU for three days
	Vitamin B complex	
	Vitamin C	
	Vitamin E	
	Water	

*See note, p. 166.

ACNE

Acne is a common disorder of the oil glands in the skin characterized by the recurring formation of blackheads, whiteheads, and pimples. Acne occurs primarily on the face and sometimes on the back, shoulders, chest, and arms. The incidence of acne is greatest during puberty and adolescence, when hormones influencing the secretion of the oil glands are at their peak level of activity.

Proper nutrition and skin cleanliness, together with adequate rest, exercise, fresh air, and sunlight, are helpful in the treatment of acne. Many authorities believe overindulgence in carbohydrates and foods with high fat content should be avoided. Candy, sweetened soft drinks, fried foods, and nuts should be avoided. An excess of oxalic acid found in chocolate, cocoa, spinach, and rhubarb may inhibit the body's absorption of calcium. Calcium helps maintain the acid-alkali balance of the blood necessary for a clear complexion.

Vitamin A is especially beneficial for clear, healthy skin. The B-complex vitamins, especially riboflavin, pyridoxine, and pantothenic acid, help reduce facial oiliness and blackhead formation. Vitamin C aids in resisting the spread of acne infection, and vitamin D guards the body's store of calcium from excretion. Vitamin E has been found helpful in the prevention of scarring.[1]

NUTRIENTS THAT MAY BE BENEFICIAL IN TREATMENT OF ACNE

Body Member	Nutrients	Quantity*
Skin	Vitamin A	50,000-100,000 IU daily for one month
	Vitamin B complex	
	Vitamin B_2	5-15 mg
	Vitamin B_6	
	Niacin	100 mg three times daily
	Pantothenic acid	300 mg
	Vitamin C	1,000 mg
	Vitamin D	200-400 mg
	Vitamin E	
	Vitamin F	
	Calcium	
	Potassium	

*See note, p. 166.

ADRENAL EXHAUSTION

Adrenal exhaustion is the progressive lessening of activity of the adrenal glands, which may eventually lead to complete functional failure. It is characterized by a low energy level in the morning which gradually rises, being highest late at night. The person retires but cannot fall asleep right away, then sleeps soundly but arises exhausted. Adrenal exhaustion is often categorized with insomnia.

The vitamins B_2, B_{12}, folic acid, and pantothenic acid with potassium and sodium stabilize the activity of the adrenal glands.

NUTRIENTS THAT MAY BE BENEFICIAL IN TREATMENT OF ADRENAL EXHAUSTION

Body Member	Nutrients	Quantity
Glands	Vitamin B complex	
	Vitamin B_2	

[1] Adelle Davis, *Let's Get Well* (New York: Harcourt, Brace & World, 1965), p. 161.

Body Member	Nutrients	Quantity
	Vitamin B$_{12}$	
	Folic acid	
	Pantothenic acid	
	Vitamin C	
	Potassium	
	Sodium	

ALCOHOLISM

Alcoholism is a dependence on or addiction to alcohol. The body's outward reaction to alcohol suggests that it acts as a stimulant by producing aggressive social behavior such as loss of inhibitions, increased boldness, and sociability associated with drinking. In fact, alcohol is a depressant that acts to decrease the basic speed of all bodily functions, including muscle contractions, speed of reaction, digestion, and thinking processes.

Prolonged dependence upon this drug may result in severe problems in the pancreas and gastrointestinal tract as well as the emotional and mental problems associated with alcoholism. Severe deficiencies of many nutrients occur because the alcohol itself satisfies the body's caloric needs. (Alcohol contains about 70 calories per ounce.)

As the alcohol enters the bloodstream directly through the walls of the stomach, it begins to act upon the central nervous system by changing the most basic mental functions and by destroying brain cells. Cells are destroyed by the withdrawal of necessary water from the tissues and cells. The liver works to neutralize the effects of alcohol upon the body by breaking down the composition of the alcohol. Under normal circumstances, especially if there is food in the stomach, the liver can effectively perform the function of breaking down the alcohol if not more than one drink per hour is consumed. However, when the liver is overworked, it must compensate by creating an increased tolerance for alcohol. After a time the liver compensates less rapidly, becomes fatty, and is less able to decompose the alcohol. As a result, the alcoholic develops a decreased tolerance for alcohol and less is needed to produce intoxication. As drinking continues over a period of time, the liver cells die and are replaced with scar tissue. This condition is known as cirrhosis of the liver.

Diet and nutrient supplements are very important in the treatment of alcoholism. In some cases, a strict diet adequate in calories and high in protein, which contains all the vitamins and minerals and is especially high in B vitamins, reduced the alcoholic's desire to drink. Protein is necessary for tissue regeneration, particularly when cirrhosis of the liver occurs. Vitamin A is an anti-infective agent for upper respiratory infections such as tuberculosis and pneumonia which are common in alcoholics. The vitamin B complex is essential for the prevention and treatment of alcoholic neuritis, pellagra, and delirium tremens. Vitamin C, which is often deficient in alcoholics, is needed to prevent scurvy. A zinc deficiency may occur, making the alcoholic more prone to cirrhosis of the liver and preventing vitamin K from being absorbed into the body. Iron is needed to correct the anemia that often develops. A magnesium deficiency can contribute to the occurrence of delirium tremens. A deficiency of potassium may also occur in alcoholics, and supplements may be necessary. Choline aids in the decomposition of fat in the liver and helps maintain healthy kidneys jeopardized by heavy drinking.

NUTRIENTS THAT MAY BE BENEFICIAL IN TREATMENT OF ALCOHOLISM

Body Member	Nutrients	Quantity*
Brain/Nervous system	Vitamin A	25,000 IU
	Vitamin B complex	
	Vitamin B$_1$	
	Vitamin B$_2$	
	Vitamin B$_6$	100 mg
	Vitamin B$_{12}$	
	Choline	
	Folic acid	
	Niacin	100 mg in the form of niacinamide
	Pangamic acid	
	Pantothenic acid	
	Vitamin C	Up to 3,000 mg
	Vitamin D	1,000 IU
	Vitamin E	Up to 1,200 IU
	Vitamin K	
	Iron	
	Magnesium	Up to 1,000 mg
	Zinc	

*See note, p. 166.

ALLERGIES

An allergy is a sensitivity to some particular substance known as an allergen. The allergen may be harmless to some people but can cause a reaction in others. Almost any food may be an allergen to some people. The allergic reaction may be hay fever, asthma, hives, high blood pressure, abnormal fatigue, constipation, stomach ulcers, dizziness, headache, or mental depression.

NUTRIENTS THAT MAY BE BENEFICIAL IN TREATMENT OF ALLERGIES

Body Member	Nutrients	Quantity*
General	Vitamin A	10,000-25,000 IU
	Vitamin B complex	
	Vitamin B_{12}	
	Pantothenic acid	100-200 mg
	Vitamin C	250 mg four times daily; up to 5,000 mg
	Vitamin D	
	Vitamin E	Up to 800 IU
	Vitamin F	
	Calcium	Up to 1,000 mg
	Manganese	5 mg twice weekly for 10 weeks
	Potassium	

*See note, p. 166.

AMBLYOPIA

Amblyopia is an impairment of the ability of the eyes to focus. Vitamin B_1 is used to correct it.

NUTRIENTS THAT MAY BE BENEFICIAL IN TREATMENT OF AMBLYOPIA

Body Member	Nutrient	Quantity*
Eyes	Vitamin A	
	Vitamin B complex	
	Vitamin B_1	20 mg
	Vitamin C	
	Vitamin E	

*See note, p. 166.

ANEMIA

A reduction of the amount of hemoglobin in the bloodstream and/or a reduction in the number of red blood cells themselves reduces the amount of oxygen available to all body cells. Carbon dioxide accumulates in the cells, causing decreased efficiency and lower rate of body processes. When the brain cells are deprived of oxygen, dizziness may result. Additional symptoms of anemia are general weakness, fatigue, paleness, brittle nails, loss of appetite, and abdominal pain.

Anemia often arises from recurrent infections and/or diseases involving the entire body. It may also be caused by inadequate intake or impaired absorption of nutrients or by excessive losses of blood through such conditions as heavy menstruation or peptic ulcer. It has been shown that excess amounts of vitamin K in the diet during pregnancy may cause anemia in newborn infants.[2]

Iron, protein, copper, folic acid, and vitamins B_6, B_{12}, and C are all necessary for the formation of red blood cells. A deficiency in any of these nutrients can cause anemia, although iron-deficiency anemia is the most common form of the condition. Infants, adolescents, and women, particularly during pregnancy, are often deficient in iron and may require iron supplements. Vitamin C aids in the absorption and retention of iron. Vitamin E may be needed to help maintain the health of red blood cells.

NUTRIENTS THAT MAY BE BENEFICIAL IN TREATMENT OF ANEMIA

Body Member	Nutrients	Quantity*
Blood/Circulatory system	Vitamin B complex	
	Vitamin B_1	50-100 mg
	Vitamin B_6	
	Vitamin B_{12}	20-50 mcg
	Folic acid	0.5-5 mg
	PABA	Up to 50 mg
	Pantothenic acid	Up to 100 mg
	Vitamin C	500 mg
	Vitamin E	Up to 1,000 IU

*See note, p. 166.

[2]Phyllis Sullivan Howe, *Basic Nutrition in Health and Diseases* (Philadelphia: W. B. Saunders Co., 1971), p. 96.

Body Member	Nutrients	Quantity
	Calcium	
	Iron	10 mg
	Copper	
	Protein	

ANGINA PECTORIS

Angina pectoris is a condition characterized by severe pain in the heart area. It is due to insufficient supply of blood to the heart tissue which results in a lack of oxygen in these tissues. The most frequent cause of this insufficient blood supply is atherosclerosis of the arteries that supply the heart with blood. This condition is most commonly found in males over age forty-five.

Attacks are brought on by a heavy meal, unaccustomed physical exertion, stress, emotional tension, or exposure to cold. The frequency and duration of attacks vary and may range from several attacks per day to one attack every few years.

The pain varies greatly in severity from a mild pressure to an intolerable agony. It usually starts in the upper chest or throat and radiates to the left shoulder and down the left arm. The patient is pale, sweaty, and very apprehensive. These symptoms are similar to those of a heart attack but can be differentiated in that the pain lasts only for minutes and can be relieved by rest. However, if the blood supply is insufficient enough, angina pectoris can progress to a heart attack.

In the treatment of angina pectoris, effort should be made to obtain rest and to decrease the workload of the heart. Because the workload of the heart increases after meals, the diet should consist of small, frequent feedings that are salt-free and low in saturated fat and calories. Cold fluids should be avoided because they may trigger irregularities in the heart function. Protein intake should be adequate to replace protein lost from the damaged heart cells.

Preventive measures for angina pectoris include avoidance of smoking, alcohol, exposure to cold, and overweight. The B-complex vitamins and vitamin C may be helpful in maintaining the integrity and health of the heart and circulatory system in the atherosclerosis victim. Some authorities state that vitamin E and iodine may prove helpful because they open the arteries, enabling more blood to flow through the circulatory system.[3]

NUTRIENTS THAT MAY BE BENEFICIAL IN TREATMENT OF ANGINA PECTORIS

Body Member	Nutrients	Quantity*
Blood/Circulatory system	Vitamin A	25,000 IU
	Vitamin B complex	
	Vitamin B$_{12}$	25 mcg
	Choline	
	Pangamic acid	
	Vitamin C	3,000 mg
	Vitamin E	200 IU daily; gradually work up to 1,600 IU daily
	Iodine	
	Potassium	
	Protein	

*See note, p. 166.

ARTERIOSCLEROSIS AND ATHEROSCLEROSIS

A thickening and hardening of the walls of the arteries is known as arteriosclerosis. Arteriosclerosis occurs in two forms. The first type of hardening is caused by a gradual deposit of calcium in the artery walls, restricting the flow of blood to the body cells. A second, more advanced type of hardening, called atherosclerosis, is due to the buildup of cholesterol or fatty deposits in the artery walls and contributes to the degeneration of the arteries involved. Atherosclerosis usually affects the aorta, heart, and brain arteries as well as the other blood vessels of the body and extremities. It usually occurs in older people and is still considered the number one cause of death in the United States.

There are several theories as to the cause of atherosclerosis. It is often thought to be a metabolic defect involving fats. Fat molecules are normally absorbed through the artery walls. When an excess of fatty material starts to restrict blood flow, fatty streaks begin to appear on the interior of the arteries. As more and more

[3]Wilfrid E. Shute and Harold J. Taub, *Vitamin E for Ailing and Healthy Hearts* (New York: Pyramid House, 1969), p. 44.

of this fat is introduced, the artery walls thicken and plaques of cholesterol narrow the arteries. The artery walls then lose their elasticity and become hard and brittle. Hemorrhages from small vessels located in the arterial wall beneath the plaques may cause the cholesterol deposits to break free from the wall, or a clot may form as blood passes over the rough edge of a plaque. The plaques, clots, or a combination of these may cause a total block in the vessel, resulting in death.

Symptoms of atherosclerosis are hypertension, cramping or paralysis of muscles, a sensation of heaviness or pressure in the chest, and pains that radiate from the chest to the left arm and shoulder. Factors that enhance the tendency to develop atherosclerosis are obesity, lack of exercise, hypertension, smoking, heredity, stress, and poor diet. Males over forty years of age are highly susceptible, but women do not usually suffer from it until after menopause. Some researchers believe that a high intake of carbohydrates is a factor that predisposes toward atherosclerosis.[4]

Prevention and treatment measures for the disease include reducing the percentage of fat in the diet to no more than 30 to 35 percent with the ratio of unsaturates to saturates being 2 to 1 and limiting the cholesterol intake to 300 milligrams daily. If obesity is present, weight should be reduced to a normal level. Physical exercise is necessary for stimulating circulation and strengthening the heart muscles. Reducing salt intake is important if hypertension is present.

The B complex helps in the prevention of atherosclerosis by reducing blood cholesterol levels. Vitamin C is necessary to help maintain health of the arteries and prevent hemorrhaging. Some researchers indicate that vitamin E may help prevent clot formation.[5]

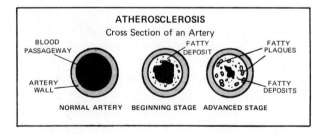

ATHEROSCLEROSIS
Cross Section of an Artery

BLOOD PASSAGEWAY   FATTY DEPOSIT   FATTY PLAQUES

ARTERY WALL   FATTY DEPOSITS

NORMAL ARTERY   BEGINNING STAGE   ADVANCED STAGE

[4] J. I. Rodale, *The Encyclopedia for Healthful Living* (Emmaus, Pa.: Rodale Books, 1970), p. 733.
[5] Linda Clark, *Get Well Naturally* (New York: Dev.n-Adair, 1963), p. 325.

NUTRIENTS THAT MAY BE BENEFICIAL IN TREATMENT OF ARTERIOSCLEROSIS AND ATHEROSCLEROSIS

Body Member	Nutrients	Quantity*
Blood/Heart	Vitamin A	20,000-100,000 IU
	Vitamin B complex	
	Vitamin B$_6$	50 mg
	Vitamin B$_{12}$	
	Choline	500 mg
	Folic acid	
	Inositol	500 mg
	Niacin	100-500 mg under doctor's supervision
	Vitamin C	Up to 3,000 mg
	Vitamin E	600-1,200 IU
	Bioflavonoids	300-600 mg
	Calcium	500 mg
	Chromium	

*See note, p. 166.

ARTHRITIS

Arthritis results in inflammation and soreness of the joints. Osteoarthritis and rheumatoid arthritis are the two main types of the disease.

Osteoarthritis, usually found in elderly people, develops as a result of the continuous wearing away of the cartilage in a joint. Cartilage, which is a smooth, soft, pearly tissue, covers the ends of the bones at the joints. It provides a smooth surface for the bones to slide against, allowing easy movement of the joints. As a result of injury or years of use, cartilage becomes thin and may disappear. When enough cartilage has worn away, the rough surfaces of the bones rub together, causing pain and stiffness. Osteoarthritis usually affects the weight-bearing joints, such as the hips and knees. Symptoms of osteoarthritis include body stiffness and pain in the joints, especially during damp weather, in the morning, or after strenuous activity.

Rheumatoid arthritis affects the entire body instead of just one joint. Onset of the disease is often associated with physical or emotional stress and usually occurs between the ages of thirty and forty. Rheumatoid arthritis destroys the cartilage and tissues in and around the joints and often the bone surfaces themselves. The body replaces the damaged tissue with scar tissue, causing the spaces between the joints to become narrow and fuse together. This causes the stiffening and crippling onset of the disease. Symptoms of rheumatoid arthritis include swelling and pain in the joints, fatigue, anemia, weight loss, and fever. These symptoms often disappear and recur at a later date.

Exercise is important in both the prevention and treatment of arthritis because unused joints tend to stiffen. Good posture is also important to prevent stiffness and crippling. Poor posture can cause body weight to be distributed unevenly, placing more stress on certain joints, thus resulting in unnecessary pain for the arthritic person.

Many nutritional cures for arthritis have been claimed, upon which research still continues. It is recommended that the arthritic have a well-balanced diet in order to provide his body with all the nutrients it needs for repair. If the arthritic is overweight he or she should lose weight in order to reduce the stress on weight-bearing joints.

Vitamin C is necessary to prevent the capillary walls in the joints from breaking down and causing bleeding, swelling, and pain. Folic acid, vitamin B_{12}, and iron may be helpful in treating the anemia that can accompany arthritis. The frequency of liver disorders in arthritic patients may deter the conversion of carotene into vitamin A. Difficulty in assimilating carbohydrates suggests vitamin B deficiency. Treatment involves a diet high in raw fruits and vegetables low in sodium (salt).

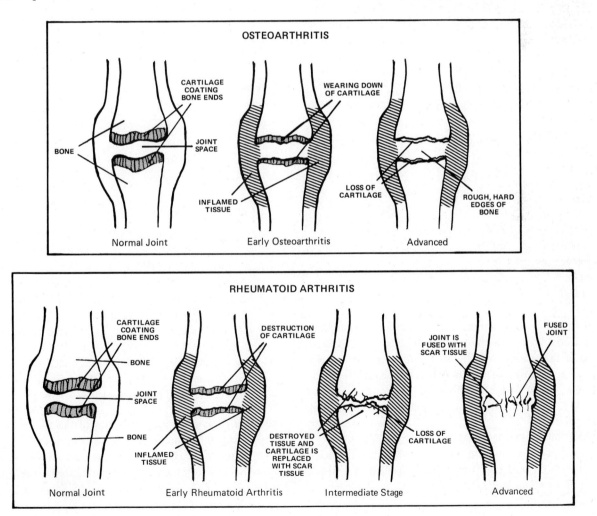

NUTRIENTS THAT MAY BE BENEFICIAL IN TREATMENT OF ARTHRITIS

Body Member	Nutrients	Quantity*
Joints	Vitamin A	
	Vitamin B complex	
	Vitamin B_2	1,000 mg under doctor's supervision
	Vitamin B_6	50-100 mg
	Vitamin B_{12}	30-900 mcg per week
	Folic acid	
	Niacin	Up to 1,000 mg under doctor's supervision
	Pantothenic acid	100 mg
	Vitamin C	3,000-5,000 mg; children, 600 mg
	Vitamin D	
	Vitamin E	600-1,000 IU
	Vitamin F	
	Bioflavonoids	3,000 mg
	Calcium	500 mg
	Iodine	
	Lecithin	
	Magnesium	500 mg
	Phosphorus	
	Potassium	500 mg
	Sulfur	
	Protein	

*See note, p. 166.

ASTHMA

Asthma is a chronic respiratory condition characterized by difficulty in breathing, frequent coughing, and a feeling of suffocation. An attack of asthma is often precipitated by physical or emotional stress, respiratory infections, air pollution, changes in temperature or humidity, and exposure to fumes such as those of gasoline or paint. It may also be related to low blood sugar, disorders of the adrenal glands, or specific allergies.

Symptoms of asthma are tightness in the chest and difficulty in breathing, usually accompanied by a wheezing or whistling sound. Violent coughing often occurs as the lungs attempt to expel mucus. An attack can last from several minutes to several days depending on individual situations and causative agents.

Skin tests are often given to pinpoint the patient's allergic tendencies. Common offenders are pollen, animal hair, dust, and certain foods. Proper nutrition is necessary, and the asthmatic should eliminate from the diet those foods that may bring on an attack. A high fluid intake and the inhalation of steam may help to liquefy mucus and make it easier to expel it from the air passages. Vitamin A is necessary for general health of the lungs and, together with vitamin E, guards against visible and invisible air pollutants. The person should have a diet sufficient in the vitamin B complex to avoid deficiency symptoms of nervousness, which might bring on an asthma attack. The need for vitamin C is increased by stress and exposure to hot or cold weather, cigarette smoking, and industrial air pollution.

NUTRIENTS THAT MAY BE BENEFICIAL IN TREATMENT OF ASTHMA

Body Member	Nutrients	Quantity*
Lungs/ Respiratory system	Vitamin A	Up to 50,000 IU
	Vitamin B complex	
	Vitamin B_6	50 mg
	Vitamin B_{12}	30 mcg
	Choline	
	Inositol	
	Pangamic acid	
	Pantothenic acid	100 mg
	Vitamin C	600 mg
	Vitamin D	800 IU
	Vitamin E	600 IU; 32 IU for children
	Vitamin F	
	Manganese	5 mg twice daily for 10 weeks

*See note, p. 166.

ATHLETE'S FOOT (TINEA PEDIS)

Athlete's foot is a fungus infection of the foot. It may occur as an inflammation, rash, or scaling of the skin. If the toenails are affected, they become brittle and discolored. Athlete's foot is most common in young adult males.

Athlete's foot is commonly transmitted from person to person through towels and locker room or bathroom floors because fungi thrive in these moist conditions. The frequent changing of socks and the use of foot powder are helpful in the prevention and treatment of athlete's foot. Vitamin A is necessary for the general health of the skin, and many enzymes that are effective in the healing of athlete's foot are activated by vitamin C.

NUTRIENTS THAT MAY BE BENEFICIAL IN TREATMENT OF ATHLETE'S FOOT

Body Member	Nutrients	Quantity
Skin	Vitamin A	
	Vitamin C	
	Vitamin E	

BACKACHE

Backache may be a symptom of a variety of disturbances in the muscles, tendons, ligaments, bones, or underlying organs. "Lumbago" is a general term frequently used to describe pain in the lower back.

A few of the many underlying causes of backache, or lumbago, are arthritis, osteoporosis, infection and fever, tumor, peptic ulcer, emotional tension or stress, slipped disc or other spinal cord injury, and disorders of the urinary system. Muscle strain or sprain as a cause of backache is quite frequent and commonly results from excessive or improper physical exertion, incorrect posture, sleeping on soft beds, or incorrect lifting. A backache that is accompanied by fever or headache should receive medical diagnosis.

Nutritional therapy for backaches varies with the disorder, but certain nutrients are essential for maintaining a healthy back. Protein is necessary for firm supporting tissue. The B-complex vitamins, especially niacin, provide strength and health for nerve tissues. Backache prevention includes exercise, good posture, proper lifting (by bending at the knees instead of the waist), and avoidance of unnecessary physical or emotional stress or strain.

Vitamins C and D together with calcium are important in the development and maintenance of bones and nerve function.

NUTRIENTS THAT MAY BE BENEFICIAL IN TREATMENT OF BACKACHE

Body Member	Nutrients	Quantity*
Bones/Spine	Vitamin B complex	
	Niacin	
	Vitamin C	500 mg
	Vitamin D	
	Vitamin E	50 IU
	Calcium	1-2 g
	Magnesium	50 IU
	Phosphorus	
	Protein	

*See note, p. 166.

BALDNESS (ALOPECIA)

Baldness is the partial or complete loss of hair, most commonly in the scalp, resulting from heredity, hormonal factors, aging, or local or systematic diseases. Hair loss and thinning not due to scarring is most frequently found in males but may occur in females. No satisfactory treatment is known, but transplants from hairy areas are popular.

NUTRIENTS THAT MAY BE BENEFICIAL IN TREATMENT OF BALDNESS

Body Member	Nutrients	Quantity*
Hair/Scalp	Vitamin B complex	
	Vitamin B_2	
	Vitamin B_6	50 mg
	Biotin	25 mg
	Choline	500-1,000 mg
	Folic acid	1 mg
	Inositol	500-1,000 mg
	Niacin	50 mg
	PABA	50 mg
	Pantothenic acid	50 mg
	Vitamin C	1,000 mg
	Vitamin E	Up to 1,200 IU
	Bioflavonoids	50-100 mg
	Copper	

*See note, p. 166.

BEDSORES

A bedsore forms when pressure on a bony area of the body, such as the elbow, heel, or hip, cuts off the blood supply to that area. The affected area is thus deprived of essential nutrients, and therefore tissue is destroyed.

The most effective prevention for bedsores is relieving pressure on the vulnerable areas of the body by using protective padding, massaging the skin to stimulate circulation, and keeping the skin dry and clean. Treatment for bedsores includes a well-balanced diet high in protein, calories, and vitamins. In some cases, direct applications of vitamins C and E to the wound have been beneficial.[6] Ointments containing vitamins A and D are also often used in treating bedsores.

NUTRIENTS THAT MAY BE BENEFICIAL IN TREATMENT OF BEDSORES

Body Member	Nutrients	Quantity*
Skin	Vitamin A	
	Vitamin B complex	
	Vitamin B_2	5 mg daily
	Vitamin C	
	Vitamin D	
	Vitamin E	
	Copper	
	Protein	

*See note, p. 166.

BELL'S PALSY (SEE ALSO "NEURITIS")

Bell's palsy is a type of paralysis characterized by distortion of the face due to a lesion of the facial nerve. It is accompanied by pain, weakness, and a sensation of pricking, tingling, or creeping on the skin, which may be a result of injury or irritation of a sensory nerve or nerve root.

NUTRIENTS THAT MAY BE BENEFICIAL IN TREATMENT OF BELL'S PALSY

Body Member	Nutrients	Quantity*
Brain/Nervous system	Vitamin B complex	
	Vitamin B_1	100-200 mg
	Vitamin C	
	Protein	

*See note, p. 166.

[6] J. I. Rodale, *The Complete Book of Vitamins* (Emmaus, Pa.: Rodale Books, 1968), pp. 355 and 651.

BERIBERI

Beriberi is a disease caused by a deficiency of thiamine. The disease seldom occurs outside the Far East, where the principal diet consists mainly of polished rice, which does not supply sufficient thiamine. Rare cases of beriberi in the United States are usually associated with stressful conditions, such as hypothyroidism, infections, pregnancy, lactation, and chronic alcoholism, which increase the body's need for thiamine.

Symptoms of beriberi in infants are convulsions; respiratory difficulties; and gastrointestinal problems, such as nausea, vomiting, constipation, diarrhea, and abdominal discomfort. Adult symptoms are fatigue, diarrhea, appetite and weight loss, disturbed nerve function causing paralysis and wasting of the limbs, edema, and heart failure.

The administration of thiamine will prevent and cure the disease. Because of the diarrhea that accompanies beriberi, the diet must be rich in all nutrients.

NUTRIENTS THAT MAY BE BENEFICIAL IN TREATMENT OF BERIBERI

Body Member	Nutrients	Quantity
General	Vitamin B complex	
	Vitamin B_1	
	Vitamin C	

BITOT'S SPOTS

Bitot's spots are characterized by white, foamy, elevated, and sharply outlined patches on the white of the eyes, caused by a deficiency of vitamin A.

NUTRIENTS THAT MAY BE BENEFICIAL IN TREATMENT OF BITOT'S SPOTS

Body Member	Nutrients	Quantity*
Eyes	Vitamin A	50,000 IU
	Vitamin D	
	Protein	

*See note, p. 166.

BOIL (FURUNCLE)

A boil, or furuncle, is an infected nodule on the skin with a central core of pus surrounded by inflamed and swollen tissue. A boil forms when skin tissue is weakened by chafing, lowered resistance due to disease, or inadequate nutrition. Boil symptoms include itching, mild pain, and localized swelling.

Proper hygiene is essential for the treatment of boils. The infected areas should be washed several times daily and swabbed with antiseptic. Hot compresses can relieve pain and promote healing. The person should receive adequate rest and pay special attention to eating a well-balanced diet. Vitamins A, C, and E are necessary for health of the skin.

NUTRIENTS THAT MAY BE BENEFICIAL IN TREATMENT OF BOILS

Body Member	Nutrients	Quantity
Skin	Vitamin A	Applied locally
	Vitamin C	
	Vitamin E	

BRONCHITIS

Bronchitis is an inflammation of the tissues lining the air passage leading to the lungs. Factors that increase susceptibility to bronchitis are asthma and other respiratory diseases, air pollution, cigarette smoking, fatigue, chilling, and malnutrition. Symptoms of bronchitis are a slight fever, back and muscle pain, and sore throat. A dry cough is followed by the coughing up of mucus as the inflammation becomes more severe.

Treatment for bronchitis includes rest, adequate fluid intake, and a well-balanced diet high in vitamins A and C. Vitamin A is essential to the health of the lung tissues; vitamin C helps fight infection and promotes healing. If the bronchitis victim is suffering from malnutrition, special attention should be paid to the adequate intake of protein and all other nutrients.

NUTRIENTS THAT MAY BE BENEFICIAL IN TREATMENT OF BRONCHITIS

Body Member	Nutrients	Quantity
Lungs/Respiratory system	Vitamin A	
	Vitamin C	
	Vitamin D	
	Vitamin E	
	Vitamin F	
	Protein	
	Water	

BRUISES

A bruise is an injury that involves the rupture of small blood vessels, causing discoloration of underlying tissues without a break in the overlying skin. Bruises are frequently the result of falling or bumping into objects.

Factors that make one susceptible to bruising are overweight, anemia, and time of menstrual period. Frequent bruising without apparent cause may signal that the materials needed for clotting may not be present in the blood. Leukemia and excessive doses of anticlotting drugs can also cause frequent or large bruises.

Excessive bruising may indicate a lack of vitamin D, a natural blood-clotting agent. Also, vitamin C and bioflavonoid deficiencies may be characterized by a weakening of the small blood vessels, resulting in easier bruising. If the cause of bruising is anemia, there should be an increased intake of iron in the diet. If obesity appears to be a cause of bruising, a well-balanced reducing diet is indicated. Frequent bruising with no apparent cause, or a bruise that applies pressure to a neighboring portion of the body, requires medical attention.

NUTRIENTS THAT MAY BE BENEFICIAL IN TREATMENT OF BRUISES

Body Member	Nutrients	Quantity
Blood/Circulatory system	Vitamin B complex	
	Folic acid	
	Vitamin C	
	Vitamin D	
	Vitamin K	
	Bioflavonoids	
	Iron	

BURNS

A burn is a tissue injury caused by heat, electricity, radiation, or chemicals. There are three degrees of burn severity. A first-degree burn appears reddened, a second-degree burn includes blister formation, and a third-degree burn involves destruction of the entire thickness of skin and possibly of the underlying muscle.

Because of tissue destruction, massive losses of body fluids, proteins, sodium, potassium, and nitrogen can occur. Because large amounts of fluids are lost in extensive burns, the possibility of shock exists. Infection is another threat to the burn victim.

Immediate treatment measures for burns include cold applications to reduce pain and swelling and cleansing and covering of the burn to minimize the possibility of bacterial infection. Ointments, salves, or butter should not be applied to burns. They tend to promote infection and prevent circulation of air to the wound by retaining heat within the body. Treatment of chemical burns may include application of an antidote specific to the offending agent.

Diet is very important to burn victims, especially to those with extensive burns. The diet should be high in calories for energy and high in protein for tissue repair. Adequate intake of fluids in proportion to the amount of fluids lost is also essential. Vitamin C may be helpful for healing the wound, and the B vitamins are necessary to meet the body's increased metabolic demands. Intake of vitamin A, necessary for the health of the skin, should be increased, as well as intake of potassium. Some authorities indicate that vitamin E relieves pain and promotes healing in burns.[7]

NUTRIENTS THAT MAY BE BENEFICIAL IN TREATMENT OF BURNS

Body Member	Nutrients	Quantity*
Skin	Vitamin A	
	Vitamin B complex	
	PABA	
	Vitamin C	
	Vitamin D	
	Vitamin E	200 IU after each meal; ointment
	Vitamin F	
	Potassium	
	Zinc	
	Protein	
	Water	

*See note, p. 166.

BURSITIS

Bursitis arises from an inflammation of the liquid-filled sac, called a bursa, found within the joints, muscles, tendons, and bones, which helps to promote muscular move-

[7]Evan Shute, *The Heart and Vitamin E* (London: Shute Foundation for Medical Research, 1963), pp. 96-97.

ment and reduce friction. The affliction is commonly found in the hip or shoulder joints, elbows, or feet and is more commonly known as "frozen shoulder," "tennis elbow," or bunion.

Bursitis may be caused by stretched muscles, shoes that are too tight, injury such as a bump or bruise, or irritation from calcium deposits found in the bursa wall. Bursitis symptoms include swelling, tenderness, and agonizing pain in the affected area which frequently limits motion. Treatment involves removing the cause of the injury, clearing up any underlying infection, and possibly, surgically removing calcium deposits. Other measures include rest and immobilization of the affected part.

Vitamin B_{12} is beneficial to the normal functioning of body cells in the bone marrow. Vitamin E has also been found to be beneficial in the treatment of bursitis. The need for protein and vitamins A and C increases during infection, and extra amounts of these nutrients are required for bursitis victims.

NUTRIENTS THAT MAY BE BENEFICIAL IN TREATMENT OF BURSITIS

Body Member	Nutrients	Quantity*
Bones/ Muscles/ Joints	Vitamin A	
	Vitamin B complex	
	Vitamin B_{12}	1,000 mcg daily for first 7-10 days; three times per week for next 2-3 weeks; one to two times per week for next 2-3 weeks
	Vitamin C	
	Vitamin E	
	Protein	

*See note, p. 166.

CANCER

Cancer cells appear as young, rapidly growing cells that do not fulfill their natural functions and invade surrounding tissue. These cells rob neighboring normal cells of their essential nutrients, causing a severe wasting away of the cancer patient. Cancer cells are capable of migrating and planting themselves in any part of the body, causing abnormal growths or tumors. Cancers are categorized according to the type of tissue they invade.

The importance of early detection in treatment of cancer cannot be overemphasized. This is the only chance for successful treatment of the disease. One must be always alert to the American Cancer Society's seven warning signs: unusual bleeding or discharge, appearance of a lump or swelling, hoarseness of cough, indigestion or difficulty in swallowing, change in bowel or bladder habits, a sore that does not heal, or a change in a wart or mole. Symptoms and their severity vary with the type and location of the cancer.

For the treatment of cancerous growths or tumors, surgery, radiation, amygdalin or laetrile, and certain drugs have proved beneficial. Surgical operations remove the original growth and any secondary ones. Drugs, although unable to completely cure cancer, are used to reduce the growth or to delay the appearance of secondary growths. Radiation is often used to destroy cancer cells and to prevent them from spreading.

The following vitamins and minerals have been found to possess properties that promote protection against cancer and aid in its healing. Vitamin A is essential because a deficiency can definitely contribute to cancer development. Vitamin C is a potent antitoxin that can neutralize or minimize the effect of many chemical carcinogens in food and in the environment. Vitamins E and C help to inhibit the activity of a growth substance, or catalyst, which is found in cancerous tissue. Vitamin E increases oxygen-holding abilities of cells. The B vitamins are important for prevention of cirrhosis of the liver, which carries a 60 percent greater risk of developing cancer than does a normal liver. Riboflavin, niacin, and pantothenic acid help tissues resist the effects cancer produces.[8] Potassium deficiency is thought by some to be a contributing cause of cancer.

For the terminally ill cancer patient, the specific food needs depend on the location of the tumor. Generally, however, a high-protein, high-calorie diet is necessary to maintain and help restore normal cells. Iron is essential to the diet in order to prevent anemia, which is a frequent complication of cancer.

[8]J.I. Rodale, *The Encyclopedia of Common Diseases* (Emmaus, Pa.: Rodale Books, 1969), p. 239.

Vitamin K has been found to protect against certain cancer-causing substances.

NUTRIENTS THAT MAY BE BENEFICIAL IN TREATMENT OF CANCER

Body Member	Nutrients	Quantity*
General	Vitamin A	50,000 IU
	Vitamin B complex	
	Vitamin B_2	
	Laetrile	
	Niacin	100 mg
	Pangamic acid	50 mg twice daily
	Pantothenic acid	50 mg
	Choline	500-1,000 mg
	Vitamin C	Up to 5,000 mg
	Vitamin D	
	Vitamin E	Up to 1,200 IU
	Vitamin K	
	Iron	
	Phosphorus	
	Potassium	
	Protein	

*See note, p. 166.

CANKER SORES

Canker sores are shallow open sores found anywhere on the mouth. They are usually located on the mucous membrane inside the lips and cheeks.

A canker sore is identified by a sensation of burning and tingling and a slight swelling of the mucous membrane. The sore, a white center surrounded by a red border, is tender to pressure and is painful when acids or spicy foods are eaten. The sore lasts from 4 to 20 days and heals spontaneously, leaving no scar.

The specific cause of canker sores is unknown, although they appear to be brought on by anxiety, other emotional stress, or sensitivity to various foods and substances that produce allergic-type reactions. Because canker sores heal spontaneously, there is no prescribed treatment for them. Application of a mild astringent and avoidance of foods that further irritate the canker sores can be useful for providing relief from the accompanying pain. Vitamin A is necessary for maintaining the condition of mouth tissue. Niacin helps in the general condition of the skin, tongue, and digestive system. A well-balanced diet that provides adequate amounts of these vitamins protects against the formation of canker sores.

**NUTRIENTS THAT MAY BE BENEFICIAL
IN TREATMENT OF CANKER SORES**

Body Member	Nutrients	Quantity*
Mouth	Vitamin A	Applied locally
	Vitamin B complex	
	Niacin	100 mg after each meal
	Vitamin C	
	Vitamin D	

*See note, p. 166.

CARBUNCLE

A painful, localized infection producing pus-filled areas in the deeper layers of the skin tissues under the skin is known as a carbuncle. It commonly appears as a group of boils but is usually more painful, deeper, and slower-healing than an ordinary boil. Carbuncles are formed when bacteria enter lesions in the skin, causing infection. Symptoms of carbuncles include fever and chills, fatigue, and weight loss.

Treatment for carbuncles demands proper hygiene, including frequent washing of the infected area with soap and water, and application of an antiseptic. Hot compresses can relieve pain and promote healing. Bed rest is beneficial, and a well-balanced diet is essential. Vitamins A and C are necessary for health of the skin. If a fever is present, vitamin E may reduce scarring. Calorie and nutrient levels should be increased.

**NUTRIENTS THAT MAY BE BENEFICIAL
IN TREATMENT OF CARBUNCLES**

Body Member	Nutrients	Quantity
Skin	Vitamin A	Applied locally
	Vitamin C	
	Vitamin D	
	Vitamin E	

CATARACTS

A leading cause of blindness, a cataract is a condition in which the lens of the eye, that part of the eye which focuses and allows us to see objects both near and far, becomes clouded or opaque. Cataracts may occur at any time in life but are usually associated with the degenerative changes that occur with age. Cataracts in young people are usually congenital but may be caused by a nutritional disorder or inflammatory condition in the eye. There is a high incidence of cataracts among diabetics.

Symptoms of cataracts include painless, progressive blurring and loss of vision, sensitivity to bright light, and the appearance of halos around lights. Surgical removal of the lens is necessary to restore normal vision and prevent blindness.[9]

Research has shown that a reduction of vitamin C and riboflavin in the lens of the eye may contribute to the development of cataracts. High blood sugar levels, as in diabetes, can cause cataract formation. Low levels of calcium in the blood can also cause cataracts. Maintaining an adequate intake of vitamin C, riboflavin, and calcium may be useful in preventing cataract formation.

**NUTRIENTS THAT MAY BE BENEFICIAL
IN TREATMENT OF CATARACTS**

Body Member	Nutrients	Quantity*
Eye	Vitamin A	100,000 IU
	Vitamin B complex	
	Vitamin B_2	
	Pantothenic acid	
	Vitamin C	500-15,000 mg
	Vitamin D	
	Vitamin E	400-600 IU
	Calcium	
	Protein	

*See note, p. 166.

CELIAC DISEASE

Celiac disease is an intestinal disorder caused by the intolerance of some individuals to gluten, a protein in

[9]David Holvey, *The Merck Manual*, 12th ed. (Rahway, N.J.: Merck and Co., 1972), p. 1015.

wheat, rye, and barley. Ingestion of gluten irritates the intestinal lining, interfering with the absorption of nutrients and water.

Symptoms of celiac disease are weight loss, diarrhea, gas, abdominal pain, and anemia. Malnutrition often accompanies this disorder because of the greatly reduced absorption of nutrients.

Treatment for celiac disease includes eating a well-balanced, gluten-free diet that is high in calories and proteins and normal in fats. The diet excludes all cereal grains except rice and corn. Common nutrient deficiencies that occur with celiac disease and that should be corrected include deficiencies in calcium, vitamin B complex, and vitamins A, C, D, K, and E. Iron, folic acid, and vitamin B_{12} can be used to correct the anemia that usually accompanies celiac disease.

NUTRIENTS THAT MAY BE BENEFICIAL IN TREATMENT OF CELIAC DISEASE

Body Member	Nutrients	Quantity*
Intestine	Vitamin A	
	Vitamin B complex	
	Vitamin B_6	30 mg
	Vitamin B_{12}	
	Folic acid	
	Vitamin C	
	Vitamin D	
	Vitamin E	
	Vitamin K	
	Calcium	
	Iron	
	Magnesium	
	Proteins (no gluten)	

*See note, p. 166.

CEREBROVASCULAR ACCIDENT (CVA, OR STROKE)

A stroke, or cerebrovascular accident, occurs when the blood supply of an area of brain cells is cut off for a long period of time, resulting in the death of the deprived cells due to lack of oxygen and nutrients essential for the proper function of the brain. The blood vessels may be blocked by atherosclerosis, clotting, or hemorrhaging. The process is similar to that of a heart attack, the difference being cell death in the brain during a stroke.

Typical symptoms include impaired memory and attention span, tingling or lack of feeling in limbs, a feeling of heaviness in the limbs, and loss of movement. Symptoms are often restricted to one side of the body, as seen in the frequent right- or left-sided paralysis. Strokes may be so small that they are not even noticed or so severe as to be fatal. It is difficult to tell the extent of injury or cell death at the time the stroke occurs, and the long-term outlook therefore depends upon the area and extent of the brain damage. Physical and speech therapy are often helpful in rehabilitating the patient.

Predisposing factors are prolonged high blood pressure, atherosclerosis, diabetes, old age, obesity, and cigarette smoking. Preventive dietary measures include restricting sodium intake to reduce high blood pressure and reducing cholesterol intake to prevent further cholesterol buildup in blood vessels. The diet should be well

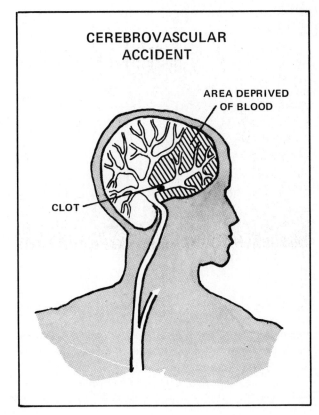

CEREBROVASCULAR ACCIDENT

AREA DEPRIVED OF BLOOD

CLOT

balanced, with special emphasis on B vitamins and vitamin C because they are needed for general health of the blood vessels. Vitamin E can be of help to prevent clots. Reduction of overweight by sensible dieting is of the utmost importance.

The diet for a patient recovering from a stroke should be well balanced and easily digested. Easily digested meals are usually light and low in roughage and gas-producing foods. Roughage comes from the carbohydrate cellulose. Caloric intake should be adjusted to the altered activity of the person.

NUTRIENTS THAT MAY BE BENEFICIAL IN TREATMENT OF CEREBROVASCULAR ACCIDENT

Body Member	Nutrients	Quantity*
Blood	Vitamin B complex	
	Choline	
	Inositol	
	Vitamin C	
	Vitamin E	300 IU
	Bioflavonoids	
	Lecithin	
	Potassium	
	Low sodium (salt)	
	Low cholesterol	
	Protein	

*See note, p. 166.

CHICKEN POX

Chicken pox is a highly contagious viral disease in which the chief symptom is generalized skin eruptions. One attack usually protects against the disease for life.

About 24 to 36 hours before the first series of eruptions, the patient may have a headache and a low fever. The rash appears as red bumps containing drops of clear fluid, usually on the face and trunk of the body. The fluid breaks out, forming a crust, and the eruptions continue in cycles for three or four days. Soothing lotions may be applied for relief of itching, and fingernails should be cut short to prevent scratching. The patient should be kept clean and should be frequently bathed with soap and water.

Fevers increase the body's need for calories and vitamins A and C. Extra protein is needed for the repair of

tissues. The patient should be isolated for 10 to 14 days to prevent the spread of the infection.

NUTRIENTS THAT MAY BE BENEFICIAL IN TREATMENT OF CHICKEN POX

Body Member	Nutrients	Quantity
Skin	Vitamin A	
	Vitamin C	
	Protein	

CHOLESTEROL LEVEL, HIGH

Cholesterol is a fatty substance manufactured by the liver. It is found only in animal fat; it is not contained in vegetable fat. Cholesterol is needed to form sex and adrenal hormones, vitamin D, and bile salts. It also has a vital function in the brain and nerves.

Some researchers believe that when cholesterol levels in the blood become abnormally high, fatty deposits composed of cholesterol and calcium tend to accumulate in the arteries, including those of the heart, increasing the susceptibility to heart attacks. Cholesterol deposits occur mostly in parts of the blood vessels which have been weakened by high blood pressure or undue strain. Cholesterol in the blood must be kept in solution to prevent deposits from forming; lecithin seems to help the bile do this. Lecithin is contained in many fatty foods, but when these fats are hydrogenated, the lecithin is lost. Adequate supplies of unsaturated fatty acids (vitamin F, especially linoleic acid) and vitamin E seem to help control the cholesterol level of the blood and prevent atherosclerosis.

NUTRIENTS THAT MAY BE BENEFICIAL IN TREATMENT OF HIGH CHOLESTEROL LEVEL

Body Member	Nutrients	Quantity*
Blood	Vitamin B complex	
	Vitamin B_6	
	Choline	
	Inositol	
	Niacin	
	Pangamic acid	
	Vitamin C	500 mg

*See note, p. 166.

Body Member	Nutrients	Quantity
	Vitamin D	
	Vitamin E	
	Vitamin F	4-5 tbsp
	Bioflavonoids	
	Lecithin	
	Magnesium	500 mg
	Zinc	

CIRRHOSIS OF THE LIVER

Cirrhosis of the liver is a chronic disease characterized by degeneration and hardening of liver cells. Scarring of the liver tissue causes improper functioning and may result from alcoholism, malnutrition, viral hepatitis, or chronic inflammation or obstruction of certain ducts in the liver.

Early signs of the disease include fever, indigestion, diarrhea or constipation, and jaundice. Later symptoms include edema, anemia, and bleeding disorders characterized by the presence of spider-shaped bruises. A deficiency of the B complex and vitamins A, C, and K may also occur.

Optimal nutrition provides the key to recovery from the disease. A high-protein diet (1 gram of protein per kilogram of body weight, or approximately 75 to 100 grams of protein per day) is prescribed to promote regeneration of the liver cells. In the case of coma, however, protein should be restricted. A high-calorie (2500 to 3000 calories per day) and high-carbohydrate (300 to 400 grams per day) diet is needed to increase the storage of glycogen, to ensure that protein is used for regeneration, and to compensate for weight losses caused by fever. If nausea is present frequently, small meals are better tolerated than three large meals.

A common complication of cirrhosis is the failure of the liver to make vitamins available in an active form in the body. For this reason, the diet should be high in the B complex and vitamins A (not in the form of carotene), C, D, and K. If jaundice is present, special attention should be paid to the fat-soluble vitamins, A, D, E, and K, because some kinds of jaundice interfere with the absorption of these nutrients. If edema is present, sodium, which causes the body to retain water, should be restricted. All alcohol should be strictly avoided.

NUTRIENTS THAT MAY BE BENEFICIAL IN TREATMENT OF CIRRHOSIS OF THE LIVER

Body Member	Nutrients	Quantity*
Liver	Vitamin A	50,000 to 100,000 IU
	Vitamin B complex	
	Vitamin B_{12}	
	Choline	1-5 g
	Inositol	
	Pangamic acid	
	Vitamin C	
	Vitamin D	
	Vitamin E	
	Vitamin F	
	Vitamin K	
	Magnesium	
	Zinc	
	Carbohydrates	
	Protein	

*See note, p. 166.

COLITIS

Colitis is a disease in which the lining of part of the colon, or large intestine, is inflamed. There are several types of colitis, all of which are determined by the extent of the inflammation, the amount of the colon involved, and the degree of severity of the colitis symptoms. Although the cause of the disease is unknown, there is usually always a correlation between colitis and depression or anxiety. The degree of a person's emotional stress will often indicate the severity of his colitis.

In early stages, colitis is characterized by abdominal cramps or pain, diarrhea, and the need to eliminate several times daily. These symptoms are accompanied by rectal bleeding as the condition becomes more severe. Instead of being absorbed by the body, water and minerals are rapidly expelled through the lower digestive tract, resulting in a loss of weight and, possibly, dehydration or anemia. Because of this rapid expulsion and decreased absorption of water and nutrients, the entire nutritional status of the colitis patient is in jeopardy.

A therapeutic diet for colitis should be bland and high in protein and vitamin F to restore lost or worn-down tissues. Foods high in roughage, such as raw fruits and vegetables, should be avoided to prevent further intestinal irritation. Milk is also frequently not tolerated; therefore a calcium supplement may be necessary. Iron is necessary to deter the development of anemia and vitamin C to aid in the absorption of iron.

NUTRIENTS THAT MAY BE BENEFICIAL IN TREATMENT OF COLITIS

Body Member	Nutrients	Quantity*
Bowel/Intestine/Colon	Vitamin A	
	Vitamin B$_6$	50 mg
	Vitamin C	
	Vitamin E	
	Vitamin F	
	Calcium	
	Iron	
	Magnesium	
	Phosphorus	
	Potassium	
	Protein	
	Low cellulose	

*See note, p. 166.

COMMON COLD

The common cold is a general inflammation of the mucous membranes of the respiratory passages caused by a variety of viruses. Colds are highly contagious. On the average, Americans contact two or three colds per year. Factors that lower the body's resistance to virus infection are fatigue, overexposure to cold, recent or present infections, allergic reactions, and inhalation of irritating dust or gas.

The virus is spread about two days before the symptoms appear. Symptoms include nose and throat irritations, watery eyes, headaches, fever, chills, muscle aches, and temporary loss of smell and taste.

Prevention of colds includes adequate sleep and a well-balanced diet. Treatment includes adequate fluid and protein intake to sustain the losses that occur with fever. Vitamin B$_6$ helps in the production of antibodies that defend the body against infection. Vitamin A is necessary to maintain the health of the mucous membrane of the respiratory passages. Some individuals have found that vitamin D is also helpful in the prevention of colds.[10] Vitamin F, or unsaturated fatty acids, reduces the incidence and duration of colds.

Reports on the role of vitamin C in the treatment of the common cold are contradictory. However, many authorities claim that the intake of vitamin C in amounts from 1 to 2 grams daily is effective in preventing a cold.[11] Another source indicates that at the onset of a cold, vitamin D taken in amounts of 600 to 625 milligrams every three hours may be successful for treatment.[12] The amount of vitamin C recommended for the prevention and treatment of a cold varies from individual to individual.

NUTRIENTS THAT MAY BE BENEFICIAL IN TREATMENT OF COMMON COLDS

Body Member	Nutrients	Quantity*
General	Vitamin A	50,000-150,000 IU for one month; then reduce to 25,000 IU daily
	Vitamin B complex	
	Vitamin B$_6$	100 mg
	Vitamin C	600-625 mg every three hours first three or four days, then 375-400 mg daily
	Vitamin D	
	Vitamin E	600 IU
	Vitamin F	
	Bioflavonoids	200-600 mg
	Calcium	
	Protein	
	Water	

*See note, p. 166.

CONGESTIVE HEART FAILURE

A heart that is weakened or damaged by diseases such as rheumatic fever, heart attack, hypothyroidism, arterio-

[10]Harriet Coston Moidel (ed.) et al., *Nursing Care of the Patient with Medical-Surgical Disorders* (New York: McGraw-Hill Book Co., 1971), p. 520.

[11]Helen A. Guthrie, *Introductory Nutrition*, 2d ed. (St. Louis: C. V. Mosby Co., 1971), p. 225.

[12]"Summer Cold? Vitamin C...," *Prevention*, July 1970, p. 49.

sclerosis, or beriberi is unable to properly pump the blood through the body. This inefficient circulation, which leads to congestion of many organs with blood and other tissue fluids, is congestive heart failure.

Early symptoms of congestive heart failure are abnormal fatigue and shortness of breath following work or exercise. Swelling, particularly in the ankles and feet, is a further symptom. Congestion of the abdominal organs causes nausea, lack of appetite, and gas. Fluid in the lungs impairs breathing and in some cases causes a persistent cough.

Medical treatment for congestive heart failure includes prescription of drugs that strengthen the heartbeat and reduce the amount of excess water in the body. Bed rest is necessary to lessen the heart's workload. The diet should be divided into frequent small meals of easily digested foods. Calories, fats, gas-forming foods, and sodium (salt) are restricted.

Because sodium is found in so many foods, a heart patient on a sodium-restricted diet should take particular care that all his nutritional needs are met. The diet should be adequate in potassium and thiamine.

NUTRIENTS THAT MAY BE BENEFICIAL IN TREATMENT OF CONGESTIVE HEART FAILURE

Body Member	Nutrients	Quantity
Heart	Vitamin A	
	Vitamin B complex	
	Vitamin E	
	Potassium	
	Low fat	
	Low sodium	

CONJUNCTIVITIS

Conjunctivitis is an inflammation of the mucous membrane that lines the eyelids and covers the white portion of the eye. Symptoms of conjunctivitis include redness, swelling, itching, and pus in the membrane. The condition may be caused by allergy, bacteria, virus, smoke, dust, or chemical irritants.

Deficiency of vitamin A, vitamin B_6, or riboflavin may cause conjunctivitis symptoms. The diet should be adequate in these vitamins to help prevent the condition.

NUTRIENTS THAT MAY BE BENEFICIAL IN TREATMENT OF CONJUNCTIVITIS

Body Member	Nutrients	Quantity
Eye	Vitamin A	
	Vitamin B complex	
	Vitamin B_2	
	Vitamin B_6	
	Niacin	
	Vitamin C	
	Vitamin D	

CONSTIPATION

Constipation is a disorder causing decreased frequency of bowel movements, resulting in waste matter remaining in the colon and becoming dry and difficult to expel. Constipation may stem from a variety of causes. Insufficient muscle tone in the intestinal or abdominal wall due to a lack of exercise; repeated failure to heed the signal to eliminate; or excessive fatigue, nervousness, anxiety, or excitement may result in constipation. A poor diet or a diet lacking in fluids or roughage can bring about constipation. The continued use of laxatives as a substitute for proper exercise, rest, and diet may result in dependency and merely perpetuate the problem.

Laxatives, stool softeners, or lubricants such as mineral oil may be prescribed medically for the treatment of constipation. Mineral oil should not be taken along with meals because it interferes with the absorption of fat-soluble vitamins. The diet should provide adequate fluids and roughage in the form of fruits and vegetables high in water content. Foods containing fats may be useful in the treatment of constipation because of their lubricating effect on the mucous walls of the colon.

NUTRIENTS THAT MAY BE BENEFICIAL IN TREATMENT OF CONSTIPATION

Body Member	Nutrients	Quantity*
Intestine	Vitamin A	25,000 IU
	Vitamin B complex	
	Vitamin B_1	100 mg
	Choline	500 mg
	Inositol	500 mg
	Niacin	

*See note, p. 166.

Body Member	Nutrients	Quantity
	Vitamin C	1,000 mg
	Vitamin D	
	Vitamin E	
	Vitamin F	
	Carbohydrates (in the form of cellulose)	
	Calcium	
	Potassium	
	Fats	
	Water	

CROUP

Croup encompasses a variety of conditions in which there is a high-pitched cough and difficulty in breathing. Fever may or may not accompany the disorder. Croup usually affects children under the age of five. Conditions that may bring on the symptoms of croup are virus, diphtheria, a foreign body in the throat, and swelling due to a throat infection.

Croup may vary greatly in severity depending upon its cause. Any underlying infections should be treated, and any obstruction in the throat should be removed. The breathing of warm moist air from a humidifier often brings relief from cough.

Nutritional treatment for croup involves a well-balanced diet high in protein to promote the growth and repair of tissues. If fever is present, the need for vitamins A and C is increased. Increased fluid intake is also essential, especially when croup occurs in very small children or infants.

NUTRIENTS THAT MAY BE BENEFICIAL IN TREATMENT OF CROUP

Body Member	Nutrients	Quantity
Lungs/Respiratory system	Vitamin A	
	Vitamin C	
	Protein	

CYSTIC FIBROSIS

Cystic fibrosis is a hereditary disease affecting certain glands in the body, such as the gallbladder, pancreas, and sweat glands. The disease usually begins during infancy, although symptoms may manifest themselves later in life.

The greatest danger at the onset of the disease is malnutrition due to an underproduction of digestive juices. As a result, all foods, especially fats, are poorly digested and absorbed, and a deficiency in all nutrients, particularly in the fat-soluble vitamins, occurs. In addition, the sweat glands produce an unusually salty perspiration, draining the body of salt and making the patient susceptible to heat exhaustion. The mucous glands in the lungs, which normally aid in moistening the air passages, produce a thick mucus that blocks the passages and promotes the growth of harmful bacteria.

Treatment for the malnutrition that occurs with cystic fibrosis may include medication to compensate for the lack of digestive juices. The recommended diet is 25 percent higher than normal in calories, the majority being in protein, which is easier to digest than fats, and starches, which are nutritionally better than sugars. The intake of fluids and salt should be increased, particularly during hot weather. Because of the poor absorption of nutrients, additional vitamin A, the B complex, and vitamins C, D, E, and K should be included in the diet.

NUTRIENTS THAT MAY BE BENEFICIAL IN TREATMENT OF CYSTIC FIBROSIS

Body Member	Nutrients	Quantity*
Glands	Vitamin A	
	Vitamin B complex	
	Vitamin C	
	Vitamin D	
	Vitamin E	300-1,500 mg
	Vitamin K	
	Sodium (salt)	
	Protein	

*See note, p. 166.

CYSTITIS (BLADDER INFECTION)

Cystitis is an inflammation of the urinary bladder. It is most frequently caused by bacteria that ascend from the urinary opening, but it may also be caused by infected urine sent from the kidneys to the bladder. Cystitis most frequently occurs in females.

Symptoms of cystitis are pain in the lower abdomen and back and frequent, urgent, and painful urination in which the urine may contain blood or pus. Fever may possibly accompany these symptoms. Treatment for cystitis includes increasing the fluid intake and maintaining a well-balanced diet. Vitamin B complex helps to maintain the muscle tone in the gastrointestinal tract and liver. Vitamin C helps ward off and clear up the infection. Vitamin E maintains proper functioning of the liver.

NUTRIENTS THAT MAY BE BENEFICIAL IN TREATMENT OF CYSTITIS

Body Member	Nutrients	Quantity*
Bladder	Vitamin A	25,000-50,000 IU
	Vitamin B complex	
	Vitamin B$_6$	
	Pantothenic acid	
	Vitamin C	5,000-10,000 mg
	Vitamin D	
	Vitamin E	600 IU
	Fluids (water)	

*See note, p. 166.

DANDRUFF

Dandruff (seborrhea) is a covering of dead skin that prevents new hair from growing because it cannot break through the dead skin. Dandruff may be dry and scaly or, at times, oily and is due to a dysfunction of the sebaceous glands. It often occurs in persons with oily skin who are prone to develop superficial, acute and chronic bacterial skin conditions.

It is caused primarily by a vitamin A deficiency or constipation and may be corrected by proper nutrient supplementation and cleansing with a shampoo designed to aid in the control of dandruff.

NUTRIENTS THAT MAY BE BENEFICIAL IN TREATMENT OF DANDRUFF

Body Member	Nutrients	Quantity
Skin/Scalp	Vitamin A	
	Vitamin B complex	
	Vitamin B$_6$	
	Vitamin E	
	Vitamin F	

DERMATITIS

Dermatitis is an inflammatory, usually recurring skin reaction. It is caused by contact with an irritating agent that is ingested or found in the environment. Dermatitis is usually associated with hereditary allergic tendencies and may be aggravated by emotional stress and fatigue.

A primary symptom of dermatitis is eczema. Eczema is a type of skin eruption characterized by tiny blisters that weep and crust. Chronic forms are characterized by scaling, flaking, and eventual thickening and color changes of the skin. Itching is almost always present.

If the irritating agent is a food item, it should be eliminated from the diet. Deficiency of any of the B vitamins can cause dermatitis, and these vitamins should, therefore, be present in the diet in adequate amounts. Linoleic acid (unsaturated fat) and vitamin B$_6$ have been found to cure infants who have dermatitis caused by a fat-free diet.[13] Vitamin A is also essential for maintaining healthy skin tissue. A protein deficiency can cause chronic eczema.

NUTRIENTS THAT MAY BE BENEFICIAL IN TREATMENT OF DERMATITIS

Body Member	Nutrients	Quantity*
Skin	Vitamin A	50,000-75,000 IU for two to three months; then reduce to 25,000 IU after one month
	Vitamin B complex	
	Vitamin B$_2$	
	Vitamin B$_6$	
	Biotin	
	Niacin	300 mg
	Vitamin D	
	Vitamin F	
	Potassium	
	Sulfur (ointment form)	
	Protein	

*See note, p. 166.

[13]Marie V. Krause and Martha A. Hunscher, *Food, Nutrition and Diet Therapy*, 5th ed. (Philadelphia: W. B. Saunders Co., 1972), p. 56.

DIABETES

Diabetes is a metabolic disorder characterized by decreased ability, or complete inability, of the body to utilize carbohydrates. Carbohydrates are normally broken down within the body in the form of glucose, the body's main energy source. Insulin, a hormone produced in the pancreas, is essential for the conversion of this glucose into energy. In the diabetic, there is insufficient production of insulin and therefore glucose cannot be converted to energy but instead accumulates in the blood, resulting in symptoms ranging in severity from mental confusion to coma.

The major symptoms of diabetes are excessive thirst, frequent urination, increased appetite, and loss of weight. Other symptoms, though less characteristic of the disease, are muscle cramps, impaired vision, itching of the skin, and poorly healing wounds.

The tendency to develop diabetes frequently seems to be hereditary. Other conditions that contribute to its development are pregnancy, surgery, physical or emotional stress, and obesity. Weight control through proper nutrition is an important factor in the prevention of diabetes.

Methods of medical treatment for diabetes are used in conjunction with a specific diet. In mild cases of the disease, diabetes can be regulated by diet alone. In more severe cases, regulation of the diet is accompanied by oral medication or injections to increase the pancreatic output of insulin. Exercise is a factor in diabetes treatment because it determines insulin needs.

Unless a diabetic is overweight, his caloric intake may remain the same but his calorie sources must be regulated. Since the diabetic cannot properly utilize carbohydrates, their intake must be greatly restricted. Concentrated sources of carbohydrates, such as cakes, cookies, and candy, should be avoided. The diabetic may be allowed some fruits and vegetables because their carbohydrate content is not as great as that of these foods. However, depending upon the individual diet, fruits and vegetables that have the greatest carbohydrate content may have to be avoided also. To maintain his normal caloric intake while restricting his carbohydrates, the diabetic eats a diet that is increased in amount of proteins and unsaturated fats.

Generally, a well-balanced diet rich in vitamins and minerals is one of the most important factors in the control of diabetes. Some authorities find that the diabetic is unable to convert carotene into vitamin A, while others deny such findings. It is advisable, however, for the diabetic to ingest at least the Recommended Dietary Allowance of vitamin A from a noncarotene source, such as fish-liver oil.[14] Because the diabetic, especially when on insulin therapy, loses vitamin C more readily than does the nondiabetic, daily supplementation of vitamin C is necessary. The minerals zinc, chromium, and manganese have been associated with the treatment of diabetes, although their specific effect on the disease has not yet been determined.

NUTRIENTS THAT MAY BE BENEFICIAL IN TREATMENT OF DIABETES

Body Member	Nutrients	Quantity*
Blood/ Circulatory system	Vitamin A	5,000 IU
	Vitamin B complex	
	Vitamin B$_1$	10 mg
	Vitamin B$_2$	10 mg
	Vitamin B$_6$	50-100 mg
	Vitamin B$_{12}$	25 mcg minimum
	Niacin	Up to 100 mg
	Pangamic acid	
	Vitamin C	1,000-3,000 mg
	Vitamin D	400 IU
	Vitamin E	400-1,200 IU
	Vitamin F	Six capsules or 2 tbsp of cold-pressed vegetable oil
	Calcium	
	Chromium	2 mg for six months
	Iron	
	Magnesium	500 mg
	Maganese	
	Potassium	300 mg
	Zinc	
	Protein	

*See note, p. 166.

DIARRHEA

Diarrhea is a condition causing frequent elimination of stools abnormally watery in nature. The condition is fairly common and can exist alone or as a symptom of other diseases. Diarrhea is accompanied by increased

[14]Norman Jollife (ed.), *Clinical Nutrition*, 2d ed. (New York: Harper Bros., 1962), p. 489.

thirst, abdominal cramps and bloating, intestinal rumbling, and loss of appetite.

Because of the decreased appetite associated with diarrhea and rapid expulsion of food through the lower digestive tract, an individual with diarrhea does not properly absorb nutrients and can therefore develop nutrient deficiencies. In addition, the change in consistency of the stool causes the body to lose a great amount of water, a loss that can cause dehydration as well as the loss of minerals and water-soluble vitamins.

The most frequent cause of diarrhea is the presence in the colon of bacteria foreign to the intestinal tract. Bacteria may come from poisoned, poorly refrigerated, undercooked, or partially rancid food. Emotional stress, such as anxiety, is another major cause of diarrhea. Diarrhea can also be brought about by some types of allergic reactions, the prolonged use of laxatives, or a diet that is overly abundant in roughage, which increases the movement of food through the intestines.

Medical treatment of diarrhea may include the prescription of antibiotics to combat bacterial infection or medication to relax the colon muscles. The diet of the diarrhea patient should be low in bulk to decrease the tendency for rapid expulsion but rich in protein, carbohydrates, vitamins, and minerals to compensate for the loss of all nutrients that occurs with the condition. The diet should be supplemented with the water-soluble B-complex vitamins and vitamin C as well as with sodium and potassium, which are bound closely to water and which the body always loses when it becomes dehydrated. An adequate fluid intake is the most essential aspect of the treatment for diarrhea, to replace the water that is lost in the stools, thereby preventing dehydration.

NUTRIENTS THAT MAY BE BENEFICIAL IN TREATMENT OF DIARRHEA

Body Member	Nutrients	Quantity*
Bowel	Vitamin A	25,000 IU
	Vitamin B complex	
	Vitamin B$_1$	200 mg daily reduced to 50 mg after two weeks
	Vitamin B$_2$	10 mg
	Vitamin B$_6$	50-100 mg
	Folic acid	
	Niacin	100 mg three times daily reduced to 100 mg

*See note, p. 166.

Body Member	Nutrients	Quantity
		daily after two weeks
	Pantothenic acid	100 mg
	Vitamin C	1,000-3,000 mg
Cells	Vitamin F	
	Calcium	2 g
	Chlorine	
	Iron	
	Magnesium	500 mg
	Potassium	
	Sodium	
	Carbohydrates (cellulose)	
	Protein	

DIVERTICULITIS

Diverticulitis is the inflammation of the small sacs (diverticula), or out-pouchings, that may be found along the small or large intestine (colon). When empty, the diverticula remain dormant and without complication. However, when food particles get trapped in the sacs and are digested by the bacteria normally present in the colon for this purpose, the digested food particles become stagnant, a situation that leads to inflammation and infection. Diverticulitis may be hereditary, or it may accompany old age, when the muscles of the colon are weakened from years of use.

As diverticulitis becomes more severe, the infection can spread out of the sacs to the rest of the colon and to other organs of the abdomen. In very severe cases, the disease can result in perforation of the wall of the colon, causing severe bleeding for which immediate surgical attention is necessary.

Diverticulitis can manifest itself in a short but severe attack or in a long-term, less severe problem. Symptoms of the disease include cramps and pain in the lower abdomen accompanying bowel movements, abdominal bloating, and the frequent urge to eliminate followed by constipation. If infection ensues, fever can develop.

The most effective prevention for diverticulitis is to avoid constipation. One of the best ways to accomplish this is by a marked increase in fluid intake, which helps to prevent dehydration of intestinal material. A diet moderate in roughage will prevent further accumulation of food in the diverticula. Fruits and vegetables in juice or puree form will provide the body with vitamins and minerals. Supplementing the diet with agar-agar, a sea-weed derivative, can help to increase bulk for movement through the colon.

Because some of the B vitamins are manufactured by the intestinal bacteria, a deficiency may occur if these bacteria are destroyed by the infection. It is therefore necessary that the diet provide adequate amounts of the B vitamins, especially folic acid.

NUTRIENTS THAT MAY BE BENEFICIAL IN TREATMENT OF DIVERTICULITIS

Body Member	Nutrients	Quantity*
Intestine	Vitamin B complex	
	Folic acid	1 mg
	Vitamin C	
	All minerals	
	Carbohydrates (cellulose)	
	Water	

*See note, p. 166.

DIZZINESS/VERTIGO

Dizziness is characterized by a sensation of giddiness, un-steadiness, or light-headedness. The terms "vertigo" and "dizziness" are often used interchangeably, but true vertigo is a sensation of spinning or a feeling that the floors are sinking or rising. True vertigo is usually accompanied by nausea, vomiting, perspiration, and headache.

Dizziness and vertigo both may be caused by infections of or injuries to the inner ear, which normally helps to maintain the body's sense of balance. A physical injury such as a concussion or skull fracture may injure the inner ear; in this type of injury, dizziness may occur long after the injury is supposedly healed. Brain tumors, anemia, high or low blood pressure, lack of oxygen or glucose in the blood, psychological stress, or nutritional deficiencies may be other causes of vertigo.

A deficiency of vitamin B_6 or niacin may cause dizziness. Including these B-complex vitamins in the diet may prevent and alleviate the sensation.

NUTRIENTS THAT MAY BE BENEFICIAL IN TREATMENT OF DIZZINESS/VERTIGO

Body Member	Nutrients	Quantity
Brain/Nervous system	Vitamin B complex	
	Vitamin B_1	
	Vitamin B_2	
	Vitamin B_6	
	Vitamin B_{12}	
	Choline	
	Inositol	
	Niacin	
	Vitamin C	
	Vitamin E	
	Calcium	

DRUG ABUSE OR DEPENDENCY

The use or abuse of drugs, whether illegal or legal, resulting in dependency over a prolonged period may have several detrimental effects on the general state of health of an individual. Research shows that most drugs have definite side effects, including severe depletion of essential nutrients stored in the body.

Continued use of illegal drugs, such as narcotics, stimulants, barbiturates, and hallucinogens, may result in dependency and severe mental and physical deterioration. Prolonged use may result in damage to the cells, chromosome damage, male sterility, and increased risks of cancer.

Of nearly as great a concern is the problem of indiscriminate use of legal drugs, both prescription and patent medicines. The classic example is the common aspirin tablet. Although many people consider average doses of aspirin completely harmless, researchers invariably discover that when taken in daily doses such as those used to relieve the pain of arthritis, aspirin causes irritation to the stomach lining and varying amounts of internal bleeding. This bleeding may be extensive enough to cause slight anemia. Aspirin-induced irritation of the stomach and accompanying internal bleeding may be very dangerous to ulcer sufferers. There may also be instances of severe allergic reactions to aspirin itself.

Especially dangerous is the habitual use of combinations of drugs such as sleeping pills to go to sleep, stimulants to wake up in the morning, and alcohol to calm down in the midafternoon. A person following such a daily pattern may be just as "hooked" on drugs as any recognized addict. In fact, the taking of such substances as alcohol and sleeping pills (barbiturates) together may so severely depress the body functions as to cause death.

It should be stressed that drugs may produce dietary deficiencies by destroying nutrients, preventing their absorption, and increasing their excretion. Also, many drugs depress the appetite; therefore people who become reliant upon drugs tend to eat inadequately, thus depriving themselves of the essential nutrients necessary for good health.

EAR INFECTION

An ear infection can occur in any of the three sections within the ear. The outer ear is that section which is visible, plus the ear canal, a skin-lined tube that ends at a disk known as the eardrum. The middle ear is composed of three small bones that lie on the inward side of the eardrum. These bones connect with the inner ear, which changes sound waves into nerve impulses and sends them to the brain.

Infection in the outer ear is usually caused by swimming in contaminated water or by damage to the wall of the ear canal. A symptom of the infection is severe pain, possibly accompanied by fever.

Infection in the middle ear is most frequently due to the spread of bacteria to the ear from infection in the nose and throat. Symptoms include earache, a feeling of fullness in the ear, diminished hearing, and fever.

Infection in the inner ear usually arises from meningitis or from the spread of a middle-ear infection. Symptoms include loss of hearing, dizziness, nausea, vomiting, and fever. Severe ear infections may result in permanent scarring and partial or total loss of hearing.

Medical treatment for ear infection involves rest, warmth applied to the ear, antibiotics, and surgical draining of the infected area. Nutritionally, the body's needs for vitamins A and C are increased during a fever. A well-balanced diet adequate in protein is necessary to help the body fight infection and repair damaged tissue.

NUTRIENTS THAT MAY BE BENEFICIAL IN TREATMENT OF EAR INFECTION

Body Member	Nutrient	Quantity*
Ear	Vitamin A	50,000 IU
	Vitamin C	
	Protein	

*See note, p. 166.

ECZEMA

Eczema is a skin condition characterized by inflammatory itching and the formation of scales. Sometimes eczema is related to an allergic reaction. Vitamins A and C together with the B-complex vitamins are helpful in the prevention and healing of eczema.

NUTRIENTS THAT MAY BE BENEFICIAL IN TREATMENT OF ECZEMA

Body Member	Nutrients	Quantity*
Skin	Vitamin A	50,000-75,000 IU for two to three months; 25,000 IU for next few months if condition does not clear up
	Vitamin B complex	
	Vitamin B$_6$	
	Biotin	
	Choline	
	Inositol	500 mg
	Vitamin C	Up to 1,000 mg
	Vitamin D	800 IU
	Vitamin F	
	Sulfur	Ointment

*See note, p. 166.

EDEMA (SWELLING)

Edema is a condition in which excess fluid is retained by the body, either localized in one area or generalized throughout the body. This retention of fluids appears as swelling. Swelling is most often seen in the hands, in the feet, or around the eyes, but it may be located in any area of the body.

Disorders that can cause edema are poor kidney functioning, congestive heart failure, protein or thiamine deficiency, varicose veins, phlebitis, or sodium retention. Other factors that may cause edema are standing for long periods of time, pregnancy, premenstrual tension, the use of oral contraceptives, injury to an area of the body (such as a sprain), or allergic reactions (such as an insect bite).

If edema is the result of protein or thiamine deficiency, correction of the deficiency is essential. Sodium, as found in table salt, is often restricted in diets of individuals who are prone to edema because excess sodium causes the body to retain water. Individuals who are prone to edema should try to promote good circulation by elevating the legs while at rest, exercising regularly, avoiding restrictive clothing, and refraining from crossing the legs.

An increase in vitamin B_6 intake reduces fluid retention. The recommended supplemental source of B_6 is dessicated liver.

NUTRIENTS THAT MAY BE BENEFICIAL IN TREATMENT OF EDEMA

Body Member	Nutrient	Quantity*
General	Vitamin B complex	
	Vitamin B_1	
	Vitamin B_6	50-200 mg
	Vitamin C	2,000-5,000 mg
	Vitamin E	
	Copper	
	Potassium	
	Protein	
	Low sodium	

*See note, p. 166.

EMPHYSEMA

Emphysema is characterized by abnormal swelling and destruction of the tiny air sacs of the lungs. These sacs become thin and stretch, thus losing their elasticity. This results in an accumulation of used air in the lungs and leads to a decreased ability to utilize fresh air.

Factors that may contribute to the onset of emphysema are exposure to various dusts, cigarette smoking, bronchitis, asthma, or other respiratory diseases. Symptoms of the condition include wheezing, shortness of breath and difficulty in breathing, and coughing often accompanied by mucus. Weight loss occurs as the condition progresses, and the victim may develop a characteristic "barrel chest."

Vitamins A and C provide some protection against emphysema for cigarette smokers by helping to maintain healthy tissues in the respiratory passage. The vitamin B complex and protein are necessary to strengthen the deteriorating tissue. Since the emphysema victim suffers from a lack of oxygen, many authorities suggest that vitamin E may be beneficial.[15]

[15]Spencer H. Robley, *Emphysema and Common Sense* (West Nyack, N.Y.: Parker Publ. Co., 1968), p. 144.

NUTRIENTS THAT MAY BE BENEFICIAL IN TREATMENT OF EMPHYSEMA

Body Member	Nutrients	Quantity*
Lungs/ Respiratory system	Vitamin A	50,000 IU
	Vitamin B complex	
	Folic acid	
	Pangamic acid	50 mg three times daily
	Vitamin C	3,000-5,000 mg
	Vitamin D	
	Vitamin E	Up to 16,000 IU
	Protein	

*See note, p. 166.

EPILEPSY

Epilepsy is a disease characterized by seizures. There are two forms of seizures. A sensory seizure involves only a change in sensation or a loss of consciousness, while a convulsive seizure (convulsion) involves abnormal muscular behavior. Epileptic seizures are caused by an electrical disturbance in the nerve cells in one section of the brain and may be the result of such factors as head injury or infection, rabies, tetanus, meningitis, rickets, malnutrition, hypoglycemia, or fever.

Epilepsy occurs in both sexes and at all ages. An individual may experience only one seizure in his lifetime or several seizures per day. Factors that may precipitate a seizure are fatigue, overeating or overdrinking, emotional tension or excitement, fever, new environmental stresses, or menstruation.

The epileptic should maintain a well-balanced diet and should avoid taking in excessive amounts of food or fluid at one time, because these may bring on an attack. Alcoholic beverages should also be avoided. Regular exercise and rest should be encouraged.

Anticonvulsive drugs are effective in preventing most seizures. However, for children with petite mal epilepsy—characterized by brief losses of consciousness lasting from 5 to 30 seconds, accompanied by twitching of the eyeballs—a ketogenic diet may be beneficial when there is no response to drug therapy. A ketogenic diet is used in less than 8 percent of all epilepsy cases and must be administered under medical supervision. It consists of restricting protein and carbohydrate intake and increasing fat intake, producing acid levels in the bloodstream which act to inhibit brain stimulation of seizures.

NUTRIENTS THAT MAY BE BENEFICIAL IN TREATMENT OF EPILEPSY

Body Member	Nutrients	Quantity*
Brain/ Nervous system	Vitamin A	10,000 IU (one capsule)
	Vitamin B complex	
	Vitamin B_6	100 mg under doctor's supervision, up to 300 mg
	Vitamin B_{12}	25 mcg
	Folic acid	0.5 mg
	Niacin	50 mg
	Pangamic acid	50 mg twice daily
	Pantothenic acid	50 mg twice daily
	Vitamin C	2,000 mg
	Vitamin D	1,000 IU (one capsule)
	Vitamin E	Begin dosage at 300 IU; increase up to 2,000 IU
	Calcium	1,000 mg
	Magnesium	800 mg; for children 500 mg
	Fats	
	Low carbohydrates	
	Low protein	

*See note, p. 166.

EYESTRAIN

The human eyes are marvelously adaptable and sensitive organs, but they can be abused by using them excessively in improper light. Too little light, glaring light and reflections, shadows on work areas, and flickering light such as that from some fluorescent tubes cause the eyes to make numerous unnecessary adjustments that may lead to eyestrain. Eyestrain may also be a result of uncorrected eyesight; eyes should be checked regularly by an eye specialist for any corrections or adjustments that should be made.

Frequent relaxation of the eyes, especially by changing the range of focus by looking up and away from your work towards a distant object, may alleviate strain caused by improper light and headaches caused by nervous tension.

Vitamin A, the B complex, and vitamin C are especially important in the maintenance of good eye health.

NUTRIENTS THAT MAY BE BENEFICIAL IN TREATMENT OF EYESTRAIN

Body Member	Nutrients	Quantity*
Eye	Vitamin A	
	Vitamin B complex	
	Vitamin C	Large doses
	Vitamin D	
	Vitamin E	

*See note, p. 166.

FATIGUE

Fatigue is a feeling of physical and mental weariness which may be caused by a variety of conditions, such as anemia, physical exertion, nutrient deficiency, weight loss, obesity, boredom or emotional tension, or almost any disease process. In addition to a feeling of weariness, symptoms of fatigue include headache, backache, irritability, and indigestion.

Adequate rest, exercise, and a well-balanced diet can prevent fatigue. Reducing to a normal weight is necessary when overweight is present. Deficiencies of the vitamin B complex, vitamins C and D, or iron may cause fatigue and therefore should be corrected.

NUTRIENTS THAT MAY BE BENEFICIAL IN TREATMENT OF FATIGUE

Body Member	Nutrients	Quantity
General	Vitamin A	
	Vitamin B complex	
	Folic acid	
	Vitamin C	
	Vitamin D	
	Iron	
	Manganese	
	Carbohydrate (cellulose)	

FEVER

Fever is the elevation of body temperature above normal. Normal temperature varies from individual to individual, although normal is generally considered to be within the range of 97° to 99°F. When the body temperature is raised not more than 5°, the rise does not completely interfere with bodily functions. However, when fever reaches 106°F, convulsions are common, and if fever should reach 108°F, irreversible brain damage frequently results.

Fever accompanies a wide variety of diseases ranging from mild to severe and can be considered a warning that something is wrong within the body. Symptoms associated with fever include flushed face, headache, nausea, body aches, little or no appetite, and occasionally, diarrhea or vomiting. The skin may be either hot and dry or warm to the touch with some degree of perspiring. Perspiration is the natural result of the body's attempt to lower its temperature.

Because fever increases the body's use of energy, the caloric needs are greatly increased and intake should be adjusted accordingly. Additional protein is needed to replace and rebuild the damaged body tissue and to form antibodies, substances manufactured by the body to fight infection. A high fluid intake is necessary to compensate for the loss that occurs with fever. Sodium and potassium are lost when fluid is lost; therefore their replacement is also necessary during fever. The increased energy expenditure that occurs during fever increases metabolism; because vitamin A, the B complex, and vitamin C are involved in the process of metabolism, deficiencies of these nutrients may arise also. The vitamin B complex especially should be increased during an extended fever since these vitamins may stimulate the appetite. Additional calcium may also be required because of its decreased absorption during fever.

NUTRIENTS THAT MAY BE BENEFICIAL IN TREATMENT OF FEVER

Body Member	Nutrients	Quantity
General/Head	Vitamin A	
	Vitamin B complex	
	Vitamin B_1	
	Vitamin C	
	Vitamin D	
	Calcium	
	Phosphorus	
	Potassium	
	Sodium	
	Protein	

FRACTURE (BROKEN BONE)

A fracture is any break in a bone. When the bone breaks but the skin remains intact, the fracture is called "closed" or "simple." When the bone breaks through the skin, an opening for bacteria is created and the fracture is called "open" or "compound."

Most fractures occur as the result of an accident, but some occur because of tumors, osteoporosis, or deficiencies of vitamin D or calcium. Fracture symptoms include limb deformities, limited limb functioning, shortening of the limb in fractures of long bones, pain, a grating sensation if the broken bone ends rub against each other, and swelling and discoloration of the skin overlying the fracture area.

First aid treatment for fractures should include covering any wound and immobilizing or splinting the broken part in the position it was found. Medical treatment involves replacing the bone pieces into their normal position.

In the healing process, a bridge of tissue composed largely of protein fibers grows across the ends of the broken bones. Calcium and phosphorus then deposit among these protein fibers to form a new bone. The diet must therefore be high in protein and adequate in calcium and phosphorus. However, calcium intake should not be unusually high because a high calcium intake may promote kidney stone formation during the immobile period while the cast is on. Vitamin D intake must be adequate because it is essential for the absorption of calcium and phosphorus. Potassium is required for cell formation, vitamin C is necessary for the maintenance and development of bones, and vitamin A helps to increase the rate of bone growth. The diet should be high in calories to provide the energy necessary for new bone cell formation.

NUTRIENTS THAT MAY BE BENEFICIAL IN TREATMENT OF FRACTURE

Body Member	Nutrients	Quantity*
Bones	Vitamin A	
	Pantothenic acid	

*See note, p. 166.

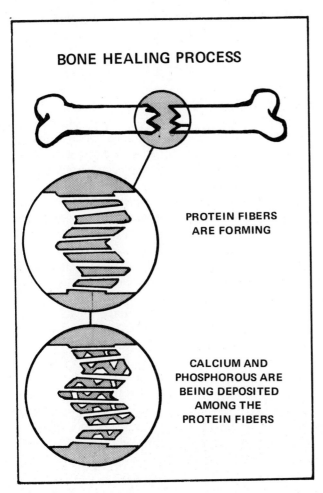

BONE HEALING PROCESS

PROTEIN FIBERS
ARE FORMING

CALCIUM AND
PHOSPHOROUS ARE
BEING DEPOSITED
AMONG THE
PROTEIN FIBERS

Body Member	Nutrients	Quantity
	Vitamin C	
	Vitamin D	
	Calcium	
	Phosphorus	
	Potassium	
	Magnesium	500 mg
	Protein	160 g

GALLSTONES

Gallstones develop when deposits of cholesterol or calcium combine with bile. Bile is a secretion produced by the liver to emulsify fats so that they can be digested. Most of the bile manufactured by the liver is stored in the gallbladder until the small intestine calls for it when fat has been ingested. However, some bile travels directly from the liver to the small intestine. Gallstones may form in the passages between liver and gallbladder, between liver and intestine, or in the gallbladder itself.

Gallstones are more frequently found in diabetics, obese persons, elderly people, and females, especially those who have had children. Although the exact reason for this stone formation is still unknown, there are certain predisposing conditions, such as any infection in the body and long periods of inactivity or bed rest.

Nearly half of all gallstone patients are without symptoms. It is when a stone obstructs any of the bile passages that symptoms occur. These symptoms characteristically include nausea, vomiting, and severe right upper abdominal pain that may radiate to the right shoulder or back. The symptoms commonly occur a few hours after eating a heavy meal of fatty or fried foods. If the stone totally obstructs one of the bile passages, jaundice (a yellowish cast to the skin and eyeballs), dark urine, clay-colored stools, and itching of the skin may also occur.

Medical treatment for gallstones may involve a modification of diet or surgery. Persons suffering from gallstones should avoid large meals, fats, and other foods that aggravate the conditions. This type of diet is helpful in avoiding the abdominal discomfort (bloating, belching, heartburn) that commonly occurs several hours after eating. A diet high in protein and carbohydrates and low in fats is generally recommended to meet the person's nutritional needs. Fluid intake should be frequent. Since the gallstone patient may have impaired absorption of fats, particular attention to the adequate ingestion of the fat-soluble vitamins A, D, E, and K is imperative to avoid their depletion and deficiency.

**NUTRIENTS THAT MAY BE BENEFICIAL
IN TREATMENT OF GALLSTONES**

Body Member	Nutrients	Quantity
Gallbladder	Vitamin A	
	Vitamin B complex	
	Vitamin C	
	Vitamin D	
	Vitamin E	
	Vitamin K	
	High carbohydrates	
	High protein	
	Low fat	

GASTRITIS

Gastritis is a disease in which the mucous lining of the stomach becomes irritated and inflamed. If gastritis is prolonged, the stomach walls become very thin, secreting almost entirely mucus and very little digestive acid. In this condition the stomach is unable to produce the intrinsic factor, a substance necessary for the absoprtion of vitamin B_{12}, which the body needs for the formation of red blood cells. Thus the gastritis patient is in danger of developing pernicious anemia.

Symptoms of gastritis include dyspepsia or indigestion, vomiting, headache, coated tongue, and abnormal increase or decrease in appetite. Diarrhea and abdominal cramps also may occur.

Although the specific cause of gastritis is unknown, it appears to result from overindulgence in alcohol, coffee, or highly seasoned or fried foods, all of which increase the activity of the stomach, thereby irritating it more. Eating rancid foods can cause bacterial infection, which may cause gastritis. Recurring cases of gastritis may be the result of ulcers or of the buildup of poisonous body wastes due to such diseases as chronic uremia or cirrhosis of the liver.

The diet in treating gastritis should be bland. Roughage, fried foods, and highly seasoned foods should be avoided. Alcohol, coffee, aspirin, and other substances that irritate the stomach lining must be eliminated. Frequent small meals are easier for the stomach to digest than fewer large meals. If gastritis is severe, iron supplements and injections of vitamin B_{12} may be helpful for preventing pernicious anemia.

NUTRIENTS THAT MAY BE BENEFICIAL IN TREATMENT OF GASTRITIS

Body Member	Nutrients	Quantity
Stomach	Vitamin A	
	Vitamin B complex	
	Vitamin B_6	
	Vitamin B_{12}	
	Folic acid	
	Inositol	
	Pantothenic acid	
	Vitamin D	
	Vitamin E	
	Lecithin	
	Linoleic acid	

Body Member	Nutrients	Qualtity
	Iron	
	Low cellulose (a carbohydrate)	

GASTROENTERITIS (STOMACH FLU)

Gastroenteritis, or stomach flu, is the inflammation of the lining of the stomach. The inflammation has a variety of causes, such as food poisoning, certain viruses, alcohol intoxication, sensitivity to drugs, and allergies. Symptoms of gastroenteritis include diarrhea, vomiting, possible fever, chills, and abdominal cramps that vary in severity, but recovery is usually within one or two days.

Treatment for stomach flu includes bed rest and abstention from food until the stomach can tolerate it. A regular well-balanced diet should then be introduced as soon as possible. Repeated vomiting and diarrhea can cause potassium and fluid loss, which should be corrected as soon as possible. If fever is present, intake of vitamins A and C should be increased.

NUTRIENTS THAT MAY BE BENEFICIAL IN TREATMENT OF GASTROENTERITIS

Body Member	Nutrients	Quantity
Stomach	Vitamin A	
	Vitamin C	
	Potassium	

GLAUCOMA

Glaucoma is characterized by an increase in pressure of the fluid within the eyeball and a hardening of the surface of the eyeball. The cause of glaucoma is currently unknown, but usually it occurs after age forty and it may be due to tumor, trauma, infection, and in one type, heredity. Glaucoma is often associated with anxiety and stress, allergy, or hormone disorders. Symptoms include eye discomfort or pain, especially in the morning, blurred vision, halos around lights, inability to adjust to a darkened room, and loss of vision at the sides. Early detection of glaucoma can substantially reduce the incidence of blindness resulting from it.

Glaucoma cannot be cured, but it can be controlled through the use of prescribed eye drops. The diet of those affected should be rich in vitamin A, essential for eye-tissue health. If the symptoms of anxiety are related to a deficiency of the B vitamins, then correction of this deficiency would decrease the susceptibility of an individual to glaucoma. Alcohol, tobacco, coffee, and tea should be avoided.

NUTRIENTS THAT MAY BE BENEFICIAL IN TREATMENT OF GLAUCOMA

Body Member	Nutrients	Quantity*
Eye	Vitamin A	25,000 IU
	Vitamin B complex	
	Vitamin B$_2$	
	Choline	Up to 2 g
	Inositol	
	Vitamin C	60-250 mg per lb of body weight
	Vitamin D	
	Bioflavonoids	

*See note, p. 166.

GOITER

A goiter is an enlargement of the thyroid gland. The thyroid gland is located at the base of the neck. Its chief function is to regulate the rate of metabolism. Goiter may be caused by a lack of iodine in the diet, inflammation of the thyroid gland due to infection, or under- or overproduction of hormones by the thyroid gland.

Symptoms of goiter are a swelling at the base of the neck, hoarseness, change in the rate of metabolism, and in extreme cases, difficulty in swallowing and breathing. Treatment of goiter varies with the cause. If goiter is due to an iodine deficiency, increasing the intake of iodine will prevent further enlargement of the gland and, in some cases, reduce its size. The use of iodized salt has helped to eliminate goiter in many places where iodine does not occur naturally in foods.

NUTRIENTS THAT MAY BE BENEFICIAL IN TREATMENT OF GOITER

Body Member	Nutrients	Quantity
Thyroid	Vitamin A	
	Vitamin C	
	Calcium	
	Iodine	

GOUT

Gout is a metabolic disturbance characterized by an excess of uric acid in the blood and deposits of uric acid salts in the tissue around the joints, especially in the fingers and the toes. It can also occur in the heel, knee, hand, ear, or any joint in the body.

Gout results when certain crystals are formed as an end product of improper protein metabolism. These crystals are deposited in a joint, forming a bump or growth that irritates the joint, causing it to become inflamed; thus an attack of gout occurs.

A gout attack begins with pain in the inflamed joint which may spread to other joints of the body. Pain is greatest in the early morning and finally abates later in the day. An attack usually lasts from 5 to 12 days and may recur months later.

Although the exact cause of gout is unknown, it most often appears to be hereditary. However, factors such as obesity, increasing age, and improper diet increase an individual's susceptibility to gout. Alcohol, a large meal, or any physical or emotional stress also may bring on an attack of gout.

Medical treatment for gout involves prescription of drugs to decrease the inflammation and pain, and encouragement of regular patterns of exercise, rest, and diet. A therapeutic diet should be moderate in protein and low in fats. Foods that have a high content of purine, forerunner of uric acid, should be avoided. One such type of food is organ meats. Because a low-purine diet is normally lacking in the vitamin B complex and vitamin E, special attention should be paid to including these vitamins in the diet. Emphasis should be placed on including adequate intake of fluids to prevent the buildup of the gout-producing crystals in the kidneys. A gradual weight-reduction program for overweight individuals will help prevent gout attacks, while a rapid weight loss may bring on attacks, due to the stressful effect on the body. Pantothenic acid especially aids in the metabolic functioning of the cells.

NUTRIENTS THAT MAY BE BENEFICIAL IN TREATMENT OF GOUT

Body Member	Nutrient	Quantity*
Joints	Vitamin A	
	Vitamin B complex	
	Pantothenic acid	
	Vitamin C	Up to 5,000 mg

*See note, p. 166.

Body Member	Nutrients	Quantity
	Vitamin E	
	Calcium	
	Iron	
	Magnesium	
	Phosphorus	
	Potassium	Two tablets

HAIR PROBLEMS

Hair is composed primarily of protein. A deficiency of protein in the diet can result in a temporary change of hair color and texture, resulting in dull, thin, dry hair. If the protein deficiency is corrected, the hair will return to its normal condition.

A deficiency of vitamin A may cause hair to become dull, dry and lusterless and eventually to fall out. However, an excess of vitamin A may cause similar problems. Deficiencies of the vitamin B complex and vitamin C have also been associated with poor appearance of hair.[16]

A well-balanced diet is important to maintain healthy hair, although hereditary graying and balding cannot be completely prevented by nutritional means.

Good hygiene is also important for healthy hair. This includes brushing the hair properly and washing it with mild shampoo. Exposure to wind and sun may cause brittle, broken hair.

NUTRIENTS THAT MAY BE BENEFICIAL IN TREATMENT OF HAIR PROBLEMS

Body Member	Nutrients	Quantity
Hair	Vitamin A	
	Vitamin B complex	
	Vitamin C	
	Iodine	
	Protein	

HALITOSIS

Halitosis is an unpleasant odor of the breath. It may be caused by improper diet, poor mouth hygiene, nose or throat infections, extensive teeth or gum decay, excessive smoking, or the presence of bacteria that are foreign to the mouth.

Treatment for halitosis involves proper mouth hy-

giene, including regular tooth brushing. Often the use of dental floss is recommended. A carefully balanced diet is essential for the prevention of halitosis. Avoiding excessive consumption of carbohydrates may help prevent tooth decay that can cause bad breath. Vitamin C is needed to prevent scurvy, which can cause the gums to bleed and become infected. Vitamin A is necessary for the overall development and health of the gums and teeth.

NUTRIENTS THAT MAY BE BENEFICIAL IN TREATMENT OF HALITOSIS

Body Member	Nutrients	Quantity*
Mouth	Vitamin A	
	Vitamin B complex	
	Vitamin B_6	50 mg
	Niacin	
	Vitamin C	1,000 or more mg

*See note, p. 166.

HAY FEVER (ALLERGIC RHINITIS)

Hay fever is a reaction of the mucous membranes of the eyes, nose, and air passages to seasonal pollens and dust, feathers, animal hair, and other irritants. Hay-fever symptoms include itching in the eyes, nose, and throat, a clear, watery discharge from the nose and eyes, frequent sneezing, and nervous irritability. Alcoholic beverages and stressful situations may precipitate an attack of hay fever.

The most effective treatment for hay fever is to avoid the irritant. Vitamin A is essential for the general health of the respiratory system. Some authorities believe that vitamin C in doses of 200 or more milligrams daily can relieve hay-fever symptoms.[17]

NUTRIENTS THAT MAY BE BENEFICIAL IN TREATMENT OF HAY FEVER

Body Member	Nutrients	Quantity*
Lungs/ Respiratory system	Vitamin A	100,000 IU for four months
	Vitamin B complex	
	Vitamin C	100-1,000 mg daily
	Vitamin E	

*See note, p. 166.

[16]Ruth Adams and Frank Murray, *Body, Mind and the B Vitamins* (New York: Larchmont Books, 1962), pp. 227-228.

[17]Guthrie, *Introductory Nutrition*, p. 225.

HEADACHE

A headache is a pain or ache in any portion of the head. It is a symptom rather than a disease in itself. Headache is most frequently a sign of emotional stress or tension. However, there are many other possible causes of headache, such as diseases of the eye, nose, or throat; trauma to the head; air pollution or poor ventilation; drugs; alcohol; tobacco; fever; generalized body infections; disturbances of the digestive tract and circulatory system; brain disorders; anemia; low blood sugar; niacin or pantothenic acid deficiency; or an overdose of vitamin A.

A migraine is a particular type of headache due to the alternating constriction and dilation of the blood vessels in the brain. The exact cause of migraine is unknown, although as in the case of most headaches, emotional stress usually plays a large role. The symptoms of migraine include either generalized or one-sided head pain and possibly nausea, vomiting, and visual disturbances. A migraine attack may last for hours or days.

Treatment for headache depends upon the underlying cause. Repeated headaches may be a symptom of a serious disorder and therefore deserve attention, or they may be the result of stress. Learning better ways of coping with stress and relieving nervous tension is often the most effective treatment for headaches and migraine. Special attention should be paid to prevent deficiencies of iron, niacin, and pantothenic acid. Vitamin A may also prove helpful to some headache victims. Treatment for migraine may include pain-relieving drugs and the entire B complex for health of the nerves.

NUTRIENTS THAT MAY BE BENEFICIAL IN TREATMENT OF HEADACHE

Body Member	Nutrients	Quantity*
Head	Vitamin A	
	Vitamin B complex	
	Vitamin B_1	
	Vitamin B_2	10 mg per meal
	Vitamin B_6	50 mg
	Niacin	100 mg three times daily
	Pangamic acid	100 mg
	Pantothenic acid	100 mg
	Vitamin C	Up to 1,000 mg
	Vitamin E	Up to 1,200 IU
	Calcium	
	Potassium	

*See note, p. 166.

HEART DISEASE

The heart is the chief organ of the circulatory system; it is the most delicate and yet the most durable because it is made of the toughest muscle fibers of the body. The heart is a very efficient pump, but over a million Americans die of heart disease each year.

Some of the major ailments connected with the heart are the following: A *coronary thrombosis* is the formation of a blood clot that blocks the artery leading to the heart. Although this type of heart disease is the greatest single killer in the world today, 50 percent of the victims of coronary thrombosis survive. Those who survive usually have damaged heart muscle because there is no replacement for the artery that flows into the heart. If a blood clot slips into the coronary artery and partially blocks the main artery, the attack is not fatal; complete blockage is fatal.

A *coronary occlusion* results if the clot blocks a small branch artery and the part of the heart that receives nourishment from that branch dies. The heart and brain are the only two organs susceptible to occlusion.

Coronary sclerosis, a restriction of the coronary blood supply to the heart muscle due to thickening and hardening of the blood vessels (sclerosis), results in the severe pain *angina pectoris*. This pain develops whenever the working demand exceeds the supply of oxygen to the heart. High blood pressure generally is an accompanying condition of coronary sclerosis.

A *stroke* occurs when the blood supply to the brain, or to some portion of it, is cut off. This usually takes place in the cerebrum, that part of the brain where nerve centers controlling sight, hearing, speech, and body movements are located. If a blockage stops blood flow to one of these control zones or to nerve fibers leading from the zones, the activity controlled by the zone will be impaired.

Some physicians believe that emotional stress is the main cause of *arteriosclerosis* (hardening of the arteries) because stress raises blood pressure. It is not normally high blood pressure, but the characteristic fluctuations in pressure caused by stress and strain, which damage the artery walls.

A nutritionally balanced diet is important for efficient operation of the heart. Protein foods and fresh fruits and vegetables should be substituted for high intake of starches, sweets, and hydrogenated fats. Protein is essential to the strength of all muscles, including the heart. An overconsumption of fat is believed to be detrimental because it may weaken arteries, reduce their elasticity, and clog them with cholesterol. Supplementary intake of vitamin E is needed as an anticoagulant to reduce arterial clots and as an oxygen conserver to keep oxygen in the blood. Vitamin E, through interaction with vitamin F, also allows for the reduction of cholesterol. This will prevent the metabolic imbalance that causes cholesterol to collect in the arteries. A deficient operation of the thyroid gland may be involved in some cases of faulty fat metabolism. Vitamin C and the B vitamins are necessary to maintain arterial health.

A pulse rate of about 70 beats per minute for men and 80 beats per minute for women is best for the heart. A pulse rate of 100 is usually considered abnormally high, although there are variations in normal rates. To lower a pulse rate, reduce the intake of food, avoid emotional stress, and curtail use of drugs, alcoholic drinks, and tobacco products. It should be remembered that substances to which one is allergic will raise the pulse rate and thus produce further stress on the heart.

Overweight can be a contributing factor to both high pulse rate and high blood pressure: excess pounds greatly tax the heart and the circulatory system in general. A properly balanced diet will lead to reduction of pounds without the adverse symptoms experienced when eating only one or two foods as is common in many fad diets.

Stress may raise blood pressure as well as pulse rate. Fluctuations of blood pressure against artery walls contribute to arterial injury and hardening. Exercise is an excellent way to deal with stress and improve muscle tone of the heart and entire body. Unless otherwise advised by your physician, begin walking for ten minutes a day and gradually increase up to one hour. Walking should be at a brisk pace but must be begun slowly. Strenuous exercise (work or recreation) to which one is not accustomed should be avoided because the heart may not be able to meet the unusual requirements made upon it. (See also "Arteriosclerosis" and "Cerebrovascular Accident.")

NUTRIENTS THAT MAY BE BENEFICIAL IN TREATMENT OF HEART DISEASE

Body Member	Nutrients	Quantity*
Heart/Blood/ Circulatory system	Vitamin B complex Vitamin B$_6$ Choline Inositol	100 mg

*See note, p. 166.

Body Member	Nutrients	Quantity
	Niacin	100 mg
	Pantothenic acid	
	Vitamin C	
	Vitamin E	300-400 IU
	Vitamin F	
	Calcium	1,000 mg
	Iodine	
	Lecithin	
	Magnesium	500 or more mg
	Phosphorus	

HEMOPHILIA

Hemophilia is a hereditary blood disease characterized by a prolonged coagulation time. The blood fails to clot, and abnormal bleeding occurs. Hemophilia is a sex-linked hereditary trait, transmitted by normal females carrying the recessive gene. This disease occurs almost exclusively in males. There is no known cure for hemophilia. Transfusion of fresh whole blood or plasma is required in emergencies to provide the necessary coagulation factors.

NUTRIENTS THAT MAY BE BENEFICIAL IN TREATMENT OF HEMOPHILIA

Body Member	Nutrients	Quantity
Blood/Circulatory system	Niacin Vitamin C Bioflavonoids Vitamin T Calcium	

HEMORRHOIDS (PILES)

Hemorrhoids are ruptured or distended veins located around the anus. The most common cause of hemorrhoids is strain on the abdominal muscles due to factors such as heavy or improper lifting, pregnancy, overweight, constipation, or an extremely sedentary life. Symptoms of hemorrhoids are local itching, pain, and the passage of bloody stools.

Treatment for severe hemorrhoids may involve surgical removal. Individuals with hemorrhoids should maintain a diet with large amounts of fluid to avoid constipation. Preventive measures include adequate exercise to strengthen abdominal muscles and avoidance of constipation.

NUTRIENTS THAT MAY BE BENEFICIAL IN TREATMENT OF HEMORRHOIDS

Body Member	Nutrients	Quantity*
Intestine	Vitamin A	25,000 IU
	Vitamin B complex	
	Vitamin B$_6$	25 mg after each meal
	Vitamin C	1,000-2,000 mg
	Vitamin E	600 IU
	Bioflavonoids	
	Calcium	
	Fluids (water)	
	Low cellulose (a carbohydrate)	

*See note, p. 166.

HEPATITIS

Hepatitis is an inflammation of the liver caused by infection or toxic agents. It begins with flulike symptoms of fever, weakness, drowsiness, abdominal discomfort, and headache, possibly accompanied by jaundice.

Infectious hepatitis is excreted in the feces two to three weeks before and up to one week after the appearance of jaundice, although many patients, particularly children, never develop jaundice. Toxic hepatitis may be caused by a wide variety of chemicals taken into the system by injection, ingestion, or skin absorption. The extent of the damage is related to the dose of the substance.

NUTRIENTS THAT MAY BE BENEFICIAL IN TREATMENT OF HEPATITIS

Body Member	Nutrients	Quantity*
General/Liver	Vitamin A	
	Pangamic acid	
	Vitamin C	10 g
	Vitamin F	

*See note, p. 166.

HYPERTENSION (HIGH BLOOD PRESSURE)

Hypertension is an abnormal elevation of blood pressure. The cause is generally unknown, but hypertension often accompanies arteriosclerosis or kidney diseases.

Symptoms of hypertension may be nonexistent, or they may include headache, nervousness, insomnia, nosebleeds, blurred vision, edema, and shortness of breath. Factors associated with the onset of hypertension are heredity, obesity, physical or emotional stress, high salt intake, cigarette smoking, and excessive use of stimulants such as coffee, tea, or drugs.

Stress is an important factor to be considered in hypertension. Many people drive themselves too hard and consequently become hypertensive. These people must learn to avoid stressful conditions by changing their lifestyle. They should take regular, unhurried meals, try to avoid worry, allow themselves plenty of leisure time, take vacations, and generally use moderation in all things. If their occupation involves excessive emotional and physical stress, they may have to consider changing it or adjusting it to make it less stressful.

Sodium is a primary cause of hypertension because it causes fluid retention, which adds additional stress to the heart and circulatory system. Increasing the potassium intake will cause the body to excrete more sodium. Vitamin C can help to maintain the health of the blood vessels that are strained by the greater pressure placed on them by hypertension.

Regular exercise is essential in preventing high blood pressure because it keeps the circulatory system healthy. Promoting a tranquil outlook on life is of primary importance in reducing and preventing hypertension.

NUTRIENTS THAT MAY BE BENEFICIAL IN TREATMENT OF HYPERTENSION

Body Member	Nutrients	Quantity*
Blood/ Circulatory system/ Heart	Vitamin B complex	
	Choline	
	Inositol	
	Niacin	
	Pangamic acid	
	Vitamin C	1,000-3,000 mg
	Vitamin E	100-600 IU
	Bioflavonoids	100-300 mg

*See note, p. 166.

Body Member	Nutrients	Quantity
	Calcium	8 g three times daily
	Lecithin	
	Magnesium	500 mg
	Protein	
	Low sodium	Less than 300 mg daily

HYPERTHYROIDISM

Hyperthyroidism is overproduction of hormones by the thyroid gland. Symptoms of the condition are nervousness, irritability, fatigue, weakness, loss of weight, goiter, and rapid pulse. Hyperthyroidism can be caused by hereditary factors, emotional stress, or other unknown factors.

The excess production of thyroid hormones speeds up all body processes. As a result, all nutrients in the body are used up at a greater rate. The diet should therefore be increased in all nutrients. If weight loss has been great, additional protein may be necessary to replace muscle tissue that may have been lost. Particular attention should be paid to the adequate intake of the vitamin B complex because it is needed for the metabolism of the extra carbohydrates and protein. Coffee and tea containing caffeine should be avoided because caffeine increases the metabolic rate, thereby resulting in more calories being expended. Nicotine and the initial effects of alcohol also increase the metabolic rate and should be avoided.

NUTRIENTS THAT MAY BE BENEFICIAL IN TREATMENT OF HYPERTHYROIDISM

Body Member	Nutrients	Quantity*
Gland, thyroid	Vitamin A	100,000 IU
	Vitamin B complex	
	Choline	
	Inositol	
	Vitamin C	
	Vitamin E	1,000 IU
	Calcium	
	Iodine	4-6 mg
	Carbohydrates	
	Protein	

*See note, p. 166.

HYPOGLYCEMIA (LOW BLOOD SUGAR)

Hypoglycemia is an abnormally low level of glucose, or sugar, in the blood caused by too much sugar in the diet, tumors in the pancreas causing an overproduction of insulin, or disorders of the liver interfering with the storage and release of sugar. An overconsumption of carbohydrates causes the blood sugar level to rise rapidly, stimulating the pancreas to secrete an excess of insulin. This excess insulin removes too much sugar from the blood, resulting in an abnormally low blood sugar level.

Symptoms of hypoglycemia include fatigue, weakness in legs, swollen feet, tightness in chest, constant hunger, eyeache, migraine, pains in various parts of the body, nervous habits, mental disturbances, and insomnia. Rapid fluctuations in blood sugar level give rise to many bizarre symptoms that may suggest mental disorder; however, a glucose tolerance test will ascertain the amount of sugar in the blood at a given time.

The therapeutic diet for hypoglycemia is high in protein, low in carbohydrates, and moderate in fat. The diet may be supplemented with high-protein between-meal snacks. Heavily sugared foods should be avoided, and foods with high natural sugar content should be restricted. When carbohydrates are unavoidable, only those that are slowly absorbed, such as fruits, vegetables, and whole-grain products, should be eaten, so that the change in the blood sugar level will be gradual. Coffee, strong tea, and cocoa should be avoided because they are capable of precipitating an attack of hypoglycemia.

There are no known drugs that specifically elevate the blood sugar. Several authorities suggest that daily ingestion of vitamin C can help prevent low blood sugar attacks.[18]

NUTRIENTS THAT MAY BE BENEFICIAL IN TREATMENT OF HYPOGLYCEMIA

Body Member	Nutrients	Quantity*
Blood/ Circulatory system	Vitamin B complex	
	Vitamin B$_6$	50 mg
	Vitamin B$_{12}$	25-50 mcg
	Pantothenic acid	100 mg
	Vitamin C	2,000-5,000 mg
	Chromium	
	High protein	

*See note, p. 166.

[18] Irvin Stone, *The Healing Factor* (New York: Grosset & Dunlap, 1972), p. 149.

Body Member	Nutrients	Quantity
	Low carbohydrates	
	Moderate fats	
	(vitamin F)	

IMPETIGO

Impetigo is a skin disease caused by bacterial infection. The disease occurs primarily in children, especially in those who are undernourished.

Impetigo is characterized by pus-filled skin lesions located mainly on the face and hands. These lesions rupture and form a honey-yellow crust over the infected area. The disease is spread by scratching the lesions and contaminating other skin areas with the fingers.

Strict hygiene is essential to prevent spread of the infection to other parts of the body or to other people. Neglected impetigo in adults may result in boils, ulcers, or other complications. Vitamin A is necessary for the health of skin tissue and may be helpful in aiding the skin in its recovery from impetigo.

NUTRIENTS THAT MAY BE BENEFICIAL IN TREATMENT OF IMPETIGO

Body Member	Nutrients	Quantity
Skin	Vitamin A	
	Vitamin C	
	Vitamin D	
	Vitamin E	

INDIGESTION (DYSPEPSIA)

Dyspepsia is imperfect or incomplete digestion, manifesting itself in a sensation of fullness or discomfort in the abdomen accompanied by pain or cramps, heartburn, nausea, and large amounts of gas in the intestines. Dyspepsia may be a symptom of a disorder in the stomach or small or large intestine, or it may be a complaint in itself. If indigestion occurs frequently and with no recognizable cause, medical investigation is advised.

The most common causes of dyspepsia are overeating or eating too rapidly; improper diet, such as a diet overabundant in carbohydrates at the expense of other nutrients; or overconsumption of stimulants such as coffee, tea, or alcohol. Lack of niacin in the diet may result in a decrease in the amount of hydrochloric acid in the stomach, consequently leading to indigestion. Smoking before or during a meal or swallowing too much air with meals, as in periods of nervousness or anxiety, can also bring about indigestion.

Dyspepsia can be prevented by avoidance of foods that produce its symptoms, especially highly seasoned foods, which tend to irritate the stomach lining, and fatty foods, which remain in the stomach longer than most foods. In treating dyspepsia, the diet should be bland and nutritionally well balanced. Special attention should be paid to the adequate intake of B vitamins, for without them carbohydrate combustion cannot take place and symptoms of indigestion can result.

NUTRIENTS THAT MAY BE BENEFICIAL IN TREATMENT OF INDIGESTION

Body Member	Nutrients	Quantity*
Stomach	Vitamin B complex	
	Vitamin B_1	50 mg
	Vitamin B_6	50 mg
	Folic acid	
	Niacin	100 mg
	Pantothenic acid	
	Low fat	

*See note, p. 166.

INFLUENZA (FLU)

Influenza is an acute viral infection of the respiratory tract. It is highly contagious and easily spread by sneezing and coughing. Symptoms of influenza include chills, high fever, sore throat, headache, abdominal pain, hoarseness, cough, enlarged lymph nodes, aching of the back and limbs, and frequent vomiting and diarrhea. Serious complications, such as pneumonia, sinus infections, and ear infections, can develop.

Influenza vaccines are available which help the body become immune to the virus. Many doctors recommend that elderly persons, pregnant women, and persons with heart, kidney, or lung disease have these vaccinations.

There is no specific treatment for influenza other than to treat its symptoms and try to prevent complications. The fever that usually accompanies influenza requires additional calories in several small feedings and additional vitamin B complex to metabolize these calories. Protein is needed for repair of tissue destroyed by fever. Infections accompanied by fever also increase the need for vitamins A and C. Vitamin A is especially important in influenza for the health of the lining of the throat. Increased fluid intake is also important in the event of fever.

NUTRIENTS THAT MAY BE BENEFICIAL IN TREATMENT OF INFLUENZA

Body Member	Nutrients	Quantity*
Lungs/ Respiratory tract	Vitamin A	
	Vitamin B complex	
	Vitamin B$_1$	50-200 mg
	Vitamin B$_2$	10 mg
	Vitamin B$_6$	50-100 mg
	Vitamin C	300-500 mg
	Niacin	50-100 mg
	Pantothenic acid	25 mg
	Protein	

*See note, p. 166.

INSOMNIA (SLEEPLESSNESS)

Insomnia is the inability to sleep soundly. It is a disturbance in the amount and depth of sleep. The need for sleep varies from person to person, but in general, it tends to decline as one grows older. The main causes of insomnia are anxiety or pain. Vigorous mental activity late at night, excitement, headache, or tired and aching muscles may also cause insomnia. In addition, caffeine, a stimulant found in coffee, tea, and cola drinks, is often responsible for keeping people awake.

Sleeplessness may be a symptom of a serious disease, but often it is a result of an individual's faulty reactions to stress. Insomnia perpetuates itself, in that thinking about the inability to sleep creates further tension in the mind and body. Only by relaxing and ceasing to worry about insomnia can a person resume sleeping and thus relieve his anxiety and tension. In learning to change his patterns of thought associated with sleep, the insomniac must establish a new bedtime routine, which might include such muscle and mind relaxers as leisurely walks, warm baths, massages, hot milk, soft music, or quiet meditation.

The well-nourished person who enjoys good health and a feeling of well-being probably will be less troubled by insomnia than one who subsists on a diet deficient in some essential nutrients. Deficiencies in the B vitamins, particularly B$_6$ and pantothenic acid, have resulted in

insomnia. In some cases, vitamin B$_{12}$ has been helpful in treating anxiety in insomniacs. Vitamin C, protein, calcium, and potassium can also calm the nerves and promote sleep. Sleeping pills or barbiturates should be used only as a last resort because they may produce dependence and other serious side effects.

NUTRIENTS THAT MAY BE BENEFICIAL IN TREATMENT OF INSOMNIA

Body Member	Nutrients	Quantity*
Brain/Nervous system	Vitamin B complex	
	Vitamin B$_6$	10 mg
	Vitamin B$_{12}$	
	Niacin	100 mg
	Pantothenic acid	
	Vitamin C	
	Vitamin D	
	Calcium	2 g taken before bedtime
	Magnesium	250 mg
	Phosphorus	
	Potassium	

*See note, p. 166.

JAUNDICE

Jaundice is a condition in which the skin, whites of the eyes, and urine become abnormally yellow because of the presence of pigments from worn-out red blood cells; the pigments accumulate in the blood because they are not being excreted as a waste product in the bile as they should be. Jaundice may indicate blood, kidney, or liver disorders; a doctor should be consulted in cases of jaundice.

NUTRIENTS THAT MAY BE BENEFICIAL IN TREATMENT OF JAUNDICE

Body Member	Nutrients	Quantity*
Blood	Vitamin A	
	Vitamin B$_6$	50 mg
	Vitamin C	1,000-1,500 mg every three hours in acute conditions, given even during

*See note, p. 166.

Body Member	Nutrients	Quantity
		fasting. In chronic conditions, 3,000-5,000 mg daily
	Vitamin D	
	Vitamin E	600 IU
	Vitamin F	
	Pantothenic acid	100 mg
	Calcium	
	Lecithin	Large amounts
	Magnesium	
	Phosphorus	
	Protein (sulfur-containing amino acids—eggs)	250 g

KIDNEY STONES (RENAL CALCULI)

Kidney stones are abnormal accumulations of mineral salts which form in the kidney but may lodge anywhere in the urinary tract. The stones are composed primarily of calcium. In the process of being filtered out of the blood by the kidneys, the calcium conglomerates into a stone. Stone formation may be due to overactivity of the parathyroid gland, which causes an elevated level of calcium in the blood. Additional conditions that increase the risk of kidney stone formation are dehydration, prolonged periods of bed rest, infections, and rarely, overingestion of vitamin D and calcium.

Symptoms of kidney stones include pain originating in the middle back which radiates around the abdomen toward the genitalia, increased urination that may contain blood or pus, nausea, and vomiting. Irritation by the stone may induce an infection in the urinary tract, giving rise to fever and chills and general discomfort.

Dietary therapy can not remove already formed kidney stones. However, to prevent further stone formation, calcium intake should be limited, although not excluded. A deficiency of vitamin B_6 and magnesium may cause stone formation; attention should therefore be paid to ensure their adequate intake. Persons whose diets are deficient in vitamin A tend toward kidney stone formation, so an adequate supply of this vitamin should be included in the diet.[19]

[19] Krause and Hunscher, *Food, Nutrition and Diet Therapy*, p. 482.

NUTRIENTS THAT MAY BE BENEFICIAL IN TREATMENT OF KIDNEY STONES

Body Member	Nutrients	Quantity*
Kidney	Vitamin A	
	Vitamin B_6	50 mg
	Vitamin C	
	Vitamin E	
	Magnesium	250-500 mg
	Restricted calcium	

*See note, p. 166.

KWASHIORKOR

Kwashiorkor is a severe malnutritional disease caused by a diet which supplies adequate calories through its carbohydrate content but which is seriously lacking protein. Kwashiorkor commonly develops in children who are between the ages of one and five and who are weaned from milk to a diet of primarily starches and sugars.

Symptoms of kwashiorkor include changes in the skin and hair, retarded growth, diarrhea, loss of appetite, nervous irritability, and edema. Severe infections and many vitamin deficiencies often accompany kwashiorkor.

The initial treatment for the disease is aimed at correcting the protein deficiency. Because of the patient's poor ability to tolerate fat, a skim-milk formula is often used in treatment. Gradually, additional foods are added until the patient progresses to a well-balanced diet. Vitamin deficiencies, if they exist, must be corrected.

NUTRIENTS THAT MAY BE BENEFICIAL IN TREATMENT OF KWASHIORKOR

Body Member	Nutrients	Quantity
Body	Vitamin A	
	Folic acid	
	Vitamin C	
	Vitamin D	
	Vitamin E	
	Chromium	
	Copper	
	Iron	
	Magnesium	
	Selenium	
	Protein	

LEG CRAMP, "CHARLEY HORSE"

A leg cramp is an involuntary contraction, or spasm, of a muscle in the leg or foot. Cramps most commonly occur at night, when the limbs are cool, particularly after a day of unusual exertion, and more frequently in the elderly, the young, and persons with arteriosclerosis. These cramps seem to be caused by unnatural positions, which impair the blood supply to the lower extremities causing the muscles to abnormally contract, thus bringing about cramps. A cramp usually lasts only a few seconds or minutes. If a cramp occurs while a person is walking, it may be a signal of seriously impaired circulation, but a cramp that occurs while a person is resting does not indicate this severity. Patients most susceptible to repeated leg cramps are those with advanced arteriosclerosis.

Leg cramps may signify a variety of nutritional deficiencies. The most common is lack of calcium, which is necessary for normal muscle contraction. Other deficiencies indicated are thiamine, pantothenic acid, biotin, and magnesium. Occasionally a sodium loss, such as occurs in heavy perspiration or diarrhea, may result in muscle cramps. A vitamin C deficiency also can be responsible for pains in the muscles and joints. Prevention and treatment for leg cramps should include an adequate diet containing sufficient amounts of these nutrients.

A "charley horse" is a pulled and bruised muscle that results in soreness and stiffness. It is usually due to a blow or to a forceful stretch of the leg during athletic activity. A person who has suffered a charley horse should have a high intake of protein to rebuild damaged tissues.

NUTRIENTS THAT MAY BE BENEFICIAL IN TREATMENT OF LEG CRAMP

Body Member	Nutrients	Quantity*
Leg	Vitamin B complex	
	Vitamin B$_1$	
	Vitamin B$_2$	
	Bioton	
	Pantothenic acid	100 mg
	Vitamin C	
	Vitamin D	
	Vitamin E	400-1,000 IU
	Vitamin F	
	Calcium	

*See note, p. 166.

Body Member	Nutrients	Quantity
	Magnesium	800 mg
	Phosphorus	
	Sodium	
	Protein	

LEUKEMIA

Leukemia is a fatal blood disease characterized by an overproduction of white blood cells. There are two basic types of leukemia. Acute leukemia usually occurs in children and young adults, and chronic leukemia is usually found only in adults.

Acute leukemia is marked by a sudden onset of symptoms. In chronic leukemia, symptoms develop more slowly. Symptoms of the disease include bleeding from the gums, nose, stomach, and rectum and abnormally easy, excessive bruising of the skin. Pain in the upper abdomen, anemia, fever, and increased susceptibility to infection are further leukemia symptoms.

The cause of leukemia is unknown. However, some theories suggest that excessive exposure to radiation, x-rays, or chemical pollution may cause the disease.

A well-balanced diet containing all vitamins is helpful in maintaining strength in the leukemia victim. Supplementing the diet with the vitamin B complex and iron may aid in the treatment of the anemia that accompanies the disease. Vitamin C may be helpful in fighting the infections that are often associated with leukemia.

NUTRIENTS THAT MAY BE BENEFICIAL IN TREATMENT OF LEUKEMIA

Body Member	Nutrients	Quantity
Blood	Vitamin B complex	
	Vitamin B$_{12}$	
	Folic acid	
	Vitamin C	
	Bioflavonoids	
	Copper	
	Iron	
	Zinc	

MEASLES

The two main varieties of measles are German measles and common measles. German measles is usually a mild illness with a rapid recovery period, alarming only to pregnant women. If a woman contracts German measles during the early months of her pregnancy, malformations such as heart defects, deafness, mental retardation, and blindness of the newborn commonly occur.

Symptoms of German measles may include fever, headache, and stiff joints, although most people seldom complain of any symptoms. A rash that lasts for about three days appears on the arms, chest, and forehead.

Since German measles is a virus that must run its course, there is little that can be done medically for its treatment. One attack of or vaccination for the disease will usually produce lifelong immunity against German measles. Lotions may be applied to the rash to relieve itching, and the patient should stay away from other people to avoid spreading the disease. A well-balanced diet rich in all nutrients is recommended.

Common measles is a highly contagious disease spread by droplets from the nose, throat, and mouth. The first symptoms of common measles are fever, cough, and inflammation of the eyes. Within 24 to 48 hours, small red spots with white centers appear on the inside of the cheeks. A rash which is first seen on the side of the neck and which then spreads to the rest of the body usually appears three to five days after the onset of the first symptoms. As the rash spreads, fever goes down. Common measles may have many serious complications, such as pneumonia, encephalitis, and injury to the nervous system.

The patient should be isolated in a well-ventilated room, which should be darkened if the patient is sensitive to light. Fevers increase the body's need for calories and vitamins A and C. Although the patient may not desire food for the first few days, he should be encouraged, but not forced, to eat. Frequent small meals and special foods may be beneficial. Increased fluid intake in any form, such as water, fruit juices, or milk, is essential to the measles patient.

MÉNIÈRE'S SYNDROME

Ménière's syndrome is a disease of the inner ear characterized by recurrent attacks of deafness, tinnitus, vertigo, nausea, and vomiting.

NUTRIENTS THAT MAY BE BENEFICIAL IN TREATMENT OF MÉNIÈRE'S SYNDROME

Body Member	Nutrients	Quantity*
Ear	Vitamin B complex	
	Vitamin B$_1$	10-25 mg four times daily for two weeks
	Vitamin B$_2$	10-25 mg four times daily for two weeks
	Niacin	100-250 mg four times daily for two weeks
	Vitamin E	
	Vitamin F	
	Calcium	

*See note, p. 166.

MENINGITIS

Meningitis occurs when the three layers of membranes lying between the skull and brain become infected by bacteria, viruses, or fungi. These infecting organisms are commonly spread via the bloodstream from acute infections of the nose and throat.

Meningitis is more commonly found in children than in adults. Symptoms include headache, stiff neck, high fever, chills, nausea, vomiting, changes in temperament, and drowsiness, which may develop into a coma.

Medical attention for meningitis should be sought promptly. The drug selected for treatment of the disease depends on the type of infecting organism. During the fever, the body's needs for vitamin A and C are increased. A well-balanced diet adequate in protein is necessary to help the body ward off infection and repair damaged tissue.

NUTRIENTS THAT MAY BE BENEFICIAL IN TREATMENT OF MEASLES

Body Member	Nutrients	Quantity
General/Skin	Vitamin A	
	Vitamin C	
	Vitamin E	
	Protein	

NUTRIENTS THAT MAY BE BENEFICIAL IN TREATMENT OF MENINGITIS

Body Member	Nutrients	Quantity
Brain	Vitamin A	
	Vitamin C	
	Vitamin D	
	Protein	

MENTAL ILLNESS

Mental illness is a serious disease that occurs when a person no longer is able to cope effectively with emotional or physical stress. The problems facing one person may not necessarily be more serious than the problems facing another person, but the mentally ill person has less ability to deal with problems and stress in a rational manner than does the mentally healthy person.

Mental illness may develop as a result of several factors. Inherited characteristics combined with certain environmental influences may trigger mental instability. Some types of mental illness may be a direct result of poor nutrition because the brain cells cannot function efficiently without proper nutrients. Deficiencies of B vitamins, ascorbic acid (vitamin C), and phosphorus are known to decrease the metabolic rate of the brain. Deficiency of niacin may cause symptoms of deep depression, often seen in psychosis. Symptoms of a severe vitamin B_6 deficiency are headache, irritability, dizziness, extreme nervousness, and inability to concentrate. Pantothenic acid is essential for the body's ability to handle stressful situations. Signs of a thiamine deficiency are lack of energy, constant fatigue, loss of appetite, and irritability. A prolonged thiamine deficiency may result in brain damage contributing to emotional upsets characterized by overreaction to normal stress. Irritability is also a symptom of vitamin C deficiency. The proper phosphorus-calcium ratio (1 to 2) is essential for nourishment of the entire nervous system. Calcium deficiency results in tenseness, insomnia, and fatigue.

A lack of oxygen is involved in many cases of mental disturbance, since the brain is dependent upon an uninterrupted supply of oxygen not only to function properly but also to stay alive. Vitamin E is an oxygen conserver and increases the amount of oxygen available to the brain. An unbalanced blood sugar level and hypothyroidism (which leads to a deficiency of thyroxine in the blood) are acknowledged causes of emotional disturbances. Shortage of thyroxine (the iodine-carrying hormone) generally results in a slowdown of both physical and mental activity. Hyperthyroidism (overactive thyroid) is related to emotional disturbances, forgetfulness, slow thought processes, and irritability.

A person with a magnesium deficiency is apt to be uncooperative, withdrawn, apathetic, or belligerent. Defective adrenal function may contribute to depression and other forms of mental illness. These disorders may be alleviated by proper dietary habits and food supplementation.

NUTRIENTS THAT MAY BE BENEFICIAL IN TREATMENT OF MENTAL ILLNESS

Body Member	Nutrients	Quantity
Brain/Nervous system	Vitamin B complex	
	Vitamin B_1	
	Vitamin B_6	
	Folic acid	
	Niacin	
	Pantothenic acid	
	Vitamin C	
	Vitamin E	
	Vitamin F	
	Calcium	
	Magnesium	
	Phosphorus	
	Protein	

MONONUCLEOSIS

Mononucleosis is an infectious disease, believed to be caused by a virus. It affects primarily the lymph tissues or glands that are located in the neck, armpits, and groin. The lymph glands remove many microscopic materials such as bacteria and viruses, thus helping to prevent the infection from spreading throughout the body. Symptoms of mononucleosis include sore throat, fever, chills, swollen glands, and fatigue.

Adequate rest, exercise, and nutrition are essential for the maintenance of general health and the prevention of mononucleosis. Protein is needed to stimulate the formation of antibodies, substances produced by the body to help protect it against other infections that may accompany or follow mononucleosis. Potassium and vitamin C supplements may be needed to compensate for the loss that occurs during fever. Vitamin A is needed for the health of the tissue lining of the throat. If there is a deficiency of thiamine, riboflavin, or biotin, supplementing these nutrients in the diet may be helpful in preventing fatigue and headaches.

NUTRIENTS THAT MAY BE BENEFICIAL IN TREATMENT OF MONONUCLEOSIS

Body Member	Nutrients	Quantity
Blood	Vitamin A	
	Vitamin B_1	
	Vitamin B_2	
	Vitamin B_6	

Body Member	Nutrients	Quantity
	Biotin	
	Choline	
	Pantothenic acid	
	Vitamin C	
	Potassium	
	Protein	

MULTIPLE SCLEROSIS

Multiple sclerosis is a chronic disease that causes the deterioration of the protective covering of the nerves in the brain and spinal cord, resulting in the hardening of various parts of the nervous system and the development of scars or lesions on the disturbed nerves. The cause of the disease is unknown, although it has been seen to follow malnutrition, emotional stress, and infections.

Multiple sclerosis usually occurs in persons between the ages of twenty-five and forty. The disease progresses slowly and may disappear for periods of time but returns intermittently, usually in a more severe form. Symptoms of the disease include visual and speech disturbances, dizziness, bowel and bladder disorders, weakness, lack of coordination, paralysis, loss of balance, and emotional instability.

Care should be taken to ensure adequate rest, exercise, and a well-balanced diet because all these are necessary for proper functioning of the nervous system. Vitamin B_{12} has been used to increase stability in standing and walking in some cases of the disease.[20] Vitamin B_{13} has been beneficial in treating multiple sclerosis.

NUTRIENTS THAT MAY BE BENEFICIAL IN TREATMENT OF MULTIPLE SCLEROSIS

Body Member	Nutrients	Quantity*
Brain/Nervous system	Vitamin B complex	
	Vitamin B_1	100 mg
	Vitamin B_2	150 mg
	Vitamin B_6	100-200 mg
	Vitamin B_{12}	
	Vitamin B_{13}	
	Choline	700-1,400 mg
	Niacin	100 mg
	Pangamic acid	

*See note, p. 166.

[20] Rodale, *The Complete Book of Vitamins*, p. 257.

Body Member	Nutrients	Quantity
	Pantothenic acid	100 mg
	Vitamin C	Up to 1,000 mg
	Vitamin E	Up to 1,800 IU
	Vitamin F	Six capsules
	Lecithin	
	Magnesium	
	Manganese	
	Protein	

MUSCULAR DYSTROPHY

Muscular dystrophy is an inherited disease that causes wasting of the muscles. Some authorities believe muscular dystrophy to be nutritional in origin, but no direct link has been found. The major symptom is great weakness in the legs and back so that the patient has trouble walking. The weakness gradually progresses throughout the muscles of the body, creating partial, then total, paralysis.

Muscular dystrophy is marked by remissions, or periods in which the disease appears to be arrested, but the disease usually returns and is more severe. A varied diet that is high in protein, vitamins, and minerals is recommended in the early stages of the disease to help arrest the muscular wasting and to prolong the remissions.

NUTRIENTS THAT MAY BE BENEFICIAL IN TREATMENT OF MUSCULAR DYSTROPHY

Body Member	Nutrients	Quantity*
Muscles	Vitamin A	
	Vitamin B_6	
	Vitamin B_{12}	
	Choline	
	Niacin	
	Pantothenic acid	
	Vitamin C	
	Vitamin E	600 IU
	Potassium	
	Protein	

*See note, p. 166.

MYOCARDIAL INFARCTION (HEART ATTACK)

When the vessels leading to the heart, known as coronary arteries, become blocked by blood clots or by the fatty deposits of atherosclerosis, a myocardial infarction, or heart attack, occurs. If a blood clot partially blocks the main artery, the attack is not fatal and the individual survives with some degree of heart damage. Complete blockage results in death.

Symptoms may begin anytime. The most frequent complaint is an excruciating pain usually starting in the lower chest or upper abdomen. The pain often spreads to the neck and shoulders, down the arms, especially to the left side, and possibly to the back. The pain increases in severity and is not relieved by rest or nitroglycerin, a medication often prescribed for patients with mild angina pectoris. The pain causes the patient to appear very restless and anxious. In 15 percent of heart attack cases, however, no pain is experienced and the attack is known as a "silent coronary."[21]

Additional heart attack symptoms include perspiration and pale skin, a decrease in blood pressure, weak and rapid pulse, and, possibly, nausea and vomiting. A moderate fever usually appears 24 to 48 hours after the onset of the attack.

Immediate medical attention is necessary and can best be obtained at a coronary care unit in a hospital setting. Usually the patient will be given an electrocardiogram, or EKG, a test designed to detect changes in heart function or damage to some part of the heart. But often this test will not show the heart damage until hours or days after the attack. A blood test is also often done to help detect if a myocardial infarction has occurred.

Conditions that increase the risk of heart attack are lack of exercise, cigarette smoking, obesity, diabetes, prolonged high blood pressure, overabundance of salt in the diet, a family history of heart attacks, or prolonged emotional stress.

During the first three weeks of treatment, the patient runs a great risk of suffering further irregularities in heart function. The immediate effort in treatment is for the patient to obtain rest to decrease the workload of the heart. Pain medication and oxygen therapy are often applied. Because the workload of the heart increases after meals, the diet during the first few days often consists of six small feedings low in sodium. Cold fluids should be avoided because they may trigger irregularities in heart function. Protein intake must be adequate to replace protein lost in damaged heart cells. By six weeks the healing is almost complete and increased amounts of activity can be tolerated.

[21] Lillian Brunner et. al., *Medical Surgical Nursing* (New York: J.B. Lippincott Co., 1959).

Dietary measures reducing the risk of heart attack include proper caloric intake to maintain or achieve normal weight and the use of unsaturated rather than saturated fats to help prevent further production of fatty deposits lining the blood vessels. Cholesterol intake should be restricted to 300 milligrams daily.[22] Many authorities suggest that refined carbohydrates, such as white sugar, play a large role in the development of heart disease and should therefore be restricted.[23] Vitamin C and the B complex help to maintain the integrity and health of the heart and circulatory system. Vitamin E may also help because of its anticlotting properties.

NUTRIENTS THAT MAY BE BENEFICIAL IN TREATMENT OF MYOCARDIAL INFARCTION

Body Member	Nutrients	Quantity*
Heart	Vitamin A	
	Vitamin B complex	
	Vitamin C	
	Vitamin E	Up to 1,600 IU
	Magnesium	
	Potassium	
	Protein	

*See note, p. 166.

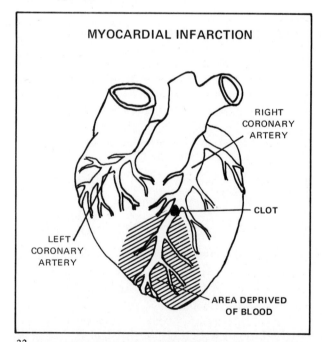

MYOCARDIAL INFARCTION

RIGHT CORONARY ARTERY

CLOT

LEFT CORONARY ARTERY

AREA DEPRIVED OF BLOOD

[22] Alberta Dent Schackelton, *Practical Nurse Nutrition Education,* 3d ed. (Philadelphia: W.B. Saunders, 1972), p. 228.
[23] Stanley Davidson, R. Passmore, and J.I. Brock, *Human Nutrition and Dietetics,* 5th ed. (Baltimore: Williams and Wilkins Co., 1972), p. 324.

NAIL PROBLEMS

Nails are composed almost entirely of protein. Abnormal or unhealthy nails may be the result of a local injury, a glandular deficiency such as hypothyroidism, or a deficiency of certain nutrients.

A severe protein deficiency can cause opaque white bands to appear on the nails or cause them to become dry and brittle. A shortage of vitamin A or calcium in the diet may also cause dryness and brittleness. A lack of the B vitamins causes nails to become fragile, with horizontal or vertical ridges appearing. An iron deficiency can disturb the growth of the nails, causing dryness, brittleness, thinning, flattening, and eventually the appearance of moon-shaped nails.

NUTRIENTS THAT MAY BE BENEFICIAL IN TREATMENT OF NAIL PROBLEMS

Body Member	Nutrients	Quantity
Nails	Vitamin A	
	Vitamin B complex	
	Folic acid	
	Calcium	
	Iron	
	Protein	

NEPHRITIS (KIDNEY INFECTION)

Nephritis is the inflammation of one or both of the kidneys. The most common form of nephritis, pyelonephritis, occurs among females, especially during childhood or pregnancy. It is caused by bacteria from the stools being introduced into the urinary opening by wiping in a forward direction. The bacteria then travel to the bladder and finally to the kidney. Another form of nephritis, glomerulonephritis, occurs as a reaction to an infection elsewhere in the body, such as an infection in the throat.

Symptoms of nephritis may be nonexistent, or they may include blood and/or albumin in the urine, fatigue, lower back or abdominal pain, fever, chills, edema, nausea and vomiting, loss of appetite, and frequent urge to urinate. Anemia and high blood pressure may accompany severe nephritis.

Medical treatment of nephritis includes antibiotics, bed rest, and increased fluid intake. Sodium, potassium, and protein are restricted in the diet. If anemia is present, the nephritis patient should be receiving iron supplements. An adequate caloric intake is essential, and a multivitamin supplement of the water-soluble vitamins is recommended.

NUTRIENTS THAT MAY BE BENEFICIAL IN TREATMENT OF NEPHRITIS

Body Member	Nutrients	Quantity*
Kidney	Vitamin A	50,000-75,000 IU
	Vitamin B complex	
	Vitamin B$_2$	25 mg
	Choline	1,000 mg
	Vitamin C	
	Vitamin E	300-600 IU
	Calcium	250 mg
	Iron	
	Magnesium	
	Water	
	Restricted protein	
	Restricted sodium	
	Restricted potassium	

*See note, p. 166.

NEURITIS

Neuritis is the inflammation or deterioration of a nerve or group of nerves. Symptoms of neuritis vary with its cause. Some symptoms are pain, tenderness, tingling and loss of the sensation of touch in the affected nerve area, redness and swelling of the affected areas, and in severe cases, convulsions.

Causes of neuritis include injury to a nerve, such as in a direct blow or a nearby bone fracture; infection involving a nerve; diseases such as diabetes, gout, and leukemia; poisons such as mercury, lead, or methyl alcohol; and dietary deficiency of the vitamin B complex, especially thiamine. A thiamine deficiency results in the impairment of nerve tissue so that it cannot properly utilize carbohydrates for energy.

Treatment for neuritis also varies with the cause. If neuritis is caused by poisons, exposure to them should be ended, and if it is caused by a specific disease or trauma, treatment should be given. When a thiamine or vitamin B complex deficiency is responsible, administration of these vitamins will result in recovery within three to four days. Adequate intake of the B vitamins is necessary even when a deficiency does not exist, since they are needed for the general health of nerve tissue.

A well-balanced diet is important to the individual with neuritis for the maintenance and repair of muscles and nerves. If infection is present, protein, calorie, and fluid intake should be increased.

NUTRIENTS THAT MAY BE BENEFICIAL IN TREATMENT OF NEURITIS

Body Member	Nutrients	Quantity*
Nervous system	Vitamin B complex	
	Vitamin B_1	
	Vitamin B_2	
	Vitamin B_6	100-300 mg
	Vitamin B_{12}	
	Niacin	
	Pantothenic acid	
	Magnesium	
	Protein	

*See note, p. 166.

NIGHT BLINDNESS

Night blindness is the inability to see well in dim or dark light. The major cause of night blindness is deficiency of vitamin A. Vitamin A is necessary for the formation of visual purple, the substance in the eyes which enables them to adjust from bright light to darkness. Other causes of night blindness are fatigue, emotional disturbances, or hereditary factors.

Adequate intake of vitamin A will protect against night blindness. The Recommended Dietary Allowance of 5,000 units is necessary for normal and healthy vision. Riboflavin, niacin, and thiamine have been reported to relieve night blindness when vitamin A has not produced a response, and attention should therefore be paid to ensure their adequate intake.[24]

NUTRIENTS THAT MAY BE BENEFICIAL IN TREATMENT OF NIGHT BLINDNESS

Body Member	Nutrients	Quantity*
Eye	Vitamin A	
	Vitamin B complex	
	Vitamin B_1	
	Vitamin B_2	5 mg
	Niacin	

*See note, p. 166.

[24] Krause and Hunscher, *Food, Nutrition and Diet Therapy*, p. 497.

OSTEOPOROSIS (BRITTLE BONES)

Osteoporosis is a reduction in the total mass of bone, with the remaining bone being fragile or "brittle." Symptoms of the disorder include increased incidence of fractures, pains in the hip and back, and reduced height. Osteoporosis is primarily a disease of the aged, usually beginning at about age fifty.

A major cause of osteoporosis is an inadequate intake of calcium over a period of years. Other causes are inability to absorb sufficient calcium through the intestine, calcium-phosphorus imbalance, lack of exercise, or lack of certain hormones.

A diet that is adequate in protein, calcium, phosphorus, and vitamin D is the best prevention and treatment for osteoporosis. Trace amounts of fluorides from foods or drinking water also protect against bone decomposition.

NUTRIENTS THAT MAY BE BENEFICIAL IN TREATMENT OF OSTEOPOROSIS

Body Member	Nutrients	Quantity*
Bones	Vitamin B_{12}	30-900 mcg
	Vitamin C	Up to 1,000 mg
	Vitamin D	Up to 5,000 IU
	Vitamin E	600 IU
	Calcium	500 mg
	Copper	
	Fluoride	
	Magnesium	500 mg
	Phosphorus	
	Protein	

*See note, p. 166.

OVERWEIGHT AND OBESITY

Overweight and obesity are one of the major nutritional problems in America today. Statistics show that people of average weight (see the "Desirable Height and Weight Chart," p. 236), have a longer life-span, have more energy, and usually feel better than those people who are overweight. Overweight and obesity precipitate such conditions as heart disease, kidney trouble, diabetes, high blood pressure, malnutrition, complications of pregnancy, and psychological problems. Glandular malfunction, malnutrition, emotional tension, boredom, habit, and love of food are the main causes of overweight.

Calories and exercise are essential considerations in losing weight. Fat is metabolically formed in the body when more food energy or calories are consumed than the body is able to use. One pound of fatty tissue is equal to 3500 calories. When the number of calories used during the day exceeds the amount consumed, the body oxidizes its supplies of fat to produce energy, and thereby a reduction of body weight results. A daily decrease of 1000 calories results in approximately two pounds of weight loss per week.

Calories may be burned up by the basal metabolism, which includes normal body functions such as breathing and digestion. All activity, such as walking, talking, working, or playing baseball, uses up additional energy and calories. For example, one hour of average office work probably uses up only 10 to 15 calories, whereas moderate housework may require 70 calories per hour more than basal metabolism requirements. Brisk walking uses up about 110 calories per hour; driving a car uses up about 40. Strenuous exercise and hard physical labor may require more than 400 calories per hour.

In order to lose weight safely, a person must set up a sensible long-range diet plan that includes all the essential nutrients and minerals. A high-protein, low-carbohydrate, low-fat diet is generally recommended for safe, gradual weight loss. Carbohydrates should be chosen from the best nutritional sources, such as whole-grain products and fruits that contain essential nutrients. Fat intake should come primarily from sources of unsaturated fatty acids and from such animal fats as butter and whole milk, which are good sources of fat-soluble vitamins. Excess fat is hard to metabolize and can upset liver and kidney functions. In general, losing weight is a matter of consciously curbing the amount of food eaten, regulating the types of food eaten, and increasing daily activity.

NUTRIENTS THAT MAY BE BENEFICIAL IN TREATMENT OF OVERWEIGHT AND OBESITY

Body Member	Nutrients	Quantity*
	Vitamin B complex	
	Vitamin B$_6$	Up to 100 mg
	Vitamin B$_{12}$	
	Inositol	500 mg
	Vitamin C	Up to 1,000 mg
	Vitamin E	Up to 600 IU

*See note, p. 166.

Body Member	Nutrients	Quantity
	Vitamin F	
	Calcium	500 mg
	Lecithin	2 tsp
	Magnesium	500 mg
	Protein	

PARKINSON'S DISEASE

Parkinson's disease is a slowly progressive disease of the nervous system in which an essential type of nerve cell is destroyed. The cause of the disease is unknown, although it usually begins after age fifty.

Symptoms of Parkinson's disease include muscular rigidity and cramping, involuntary tremors that include a characteristic pill-rolling movement of the thumb and forefinger as they rub against each other, impaired speech, a staring facial expression, drooling, and a short, shuffling gait. Despite these symptoms, sensation and mental activity are not impaired. There is often a loss of appetite and some weight loss, giving rise to the possibility of malnutrition developing. Chronic constipation may complicate the condition.

There is no cure for the disease, although drugs may be used to alleviate the symptoms. Modification of the diet and treatment of the constipation may also be helpful. Frequent small meals will increase the patient's nutrient and caloric levels, thus preventing malnutrition. The vitamin B complex is necessary for the health of the nerves; the person with Parkinson's disease should include adequate amounts of these vitamins in his or her diet. A marked increase in fluid intake is also necessary because the normal secretions of the intestines may be lessened by some of the prescribed drugs. High-residue food will assist in alleviating constipation.

NUTRIENTS THAT MAY BE BENEFICIAL IN TREATMENT OF PARKINSON'S DISEASE

Body Member	Nutrients	Quantity*
Brain/Nervous system	Vitamin B complex	
	Vitamin B$_2$	Up to 100 mg
	Vitamin B$_6$	10-200 mg
	Niacin	
	Vitamin C	Up to 100 mg
	Vitamin E	600 IU

*See note, p. 166.

Body Member	Nutrients	Quantity
	Calcium	
	Magnesium	500 mg
	Glutamic acid	
	Protein	

PELLAGRA

Pellagra is a disease caused by a deficiency of the B vitamins, particularly riboflavin, niacin, and thiamine. The disease occurs frequently in populations whose diets consist mainly of corn. Although the disease is seldom found in the United States, its rare occurrence affects persons with gastrointestinal disturbances or chronic alcoholism.

Symptoms of pellagra are diarrhea, loss of appetite and weight, reddened and swollen tongue, weakness, depression, and anxiety. Itchy dermatitis on the hands and neck is a prominent characteristic of the disease.

A diet that is adequate in the B vitamins and protein will prevent pellagra. A diet rich in the B vitamins niacin, thiamine, riboflavin, folic acid, and vitamin B_{12} will cure the disease.

NUTRIENTS THAT MAY BE BENEFICIAL IN TREATMENT OF PELLAGRA

Body Member	Nutrients	Quantity
Skin	Vitamin B complex	
	Vitamin B_1	
	Vitamin B_2	
	Vitamin B_{12}	
	Folic acid	
	Niacin	
	Protein	

PERNICIOUS ANEMIA

Pernicious anemia is a form of anemia resulting from a deficiency of vitamin B_{12}. It is a severe form of anemia in which there is a gradual reduction in the number of blood cells because the bone marrow fails to produce mature red blood cells. Pernicious anemia probably arises from an inheritable inability of the stomach to secrete a substance called the "intrinsic factor" which is necessary for the intestinal absorption of vitamin B_{12}.

Pernicious anemia occurs in both sexes. Its occurrence is rare in persons under the age of thirty, but susceptibility increases with age. Symptoms of pernicious anemia include weakness and gastrointestinal disturbances causing a sore tongue, slight yellowing of the skin, and tingling of extremities. In addition, disturbances of the nervous system, such as partial loss of coordination of the fingers, feet, and legs; some nerve deterioration; and disturbances of the digestive tract, such as diarrhea and loss of appetite, may occur.

Pernicious anemia may be fatal without treatment. Vitamin B_{12} injections together with a highly nutritious diet supplemented with large amounts of desiccated liver are the recommended treatment. Intake of the entire vitamin B complex will help maintain the health of the nervous system, although folic acid should not be taken in amounts exceeding 0.1 milligram daily. Folic acid has the effect of concealing the symptoms of pernicious anemia, allowing the unseen destruction of the nervous system to continue until irreparable damage is done. A diet rich in protein, calcium, vitamin C, vitamin E, and iron is recommended.

NUTRIENTS THAT MAY BE BENEFICIAL IN TREATMENT OF PERNICIOUS ANEMIA

Body Member	Nutrients	Quantity*
Blood/ Circulatory system	Vitamin B complex	
	Vitamin B_6	50-100 mcg
	Vitamin B_{12}	50-100 mcg in injections
	Folic acid	
	Vitamin C	
	Vitamin E	
	Calcium	
	Cobalt	
	Protein	

*See note, p. 166.

PHLEBITIS

Phlebitis, the inflammation of a vein wall, is usually found in the legs and can be a complication of varicose veins. Symptoms of phlebitis include reddening and cordlike swelling of the vein, increased pulse rate, slight fever, and pain accompanying movement of the afflicted area.

A complication that may occur in individuals with phlebitis is thrombophlebitis, the formation of a clot in the inflamed vein. If this clot should break loose from the vein wall and lodge in a blood vessel that supplies some vital area with blood, serious and possibly fatal damage may occur. In some cases, the use of oral contraceptives has been related to the occurrence of thrombophlebitis.

Factors that seem to encourage the onset of the phlebitis are operations, especially in the lower abdomen, childbirth, and infections resulting from injuries to veins. Phlebitis can be prevented by the treatment of varicose veins so that inflammation does not set in. Infections in the legs or feet, especially fungus infections of the toes, should be given immediate attention as a safeguard against phlebitis. Regular exercise is a further preventive measure.

Supplementing the diet with niacin, part of the vitamin B complex, may be useful to help prevent clot formation.[25] Vitamin C can help strengthen the blood vessel walls. Some research indicates that vitamin E may dilate blood vessels, thus discouraging the formation of varicose veins and phlebitis.

NUTRIENTS THAT MAY BE BENEFICIAL IN TREATMENT OF PHLEBITIS

Body Member	Nutrients	Quantity*
Blood/Circulatory system/Legs	Vitamin B complex	
	Niacin	
	Pantothenic acid	100 mg
	Vitamin C	5-25 g
	Vitamin E	200-600 IU

*See note, p. 166.

PNEUMONIA

Pneumonia is an ailment in which the tiny air sacs in the lungs become inflamed and filled with mucous and pus. The primary causes of pneumonia are bacteria, viruses, chemical irritants, and allergies. Factors that contribute to the onset of pneumonia are colds, alcoholism, malnutrition, and foreign matter in the respiratory passages. Symptoms of the disease vary from mild to severe, but they usually include sharp pains in the chest, fever and chills, fatigue, rapid respiration, and cough.

Vitamin A is necessary for maintaining the health of the lining of the respiratory passages. A deficiency of the vitamin increases susceptibility to respiratory infections, which in turn can lead to pneumonia. Since protein loss accompanies high fever and because protein is necessary for the repair of body tissue, its intake should be increased during pneumonia. Water and fluid intake should be increased to prevent dehydration that can result from fever and perspiration. Vitamin C intake is required to fight infection. Because deficiency of the vitamin B complex usually occurs with pneumonia, an increased intake is necessary. Some research shows a correlation between vitamin E deficiency and lung disease.[26]

NUTRIENTS THAT MAY BE BENEFICIAL IN TREATMENT OF PNEUMONIA

Body Member	Nutrients	Quantity*
Lungs/ Respiratory system	Vitamin A	
	Vitamin B complex	
	Vitamin C	500 mg every 90 minutes
	Vitamin D	
	Vitamin E	
	Bioflavonoids	
	Protein	

*See note, p. 166.

POLIO

Polio is a virus infection of the spinal cord which destroys the nerves controlling muscular movement, resulting in paralysis of certain muscles. There are two stages of this disease: the infectious stage, when the virus is active, and the noninfectious, or recovery, stage. Symptoms of the infectious stage include fever, nausea, diarrhea, headache, and irritability.

During the infectious stage, the diet of the polio patient should be high in protein and potassium to replace that which is lost because of the rapid tissue destruction. Caloric intake should also be increased because of the

---

[25] Carlton Fredericks, *Eating Right for You* (New York: Grosset & Dunlap, 1972), p. 262.

[26] Martin Ebon, *The Truth about Vitamin E* (New York: Bantam Books, 1972), p. 34.

increased energy expenditure during fever, and additional B vitamins are necessary to help metabolize the additional calories. Fever creates the need for additional sodium because of the loss that occurs with perspiration. Fluid intake should also be increased during fever to compensate for loss and to dilute the toxic substances produced by the virus. Fever and the accompanying increase in metabolism also increase the need for vitamins A and C, and attention should be paid to their intake. The intake of calcium and phosphorus should be lowered to reduce the risk of kidney or gallstone formation during prolonged periods of immobilization or bed rest.

NUTRIENTS THAT MAY BE BENEFICIAL IN TREATMENT OF POLIO

Body Member	Nutrients	Quantity
Brain/Nervous system	Vitamin A	
	Vitamin B complex	
	Vitamin C	
	Potassium	
	Sodium	
	Protein	

PROSTATITIS

Prostatitis is the inflammation of the prostate, a male sex gland. The usual cause of prostatitis in young men is a bacterial infection from another area of the body which has invaded the prostate. Prostatic enlargement, which is usually found in older males, is often due to gradual enlargement over a period of several years.

Symptoms of acute prostatitis are pain between the scrotum and rectum, fever, frequent urination accompanied by a burning sensation, and blood or pus in the urine. Symptoms of long-term prostatitis are frequent and burning urination, lower back pain, and premature ejaculation, or loss of potency. As prostatitis becomes more advanced, urination becomes increasingly difficult.

Treatment for prostatitis involves increasing the fluid intake to meet the increased needs during infection and to stimulate urine flow, thus preventing retention of urine. Urinary retention can result in cystitis and possibly in a kidney infection. Increased protein and calories are needed during fever and infection, to replace lost body tissues and energy. A well-balanced diet rich in vitamin A, the B complex, and vitamin C is also important during fever and infection. Some sources advocate the avoidance

of alcoholic beverages, spicy foods, and exposure to very cold weather if prostatitis is present.[27]

NUTRIENTS THAT MAY BE BENEFICIAL IN TREATMENT OF PROSTATITIS

Body Member	Nutrients	Quantity*
Gland, prostate	Vitamin A	
	Vitamin B complex	
	Vitamin B$_6$	
	Vitamin C	100-5,000 mg
	Vitamin E	600 IU
	Vitamin F	Six capsules
	Zinc	
	Protein	
	Water	

*See note, p. 166.

PSORIASIS

Psoriasis, a recurring disease, is characterized by eruptions on the skin of red circular patches of all sizes covered with dry, silvery scales. The patches enlarge slowly, forming more extensive patches. Psoriasis appears mainly on the legs, arms, scalp, ears, and lower back. The cause is unknown, although its occurrence correlates highly with heredity.

Exposure to sunlight or ultraviolet light reduces the scaling and redness of psoriasis. An increased intake of animal protein can spread the disease, while a reduction in animal protein and fat intake can be useful for treating psoriasis. Vitamin A, the B complex, vitamin C, and vitamin D, all of which play a part in skin health, have been found to be useful in treating some cases of the disease. Some researchers have also found vitamin E to be effective in healing psoriasis.[28]

NUTRIENTS THAT MAY BE BENEFICIAL IN TREATMENT OF PSORIASIS

Body Member	Nutrients	Quantity*
Skin	Vitamin A	Up to 100,000 IU during first week; reduce

*See note, p. 166.

[27] Robert E. Rothenberg, *Health in the Later Years*, rev. ed. (New York: Signet Books, 1972), p. 499.
[28] Rodale, *The Complete Book of Vitamins*, p. 389.

Body Member	Nutrients	Quantity
		to 25,000 IU for three months; repeat
	Vitamin B complex	
	Vitamin B$_2$	
	Vitamin B$_6$	100-200 mg
	Vitamin B$_{12}$	
	Folic acid	
	Pantothenic acid	
	Vitamin C	Up to 3,000 mg
	Vitamin D	
	Vitamin E	Up to 1,600 IU
	Vitamin F	2 tbsp
	Bioflavonoids	
	Lecithin	3,500 mg
	Magnesium	
	Sulfur	Ointment
	Low fat	
	Low animal protein	

PYORRHEA (SORE GUMS)

Pyorrhea is an infectious disease of the gums and tooth sockets characterized by the formation of pus and usually by loosening of the teeth. Gum disorders such as puffiness, tenderness, soreness, and bleeding are often related to vitamin C and bioflavonoid deficiencies that cause increased capillary fragility. Sore gums may also indicate a niacin deficiency. One form of gum inflammation is gingivitis.

NUTRIENTS THAT MAY BE BENEFICIAL IN TREATMENT OF PYORRHEA

Body Member	Nutrients	Quantity*
Teeth/Gums	Vitamin A	
	Vitamin B complex	
	Vitamin B$_6$	
	Niacin	300 mg
	Vitamin C	300 mg
	Bioflavonoids	300 mg
	Calcium	

*See note, p. 166.

RHEUMATIC FEVER

Rheumatic fever is an infection, caused by streptococcal bacteria in the body, which occurs most frequently in children between the ages of four and eighteen. It affects one or more of the following body members: joints (arthritis), brain (chorea), heart (carius), tissues (nodules), and skin (erythema marginatum). Residual heart disease is a possible complication.

A salt-restricted diet containing all essential nutrients, together with a planned exercise program to relieve joint pain is recommended. Bioflavonoids have been found valuable for treating and preventing rheumatic fever.

NUTRIENTS THAT MAY BE BENEFICIAL IN TREATMENT OF RHEUMATIC FEVER

Body Member	Nutrients	Quantity*
General	Vitamin A	
	Pangamic acid	
	Vitamin C	1-10 g
	Vitamin D	
	Vitamin E	
	Bioflavonoids	

*See note, p. 166.

RHEUMATISM

Rheumatism is a general term referring to acute and chronic conditions characterized by stiffness of muscles and pain in the joints. Rheumatism includes such conditions as arthritis and bursitis, as well as other diseases.

NUTRIENTS THAT MAY BE BENEFICIAL IN TREATMENT OF RHEUMATISM

Body Member	Nutrients	Quantity
Muscles/Joints	Vitamin B$_6$	
	Pangamic acid	
	Vitamin C	
	Vitamin E	
	Bioflavonoids	
	Calcium	
	Phosphorus	
	Potassium	
	Protein	

RICKETS AND OSTEOMALACIA

Rickets is primarily a childhood disease of malnutrition in which there is a deficiency of vitamin D, calcium, and/or phosphorus. The chief symptom of rickets is an inability of the bones to retain calcium. This causes them to become soft, which results in deformities when the bones are called upon to support weight that they are too weak to support. Such deformities include bowlegs, knock-knees, protruding breast bone, narrowed rib cage, and bony beads along the ribs. Other symptoms of rickets include tetany and easily decaying teeth. However, weight gain and growth are generally normal in children with rickets.

The adult form of rickets is known as osteomalacia. It is most likely to occur at times of bodily stress such as pregnancy or during breast-feeding. Its causes may be a kidney defect or disease, a deficiency of calcium or phosphorus, or an inability to use vitamin D. In addition to the symptoms of rickets, aching of joints and generalized weakness occur. Vitamin D, calcium, and phosphorus work together to form strong bones; if one of these nutrients is missing, the result is rickets or osteomalacia. Vitamin D is needed for proper absorption and use of calcium and phosphorus, which hardens the bones. A deficiency of vitamin C can make the bones less able to retain calcium and phosphorus. Therefore the diet must be adequate in vitamin C, calcium, and phosphorus.

NUTRIENTS THAT MAY BE BENEFICIAL IN TREATMENT OF RICKETS AND OSTEOMALACIA

Body Member	Nutrients	Quantity
Bones	Vitamin A	
	Vitamin C	
	Vitamin D	
	Calcium	
	Magnesium	
	Phosphorus	

RHINITIS

Rhinitis is the inflammation of the nasal mucosa causing nasal congestion with increased secretion of mucus.

No specific treatment is known; general measures include rest, adequate fluid intake, and a well-balanced diet. Vitamin A has been used successfully in the treatment of rhinitis. Sulfonamides and antibiotics are of no value and should not be administered.

NUTRIENTS THAT MAY BE BENEFICIAL IN TREATMENT OF RHINITIS

Body Member	Nutrients	Quantity
Mucous membrane	Vitamin A	
	Protein	

SCIATICA

Sciatica refers to severely painful spasms along the sciatic nerve of the leg. This nerve runs from the back of the thigh, down the inside of the leg, to the ankle. Among the possible causes of sciatica are trauma or inflammation of the nerve itself, sprained joints in the lower back, rupture of a disk between the spinal bones, or neuritis.

Treatment for sciatica includes rest and hot, wet applications to the affected leg for the relief of pain and inflammation. The vitamin B complex is essential for the health of nerve tissue.

NUTRIENTS THAT MAY BE BENEFICIAL IN TREATMENT OF SCIATICA

Body Member	Nutrients	Quantity*
Leg/Nervous system	Vitamin B complex	
	Vitamin B_1	25 mg/cc (injections)
	Vitamin D	
	Vitamin E	

*See note, p. 166.

SCURVY

Scurvy is a malnutrition disease caused by a diet that is deficient in vitamin C. Symptoms of adult scurvy include swelling and bleeding of the gums, tenderness of joints and muscles, rough, dry, discolored skin, poor healing of wounds, and increased susceptibility to bruising and infection. Because vitamin C facilitates the absorption of iron, scurvy may be complicated by anemia.

An infant with scurvy experiences joint pain that causes him to assume a position called the "scrobutic pose" in which he is comfortable only when lying on his back with his knees partially bent and his thighs turned outward. The vitamin C deficiency makes the infant's bones less capable of retaining calcium and phosphorus, causing them to become weak and eventually brittle.

Scurvy responds dramatically, usually in two or three days' time, to the daily administration of 100 to 200 milligrams of vitamin C. In treating complications such as anemia and bone changes, a well-balanced diet high in protein and iron is also necessary to promote tissue repair.

NUTRIENTS THAT MAY BE BENEFICIAL IN TREATMENT OF SCURVY

Body Member	Nutrients	Quantity*
General	Vitamin A	
	Folic acid	
	Vitamin C	300-500 mg
	Bioflavonoids	
	Iron	
	Protein	

*See note, p. 166.

SHINGLES (HERPES ZOSTER)

Shingles (herpes zoster) is an infection caused by a virus of the nerve endings in the skin. The disease is characterized by blister and crust formation and severe pain along the involved nerve which may last for several weeks. The infection commonly occurs on the chest or abdomen, although it may occur on the face around the eyes.

The B vitamins are necessary for the proper functioning of the nerves. Intramuscular injections of thiamine hydrochloride and vitamin B_{12} are sometimes used in the treatment of herpes zoster. Vitamins A and C help promote healing of the skin lesions characteristic of the disease.

NUTRIENTS THAT MAY BE BENEFICIAL IN TREATMENT OF SHINGLES

Body Member	Nutrients	Quantity*
Skin	Vitamin A	
	Vitamin B complex	
	Vitamin B_1	200-300 mg
	Vitamin B_6	
	Vitamin B_{12}	
	Vitamin C	
	Vitamin D	

*See note. p. 166.

SINUSITIS

Sinusitis is the inflammation of one or more of the sinus cavities, or passages. Sinusitis usually occurs in the nasal sinuses, which are located in the bones surrounding the eyes and nose. Symptoms of the inflammation include nasal congestion and discharge, fatigue, headache, earache, pain around the eyes, mild fever, cough, and an increased susceptibility to infection.

Sinusitis may be the result of a cold, sore throat, tonsilitis, or poor mouth hygiene. Recent studies indicate that a deficiency of vitamin A, which helps maintain the health of the mucous membrane of the nose and throat, may cause the condition. Smoking, damp weather, or the ingestion of spicy foods or alcohol may aggravate sinusitis.

Adequate intake of vitamin A may be useful in the treatment of sinusitis, especially if a deficiency exists. Vitamin C can help fight the infections that may occur with this condition, and protein will help restore damaged sinus tissues.

NUTRIENTS THAT MAY BE BENEFICIAL IN TREATMENT OF SINUSITIS

Body Member	Nutrients	Quantity
Sinuses	Vitamin A	
	Vitamin C	
	Vitamin E	
	Protein	

STOMACH ULCER (PEPTIC)

There are several conflicting views on dietary treatment for ulcer patients. Many physicians initially put patients with severe ulcers on a diet of milk and cream, given in hourly feedings, to reduce the acidity of the gastric juices. Other sources state that frequent small feedings of protein snacks or skim milk should be used but that cream should be avoided, particularly in patients with atherosclerosis or obesity. Further sources indicate that the patient himself should decide which foods seem to agree best with him.

Vitamin A is important for the ulcer patient for maintenance of the tissue that lines the stomach. Fruits and vegetables, sources of vitamins and minerals, should be served in puree form to eliminate hard-to-digest fiber from the diet. Citrus fruit juices, although acidic, are high in vitamin C content and may be used if they are diluted. Eggs and lean meats are good sources of iron, which the ulcer patient requires. A vitamin B complex deficiency may occur with peptic ulcers, and supplementation may therefore be necessary.

NUTRIENTS THAT MAY BE BENEFICIAL IN TREATMENT OF STOMACH ULCER (PEPTIC)

Body Member	Nutrients	Quantity*
Stomach	Vitamin A	25,000-50,000 IU
	Vitamin B complex	
	Vitamin B_2	5 mg three times daily
	Vitamin B_{12}	
	Vitamin C	
	Vitamin E	600-1,200 IU
	Calcium	
	Iron	
	Protein	

*See note, p. 166.

STRESS

Stress is any physical or emotional strain on the body or mind. Physical stress occurs when an external or natural change or force acts upon the body. Extreme heat or cold, overwork, injuries, malnutrition, and exposure to drugs and poisons are example of physical stress. Emotional stress may be a result of fear, hate, love, anger, tension, grief, joy, frustration, and/or anxiety. Physical and emotional stress can overlap, as in special body conditions such as pregnancy, adolescence, and aging. During these times, body metabolism is increased or lowered, changing the body's physical functions, which, in turn, affect the person's mental and emotional outlook on life. A certain amount of stress is useful as a motivating factor, but when it occurs in excess or is of the wrong kind, the effect can be detrimental.

The metabolic response of the body to either physical or emotional stress is to produce more adrenal hormones. These adrenal hormones are secreted by glands that lie above the kidneys. When released into the blood, these hormones prepare the body for action by increasing blood pressure and heartbeat and by making extra energy available. These body responses are useful when physical action is needed, but in our modern civilization there is usually little physical outlet for them, and the body must react to stress by channeling the body's responses inward to one of the organ systems, such as the digestive, circulatory, or nervous system. When this happens, the

system reacts adversely, and conditions such as ulcers, hypertension, backache, atherosclerosis, allergic reactions, asthma, fatigue, and insomnia often develop.

Anxiety, a fearful or distressful feeling, is responsible for the stress of many individuals. Anything that threatens a person's body, job, loved ones, or values may cause anxiety. If the person cannot cope with the situation, stress on the body is increased, resulting in many of the disorders associated with stress. Change in attitude or life-style may be necessary to eliminate the needless strain and allow the body to resume normal functioning.

The increase in the production of adrenal hormones which occurs with stress increases the metabolism of protein, fats, and carbohydrates, producing instant energy for the body to use. As a result of this increased metabolism, there is also an increased excretion of protein, potassium, and phosphorus and a decreased storage of calcium. Many of the disorders related to stress are not a direct result of the stress itself but a result of nutrient deficiencies caused by increased metabolic rate during periods of stress. For example, vitamin C is utilized by the adrenal gland during stressful conditions, and any stress that is sufficiently severe or prolonged will cause a depletion of vitamin C in the tissues.

People experiencing stress need to maintain a nutritious, well-balanced diet with special emphasis on replacing the nutrients that may be depleted during stress.

NUTRIENTS THAT MAY BE BENEFICIAL IN TREATMENT OF STRESS

Body Member	Nutrients	Quantity*
General	Vitamin A	
	Vitamin B complex	
	Vitamin B_1	
	Vitamin B_2	2 mg every three hours
	Vitamin B_6	2 mg every three hours
	Vitamin B_{12}	
	Folic acid	
	Niacin	
	Pantothenic acid	100 mg
	Vitamin C	500 mg every three hours
	Vitamin D	
	Vitamin E	
	Calcium	

*See note, p. 166.

Body Member	Nutrients	Quantity
	Phosphorus	
	Potassium	
	Carbohydrate	
	Fat	
	Protein	

SUNBURN

Sunburn is caused by excessive exposure to ultraviolet rays, which actually burn up surface skin and later the lower cells.

The amount of exposure to ultraviolet rays which causes burning depends basically on four things: the individual, place, time, and atmospheric conditions.

Caution should be used in exposing oneself to the sun for extended periods of time between 10:00 A.M. and 2:00 P.M., when most of the ultraviolet rays are present. Reflections from water, metal, sand, or snow may double the amount of rays one absorbs.

Burns may be classified in three degrees. First-degree sunburn causes reddening of the skin and possibly slight fever. Second-degree sunburn causes reddening of the skin accompanied by water blisters. Third-degree sunburn causes lower cell damage and the release of fluid resulting in eruptions and breaks in the skin where bacteria and infection can enter.

Cold water soaking or cold water compresses, together with additional intake of vitamins A, C, and E, are recommended for treatment of sunburn.

NUTRIENTS THAT MAY BE BENEFICIAL IN TREATMENT OF SUNBURN

Body Member	Nutrients	Quantity*
Skin	PABA	1,000 mg plus ointment
	Vitamin E	
	Calcium	

*See note, p. 166.

SWOLLEN GLANDS

Swollen glands is a term commonly used to describe enlargement of the lymph nodes, or glands of the neck, on both sides of the throat. Technically, however, it can also describe enlargement of any of the lymph glands, such as those located in the armpit or groin. The enlargement of lymph glands is usually a signal of an in-

fection in the area because the lymph glands function to filter out microscopic material, such as bacteria, in order to prevent the spread of infection.

Symptoms include enlarged or swollen glands that may be hard or soft. These symptoms may be accompanied by heat, tenderness, and reddening of the overlying skin, and fever.

Swollen glands may simply indicate a localized infection or may be a symptom of a more serious disease. Swollen gland conditions may occur with such disorders as mononucleosis, measles, chicken pox, leukemia, cancer, tuberculosis, and syphilis.

Treatment includes maintaining a well-balanced diet and fighting the particular infection that is causing the lymph node enlargement. In general, infection requires an increased intake of protein, fluids, and calories. If the infection is accompanied by fever, the diet should be rich in vitamins A and C and the B complex.

NUTRIENTS THAT MAY BE BENEFICIAL IN TREATMENT OF SWOLLEN GLANDS

Body Member	Nutrients	Quantity
Glands/Lymph nodes	Vitamin A	
	Vitamin B complex	
	Vitamin C	
	Protein	
	Water	

TONSILITIS

Tonsilitis is an inflammation of the tonsils, which are glands of lymph tissue located on either side of the entrance to the throat. Tonsilitis may be caused by virus infections when the body's resistance is lowered or by an improper diet that is high in carbohydrates and low in protein and other nutrients.

Symptoms of tonsilitis include pain, redness and swelling in the back of the mouth, difficulty in swallowing, hoarseness, and coughing. Headache, earache, fever and chills, nausea and vomiting, nasal obstruction and discharge, and enlarged lymph nodes throughout the body are additional symptoms of tonsilitis.

In cases of severe tonsil infection, surgical removal may be necessary. The most effective means of prevention for tonsilitis is maintaining a well-balanced diet that is adequate in protein, vitamins, and minerals. The regular intake of vitamin C may help prevent tonsilitis.[29]

[29] Linus Pauling, *Vitamin C and the Common Cold* (New York: Bantam Books, 1970), p. 29

NUTRIENTS THAT MAY BE BENEFICIAL IN TREATMENT OF TONSILITIS

Body Member	Nutrients	Quantity
Glands/Tonsil	Folic acid	
	Vitamin C	
	Protein	

NUTRIENTS THAT MAY BE BENEFICIAL IN TREATMENT OF TOOTH AND GUM DISORDERS

Body Member	Nutrients	Quantity*
Teeth/Gums	Vitamin A	
	Vitamin B_6	
	Niacin	
	Vitamin C	
	Vitamin D	
	Vitamin F	1 tbsp vegetable oil
	Bioflavonoids	
	Calcium	
	Fluorine	
	Iron	
	Magnesium	
	Phosphorus	
	Potassium	
	Sodium	
	Protein	

*See note, p. 166.

TOOTH AND GUM DISORDERS

Cavities (dental caries) are the primary dental problem in the United States. Most cavities are caused by persistent eating of refined sugars and starches, which mix with saliva to form an acid that erodes tooth enamel. One can control cavities by avoiding refined carbohydrate foods, eating a nutritionally balanced diet, and properly cleansing the mouth, including brushing both teeth and gums and cleansing between the teeth with dental floss following meals and snacks.

Although cavities are the major dental disease, a condition known as periodontitis accounts for the loss of more teeth than do cavities. Periodontitis, an inflammation of the gums and the bones that surround and support the teeth, can accompany mouth and upper respiratory infections, or it may be caused by poor fillings, poorly fitting dentures, improper cleansing of teeth and gums, or inadequate diet. Periodontitis begins as a condition known as gingivitis, in which the gums redden, swell, and tend to bleed. If not treated, gingivitis can lead to pyorrhea (see p. 157), characterized by further gum inflammation accompanied by a continuous discharge of pus, gum recession, and loosening of teeth.

Although all vitamins and minerals are essential for the proper formation and continued health of the teeth, an adequate vitamin C intake is especially helpful for the prevention of gingivitis and pyorrhea, while a deficiency of it causes teeth to loosen and break down. Vitamin A seems to control the development and general health of the gums; a lack of this vitamin often results in gum infection. Vitamin A is also necessary for the formation and maintenance of tooth development in children. Minerals important for healthy teeth are sodium, potassium, calcium, phosphorus, iron, and magnesium.

A varied diet of fresh fruits, green leafy vegetables, meat, and whole-grain bread will provide the teeth and gums with needed exercise and supply the body with vitamins and minerals essential for dental health.

TUBERCULOSIS

Tuberculosis is a contagious disease caused by bacterial infection. A person normally has some defense against the bacteria, but when the body is weakened or rundown, its susceptibility to infection is increased. Tuberculosis usually affects the lungs, but it may also involve other organs and tissues.

Many tuberculosis patients may exhibit mild symptoms from which they recover completely. This usually means that the body has successfully controlled the bacteria. Mild symptoms of the disease include fatigue and appetite and weight loss. As the disease becomes more severe, symptoms include fever, increased perspiration, and rapid loss of weight and strength. Coughing up blood is often the first indication of a severe form of the disease.

A tuberculosis patient should be isolated in a hospital for treatment during the contagious state. Antibiotics, adequate rest, and proper diet comprise the most effective therapy for tuberculosis.

Because malnutrition makes an individual more susceptible to tuberculosis, a patient is often treated with a high-protein, low-carbohydrate diet. Supplementation with vitamin A is necessary because the patient is less able

[30]J.I. Rodale, *The Health Seeker* (Emmaus, Pa.: Rodale Books, 1967), p. 857.

to convert carotene to vitamin A.[30] Vitamin C may also be deficient in the tuberculosis patient; thus additional intake may be necessary. Extra vitamin D is needed for the absorption of additional calcium, which the patient needs in order to form a case, or wall, around the invading bacteria. If the patient is losing blood, increased iron intake is required to rebuild the red blood cells. A diet high in protein and the necessary vitamins and minerals will help a person maintain his ideal weight and thus help prevent tuberculosis from recurring.

NUTRIENTS THAT MAY BE BENEFICIAL IN TREATMENT OF TUBERCULOSIS

Body Member	Nutrients	Quantity*
Lungs/Respiratory system	Vitamin A	10,000-40,000 IU
	Vitamin B_6	2 mg six times daily
	Vitamin B_{12}	50 mcg six times daily
	Niacin	
	Pantothenic acid	
	Vitamin C	500 mg six times daily
	Vitamin D	
	Calcium	
	Iron	
	Phosphorus	
	Protein	
	Low carbohydrate	

*See note, p. 166.

ULCER

An open sore (not wound) on the skin or mucous membrane is called an ulcer. Ulcerated sores often form pus and are characterized by the disintegration of tissue and resistance to healing.

NUTRIENTS THAT MAY BE BENEFICIAL IN TREATMENT OF ULCERS

Body Member	Nutrients	Quantity*
Skin	Vitamin A	100,000 IU for three months; then reduce to 25,000 IU

*See note, p. 166.

Body Member	Nutrients	Quantity
	Vitamin B complex	
	Vitamin B_2	400 mg
	Vitamin B_{12}	
	Folic acid	5 mg three times daily
	Vitamin C	Up to 3,000 mg
	Vitamin E	800 IU
	Vitamin K	
	Bioflavonoids	
	Iron	
	Protein	

UNDERWEIGHT

A person is underweight when he is 10 percent or more under the desired weight for his body size and build (see "Desirable Height and Weight chart," p. 236). Underweight develops when more calories are utilized by the body than are consumed. Underweight without a lack of nutrients may or may not be serious, depending upon the degree of underweight. The thin person is probably less apt to suffer from heart diseases and certain other ailments and will live longer than a person who is overweight. Malnutrition occurs when an individual is deficient in the nutrients necessary for life. Individuals with this problem are very susceptible to infections, lack nutrient reserves for times of stress, and are easily fatigued. When underweight and malnutrition are severe, there is starvation, the body's stores of nutrients and fats are depleted, and muscle tissue is broken down to provide energy for bodily functions.

Symptoms that may accompany underweight are weakness, fatigue, sensitivity to cold, hunger, dizziness, and loss of ambition. Underweight may be due to poor eating habits, a nervous condition, overactivity, illness, or metabolic and heredity problems. Underweight can be corrected by removal of the underlying causes and improvement of the diet. The diet should be well-balanced and higher in calories. Extra protein is needed to rebuild tissues. Frequent smaller feedings may be of help in weight gain. Exercise is important during weight gain, so that muscles, rather than fat, are formed. For the same reason, weight should not be gained at the rate of more than a pound a week. Any vitamin deficienceis should be corrected as quickly as possible (see "Nutrient Allowance Chart," p. 237).

NUTRIENTS THAT MAY BE BENEFICIAL IN TREATMENT OF UNDERWEIGHT

Body Member	Nutrients	Quantity
Body	Vitamin F	
	Protein	

VAGINITIS

Vaginitis is an inflammation of the vagina, usually caused by bacterial or yeast infection, excessive douching, vitamin B deficiency,[31] or intestinal worms. Symptoms of vaginitis include a burning or itching sensation and an abnormal vaginal discharge that is white or yellow. Vaginitis is common in pregnant or diabetic women and in women using antibiotics or oral contraceptives.

Adequate rest, a healthful diet, and meticulous personal hygiene with frequent bathing are important for the treatment of vaginitis. White cotton underwear is sometimes recommended because it allows for free circulation of air. Vaginal itching may be prevented by the intake of vitamin A and the B complex if a deficiency is present.

NUTRIENTS THAT MAY BE BENEFICIAL IN TREATMENT OF VAGINITIS

Body Member	Nutrients	Quantity*
Reproductive system	Vitamin A	50,000 IU
	Vitamin B complex	
	Vitamin B$_2$	6 mg
	Vitamin B$_6$	
	Vitamin D	
	Vitamin E	

*See note, p. 166.

VARICOSE VEINS

Varicose veins are veins that have become enlarged, twisted, and swollen. They may be located anywhere in the body, but they are most commonly found in the legs.

Factors that inhibit blood circulation, such as obesity, certain hereditary conditions, tight clothing, crossing of legs, and a sedentary occupation, can increase suscepti-

bility to varicose veins. A pregnant woman or a woman who has had several pregnancies is usually more prone to varicose veins than are most other women because pregnancy causes increased pressure on the legs.

It is essential that individuals who must sit for extended periods of time receive adequate exercise. Elevating the legs while resting is another preventive measure.

Adequate amounts of the B vitamins and vitamin C are necessary in the diet for the maintenance of strong blood vessels. Some research has indicated that vitamin E can dilate blood vessels and improve circulation, thus perhaps reducing the susceptibility to varicose veins.[32]

NUTRIENTS THAT MAY BE BENEFICIAL IN TREATMENT OF VARICOSE VEINS

Body Member	Nutrients	Quantity*
Leg	Vitamin B complex	
	Vitamin C	Up to 3,000 mg
	Vitamin E	600-1,000 IU
	Bioflavonoids	300-500 mg
	Protein	

*See note, p. 166.

VENEREAL DISEASE

Venereal disease is usually acquired through intimate contact with the sexual organs of an afflicted individual. The most frequent vehicle of the disease is the act of sexual intercourse or intimacy associated with sexual intercourse. Gonorrhea and syphilis are the two most common types of venereal disease.

Gonorrhea is transmitted through sexual intimacy or from the mother to the newborn infant as it passes through an infected birth canal. Within 3 to 14 days after contact, males experience burning, pain, and discharge of pus upon urination. Complications of gonorrhea in males may include prostatitis and testes infection. Females may have increased urinary frequency and a yellowish discharge from the vagina, but there are usually no immediate symptoms until the infection has included all of the reproductive organs of the pelvic region. Complications of gonorrhea may result in sterility in both sexes.

Syphilis is also most commonly spread through sexual intimacy, but it may also be received through a break in

[31] Davis, *Let's Get Well*, p. 308.

[32] Rodale, *The Complete Book of Vitamins*, p. 352.

the skin that has come in contact with a chancre, or open sore, fresh blood, semen, or a vaginal discharge from an infected individual. Syphilis can also be transmitted from the mother to the fetus via the bloodstream during pregnancy.

There are three distinct stages of syphilis. First, a chancre appears 10 to 28 days after contact at the point where the infecting organism entered the body, but it disappears in 2 to 5 weeks. Other possible symptoms of this stage include fever, weight loss, and anemia.

Six weeks to six months after appearance of the chancre, the second stage begins. It is characterized by skin rashes, hair loss, warts near the mouth or anus, fever, headache, sore throat, and possibly bone pain. The next one to several years may be without symptoms.

During the third stage the disease is no longer contagious. In this stage the organisms settle in specific body organs and destroy them. Commonly, the circulatory system and nervous system are attacked, often resulting in death.

Treatment for venereal disease includes massive injections of antibiotics, usually penicillin, to rid the body of the venereal organism. Early treatment is essential to prevent complicating tissue damage. To prevent the spread of venereal disease, an afflicted person should abstain from sexual intercourse and intimacy until the disease has been cured. In addition to obtaining medical treatment, an afflicted person should maintain a well-balanced diet high in protein to help repair the tissue damage that has occurred.

NUTRIENTS THAT MAY BE BENEFICIAL IN TREATMENT OF VENEREAL DISEASE

Body Member	Nutrients	Quantity
General	Protein	

VISION AND FOCUS DISORDERS

There are several disorders of the eyes, which may be due to hereditary factors, nutrient deficiencies, strain, or natural aging processes. Symptoms that indicate visual disorders are squinting, blurred vision, inability to see near or far, sensitivity to light, and itching and burning of the eyes and lids.

Vitamin A is essential to the health of the eyes. A deficiency of vitamin A can result in various conditions of poor sight. A riboflavin deficiency can result in sensitive and easily fatigued eyes, blurred vision, itching, and bloodshot eyes.

NUTRIENTS THAT MAY BE BENEFICIAL IN TREATMENT OF VISION AND FOCUS DISORDERS

Body Member	Nutrients	Quantity*
Eyes/General	Vitamin A	
	Vitamin B complex	
	Vitamin B$_2$	50 mg daily
	Vitamin C	500-1,500 mg
	Vitamin D	
	Vitamin E	200 IU

*See note, p. 166.

WORMS

There are several types of parasitic worms which can live in human intestines, the most common being pinworms, tapeworms, hookworms, and roundworms. Worms irritate the intestinal lining and therefore cause poor absorption of nutrients. Signs of worms often include diarrhea, hunger pains, appetite loss, weight loss, and anemia. Diagnosis can be made by examining the stools or, occasionally, by inducing the vomiting of worms. The extent of the intestinal damage is then determined by the type of worm, the size of the worm, and the number of worms present.

Pinworms are the most common parasitic worm in the United States. The chief symptom of this small, threadlike worm is rectal itching, especially at night. Pinworms are transmitted when eggs, which lodge under the fingernails when a person scratches, contaminate food. Personal hygiene is most important for the control of pinworms.

Tapeworms can be contracted from eating insufficiently cooked meats, especially beef, pork, and fish. The most common tapeworm in the United States, beef tapeworm, grows to a length of 15 to 20 feet in the intestines.

Hookworms are often found in the soil or sand in moderate climates. They can enter the body by boring holes in the skin of the bare feet or can enter by mouth if food contaminated by dirty hands is eaten.

Roundworms are most common in children. These worms can leave the intestines and settle in different areas of the body, causing diseases such as pneumonia, jaundice, or periodontitis.

When a person is afflicted with worms, the body's supply of all nutrients is depleted to the point that supplementation of all nutrients is necessary to restore normal health. Nutrients of special importance are vitamin A; the B complex, especially thiamine, riboflavin, B_6, B_{12}, and pantothenic acid; vitamins C, D, and K; and calcium, iron, and protein.

NUTRIENTS THAT MAY BE BENEFICIAL IN TREATMENT OF WORMS

Body Member	Nutrients	Quantity
Body/Intestine	Vitamin A	
	Vitamin B_1	
	Vitamin B_2	
	Vitamin B complex	
	Vitamin B_6	
	Vitamin B_{12}	
	Pantothenic acid	
	Vitamin D	
	Vitamin F	
	Vitamin K	
	Calcium	
	Iron	
	Potassium	
	Sulfur (ointment form)	
	Protein	

> **NOTE: Quantities shown are not prescriptive; some are extremely high and represent therapeutic test dosages. Individual needs and tolerances will vary according to body size, metabolism, age, diet, and ailment. Consult a physician who is familiar with nutritional therapy before taking large quantities.**

NORMAL LIFE CYCLE

PREGNANCY

Pregnancy is a stressful condition involving numerous physical and mental changes in the mother's body as the fetus develops. The tissues in the breasts and uterus increase, the blood supply increases, there is a frequent urge to urinate, there is slight nausea in the morning or even later in the day, the menstrual period is absent, and the need for sleep and fluids is increased. Because of these changes, all nutritional needs of the mother increase in preparation for the newborn baby.

A woman who has maintained a nutritionally balanced diet throughout her life has the best possible chance of bearing a healthy child. However, during pregnancy, nutritional needs are increased, and the condition of the mother and her child could be greatly improved by dietary supplementation. All known nutrients must be supplied to the expectant mother.

Protein, calcium, and iron are especially important to the development of bones, soft tissues, and blood of the body. Protein of both animal origin (meat, eggs, cheese, milk, fish, etc.) and plant origin (whole-grain cereals, nuts, peas, beans, soybeans, lentils, etc.) should be included in the diet because the body can make the fullest use of these products in combination. Protein is also needed to provide for the 20 percent increase in blood volume during pregnancy. An adequate supply of vitamin D is needed to ensure proper absorption and utilization of calcium and phosphorus.

Additional iron is essential to prevent anemia in both mother and baby and to guard the mother against excessive blood loss during birth. Adequate iron also guards against miscarriage and fetal malformation.

Vitamin C, vitamin K, and the bioflavonoids are necessary to strengthen blood vessels and to prevent excessive bleeding. In late pregnancy and postdelivery, thiamine requirements are greatly increased. Vitamin E may prevent miscarriage and toxemia. Iodine deficiency during pregnancy may cause mental retardation.[33]

In addition, the pregnant woman should take special care to ensure adequate intake of the vitamin B complex, protein, and calcium, which help to normalize emotional states that occur frequently during pregnancy. The B-complex vitamins, found in brewer's yeast or wheat germ, will also help relieve fatigue, insomnia, and nervous tension. Together with calcium, found in milk or bone meal, B vitamins may also help to relieve leg, back, and joint pains often associated with pregnancy. Nausea and morning sickness due to nervous conditions will probably respond to additional intake of B vitamins

[33]Adelle Davis, *Let's Have Healthy Children*. (New York: Harcourt, Brace and World, 1959), p. 47.

and vitamins C and K. The pregnant woman should not take baking soda or other common antacids for indigestion or heartburn because they contain sodium, which will increase fluid retention. Vitamin B_6 has been found to be effective in regulating fluid retention associated with the development of toxemia. The B-complex vitamins and enzyme supplements may relieve heartburn and digestive upsets.

A weight gain of 20 to 25 pounds is desirable and in most cases is in keeping with good health.

The end results of proper prenatal nutrition are a more comfortable pregnancy, an easier delivery, a healthier baby, and a greater chance of successfully nursing the baby.

LACTATION

Lactation is the secretion and yielding of milk by the mammary gland. Preparation for lactation begins during early pregnancy, when the increased production of the hormones estrogen and progesterone leads to the storage of maternal energy in the form of fat. After the baby is born, changes occur in the ductless glandular system of the mother's body which initiate the secretion of milk.

Human breast milk has a remarkably constant composition. It is the most nearly perfect food, but it is low in certain essential nutrients such as vitamin C, vitamin D, and iron. Efforts should be made to see that these nutrients are included in the diet, either through fortified formulas or through supplements.

Poor nutrition of a lactating mother tends to reduce the quantity rather than the quality of breast milk. The body maintains the quality of milk by drawing upon the mother's own store of nutrients. Therefore, a lactating mother, besides her normal requirements, needs extra nutrients to replace both those lost at delivery through bleeding and those she provides in the milk for her infant.

The requirements for thiamine, riboflavin, and nicotinic acid are related to the caloric intake. Since the lactating mother needs extra calories to meet the physiological cost of milk production, her needs for these vitamins become higher than at normal times. The best sources of these vitamins are whole-grain cereals, brewer's yeast, milk, meat, and eggs.

Since a lactating mother needs more calcium and vitamin D is necessary for the absorption of calcium, it is desirable that her diet contain an adequate supply of vitamin D. The best sources of vitamin D are fish-liver oils, butter, and milk. Adequate supply of iron is also needed.

INFANCY AND CHILDHOOD

The period of life from birth to maturity is one of intense growth and development. Heredity, environment, and nutrition are the major determinants of a child's growth potential. Nutrition, however, is the single most important factor in determining the healthy growth and development of a child.

Foods supply the chemicals necessary for forming all tissues, especially muscles, bones, blood, and teeth, and also for repairing tissues. Children need extra calories to provide energy for this growth and for the increased activity and metabolic rate in youth. Children require the same nutrients as adults for good nutrition, however, often in greater proportions. See the "Nutrient Allowance Chart" on p. 237 for children's Recommended Dietary Allowances.

ADOLESCENCE

Adolescence is a period when profound physiological and emotional changes occur within a young person, signifying the onset of puberty and continuing until maturation.

The physical development and rapid growth associated with adolescence make this a time when good nutrition is vitally important for the building of a strong, healthy body. The need for calories, protein, and other body-building elements increases during this period. Adolescents need protein, calcium, phosphorus, and vitamin D for proper bone formation. Protein is especially important for the development of new tissues and contains the amino acids vital for growth. Girls' diets are often seriously lacking in iron, protein, and thiamine. Boys have an increased need for vitamin D in their diets.

MENSTRUATION

Menstruation is the cyclical process that continuously prepares the uterus for pregnancy; it starts at puberty and continues through menopause. Menstruation occurs on an average of every 28 days except during pregnancy and lactation. It is characterized by a passing of the blood-rich uterine lining lasting approximately four or five days. However, individuals may differ in time between periods and duration of menstrual flow.

Women whose general health and resistance are good are apt to have less premenstrual tension or cramping than those women suffering from poor nutrition and lack of physical exercise. Symptoms of premenstrual tension include abdominal bloating, weight gain, breast tenderness, irritability, headache, depression, and, possibly, edema of the legs. Edema may be helped by limiting the salt and fluid intake a short time before the onset of the menstrual period. Vitamin A may relieve general symptoms associated with premenstrual tension.

The loss of blood which occurs during menstruation causes a loss of iron. The diet should be adequate in iron and iodine to replace loss plus vitamin C to aid in iron absorption. Cramping may be relieved with additional intake of calcium and niacin. The vitamin B complex, especially vitamin B_6 and folic acid, may relieve some of the tension associated with menstruation.

Unusually frequent, heavy, or scanty periods of menstrual flow may warrant concern. Medical attention should be sought to determine the cause.

SEX

Many people are not aware of the important role proper nutrition plays in improving sexual vitality. Adequate nourishment is needed to stimulate the hormonal production of the endocrine glands; this increased hormone secretion results in increased sexual vigor.

Endocrine glands, such as thyroid, pituitary, testes, and ovaries, can be specifically nourished by certain nutrients. For example, the B-complex vitamins enter into the cellular and tissue construction of the thyroid gland and act as "energizers" to increase the hormonal flow. An excellent way of obtaining B factors is mixing two tablespoons of brewer's yeast and two tablespoons of wheat germ with vegetable juice and drinking it with the evening meal. This combination is assimilated by the body in about an hour.

An iodine-deficient thryoid gland may cause a decreased interest in sex, because of a decreased rate of hormone production.[34]   One teaspoon of sea salt or kelp may increase the thyroid's metabolism and promote a flow of hormones. In addition, the amino acid tyrosine, from which the thyroid hormone thyroxine is made, helps activate sluggish thyroids. The combination of one tablespoon each of brewer's yeast, wheat germ, and blackstrap molasses mixed with fruit juices and taken three times daily may help the work of tyrosine.

The pituitary gland is responsible for the functioning of the male and female sex hormones, thus providing sex drive for body and mind. The B-complex vitamins are recommended to ensure against impotence and premature menopause.[35]

Zinc and vitamin E are also important in maintaining sexual powers. Zinc deficiency may cause retarded genital development (see "Zinc," p. 82). This mineral is found in highly concentrated form throughout the entire male reproductive system. Vitamin E is often referred to as the "sex vitamin." It may help restore the sexual organs, help stimulate the production of new sperm, and help rejuvenate the sex glands.

MENOPAUSE

Menopause is the period in a woman's life marked by glandular changes that denote the end of her menstrual cycle and reproductive years. Menopause usually results from a decreased production of the female sex hormones when a woman is between the ages of forty-two and fifty-two.

Poor diet, lack of exercise, and emotional stress may exaggerate the symptoms and discomfort of menopause. Some women experience severe nervous symptoms and become irritable, over excitable, or depressed. They may have headaches, abdominal pains, rushes of blood to the head and upper body known as "hot flashes," backaches, leg cramps, nosebleeds, frequent bruises, varicose veins, and even ulcers. Some women find themselves extremely fatigued or experiencing insomnia.

Usually within a period of months or a year or two, the body readjusts and the symptoms disappear. Although the menstrual periods cease, a woman's normal sexual needs remain after menopause, and she does not need to experience rapid aging.

Vitamin E (up to 1,200 IU) is especially important during menopause. The B complex, especially pantothenic acid and PABA, relieve nervous irritability. Vitamin C together with bioflavonoids increases capillary strength. The calcium-phosphorus balance should be

[34]Carlson Wade, "How Nutrition Can Boost Your Sex Powers," *Bestways,* September 1974, p. 25.

[35]Wade, "How Nutrition Can Boost Your Sex Powers," p. 25.

carefully maintained during the mature years, and an increase in protein with reduction of carbohydrates is generally recommended. Adequate intake of vitamin D, iron, and magnesium is also important.

AGING

Aging refers to the changes of the body that are related to the passage of time and is characterized by a deterioration of organs in the body and a general lowering of the body's ability to deal with externally produced stress. Aging may begin in persons twenty years old, as soon as growth hormones present during the teen-age years are no longer being produced. These processes of aging are accelerated by illness or abuse of the body.

It is important to remember that a diet that may be sufficient for a young person may be deficient for an older person because the older person cannot utilize nutrients in the same capacity as the young person. Many of the diseases associated with aging may be prevented or retarded through proper nutrition, adequate rest, and exercise. The process of aging increases the need for vitamins and minerals because nutrients are not as well absorbed by the aging digestive organs.

Ailments often associated with aging include impaired mobility of joints, loss of coordination and sense of balance, lessened muscle tone, and increased mental instability. They may be due to a deficiency of the vitamin B complex, especially vitamin B_{12} and niacin. A B_{12} deficiency may also be related to the development of abnormal fatigue often found among older persons.

Vitamin C decreases the probability of blood vessel ruptures and strokes, promotes healing of wounds, and increases the aging person's ability to withstand the stress of injury and infections.

Brittleness and fragility of bones are caused by loss of weight and density of bones arising from the loss of calcium from the bones. Iron should be taken to prevent anemia.

Many of the conditions normally associated with aging may arise from increased oxidation of cells; therefore vitamin E, which is an effective antioxidant, may help retard aging.

Foods, Beverages, and Supplementary Foods

Many factors influence eating patterns and therefore affect nutrition. For example, taste preferences, states of health, and various social and cultural customs all determine what foods a person eats. Poor nutrition may be the result of consuming too little, too much, or the wrong kinds of food, because of any number of reasons.

The foods and beverages we consume should provide our bodies with the nutrients necessary for good health. Protein builds and maintains body cells, and carbohydrates, fats, and some protein provide calories for energy. Vitamins and minerals help regulate the many chemical reactions within the body. For individual recommended dietary allowances of nutrients, see the "Nutrient Allowance Chart" on pages 237 to 238.

Fresh, raw fruits and vegetables are generally more nutritious than prepared ones, although many kinds of foods are more palatable when cooked. Studies indicate that considerable losses of nutrients, especially the B complex, vitamin C, and the bioflavonoid complex, occur during storage and cooking. It is essential to select, store, and prepare foods wisely in order to obtain these nutrients. Precautions should also be taken to avoid foodborne illnesses caused by the growth of harmful bacteria. Some basic rules for storing and preparing foods in order to retain their nutrient content and to prevent food poisoning are as follows:

Cook meats, especially pork and poultry, thoroughly in order to kill harmful bacteria.

Guard against the growth of harmful bacteria by immediately refrigerating leftovers or foods cooked for later use. Do not allow them to cool to room temperature first.

Keep perishable foods—especially chopped and processed meats, custards, pastries, and dairy products—in the refrigerator to avoid bacterial contamination.

Destroy cans that bulge or canned contents that bubble out when the can is opened, in order to avoid food poisoning.

Ensure thorough cooking of frozen foods by allowing them to thaw completely before cooking, unless otherwise stated on frozen food packages.

Avoid soaking fruits, vegetables, or meats in water to protect against the loss of water-soluble vitamins.

Store fresh foods as soon as possible to minimize nutrient loss.

Supplementary foods may be useful for further increasing the nutritional value of meals. Supplementary foods must also be stored and prepared properly in order to prevent nutrient loss.

In the following section, food groups, beverages, and supplementary foods are discussed alphabetically in terms of their nutrient content and special features. This information is intended for use with the "Table of Food Composition" on pages 185 to 219 and the "Nutrient Allowance Chart" on pages 237 to 238.

Any reference to a body disorder or disease in connection with a food or beverage is not meant to be prescriptive, but merely represents research findings.

FOODS

EGGS

Eggs are an excellent source of complete protein; they contain all essential amino acids. (One large egg contains 7 or 8 grams of first-class protein.) Also found in eggs are vitamins A, B_2, D, and E; niacin; copper; iron; phosphorus; and unsaturated fats. The egg yolk contains the richest known source of choline, found in lecithin and necessary for keeping the cholesterol within the egg emulsified. The egg yolk also contains biotin, one of the B-complex vitamins.

Eggs should be kept refrigerated at all times (at 45° to 55°F) because temperature variations will cause the whites to become thin. A soiled egg should be wiped clean with a dry cloth rather than washed, to preserve the natural protective film on the porous eggshell. This film prevents odors, flavors, molds, and bacteria from entering the egg. Eggs retain their freshness and quality better if stored large end up in their original carton.

Raw eggs should not be consumed in great quantity because the whites contain a protein called avidin, which may be harmful to the body if consumed over a long period of time, since it interferes with the use of biotin. However, avidin is inactivated by heat.

FISH

Fish are excellent sources of high-grade protein, polyunsaturated fatty acids, and minerals, especially iodine and potassium.

Fish are categorized as freshwater fish, saltwater fish, and shellfish. These types differ slightly in nutritive value. Freshwater fish provide magnesium, phosphorus, iron, and copper. Saltwater fish and shellfish are rich in iodine, fluorine, and cobalt. The unsaturated fat content of fish and shellfish varies with the species and season of year. Fatty fish, such as halibut, mackerel, and salmon, are good sources of vitamins A and D. Herring, oysters, and sardines contain vanadium and zinc. Shellfish are low in fatty acids but are relatively high in cholesterol.

Fish and shellfish may be purchased fresh, frozen, canned, salted, dried, or smoked. Because of the possibility of bacterial infection, fresh fish and shellfish should not remain at room temperature for more than two hours. They should be well wrapped, stored in the coldest part of the refrigerator, and used within two days.

Fish and shellfish are best cooked at low temperature (300° to 325°F) and should not be overcooked in order to preserve flavor, juices, and nutrients.

FRUITS

Fresh fruits are good sources of vitamins and minerals, especially vitamins A and C, carbohydrates in the form of cellulose and natural sugars, and water. They are good substitutes of such high-carbohydrate foods as candy, cookies, and cakes, which contain few nutrients.

Yellow fruits, such as apricots, cantaloupe, and persimmons, are good sources of carotene, which is converted to vitamin A. Aside from acerola cherries and rose hips, the best natural sources of vitamin C are the citrus fruits, such as oranges, grapefruit, lemons, and tangerines; other sources of vitamin C are cantaloupe, strawberries, and tomatoes.

Apples and bananas contain valuable bulk fiber in the form of indigestible cellulose, which is needed for regular bowel movement. Bananas are high in magnesium and may be useful for treatment of diarrhea, colitis, ulcers, and certain cases of protein allergies. Bananas and pears are the highest in natural sugars.

Fruits may be fresh, frozen, dried, or canned, but nutrient values will decrease if fruits are not properly stored or if they are refrigerated for extended periods of time. Fresh fruits offer the richest source of vitamins and minerals as well as appetite appeal in color, flavor, and texture. Fresh fruits purchased in season will be higher in nutrient quality and more economical in price than frozen, dried, or canned fruits. It is preferable to obtain ripe rather than green fruits, since ripe fruits contain simple sugars that are very easily assimilated by the digestive system. Fruits that are not fully ripe should be allowed to ripen at room temperature and then should be stored in a cool, dark place or in the refrigerator.

Fresh fruits should always be washed prior to eating so that any possible chemical residue is removed, and should be eaten whole or peeled thinly so that nutrients found in the skin are conserved. If fruits are to be cooked, they should be cooked quickly.

Frozen fruits compare favorably in nutrient content with fresh fruits, but some loss of nutritional value may occur in the processes of drying and canning, if done improperly. Dried fruits, rich in thiamine and iron, should be softened and cooked in the same water and then stored in a cool, dry place. Home-canned fruits should be stored in a dark place to preserve their vitamin C content. Water-packed and light-syrup fruits are preferable to those packed in heavy syrups that contain large amounts of sugar.

FRUIT JUICES

Fresh fruit juices usually have a pleasing flavor and are easily digested. Although the nutritive value of the whole fruit is somewhat higher, juice is an excellent source of vitamins and minerals.

Juice should be extracted from chilled fruit immediately prior to serving. It should not be allowed to stand for a long period of time after extraction, because vitamin C will be lost. Juices should be refrigerated in covered containers to ensure that vitamin C will not be lost through oxidation.

GRAINS

Grains are often referred to as cereals; they are the seeds of various grasses such as wheat, rye, oats, rice, and barley. Often called the "staff of life," they provide the bulk of the world's food supply. Common foods made from these grains are flours, breads, breakfast cereals, and macaroni.

Breads and Cereals

The main constituent of breads is flour. Flour is the product resulting from the milling process, which involves grinding and sifting of cleaned grains. The type of flour or grain from which it originates often determines the color, texture, flavor, and nutritive value of the bread. Cereals can be made from a variety of grains, such as corn, barley, oats, wheat, etc.

Whole-grain flour is the result of the first milling process. Whole-grain flour contains the germ of the grain, which possesses the most nutrients, and must be refrigerated to prevent rancidity. Whole-grain breads should be stored at room temperature or frozen until used. Refrigerated bread loses moisture and thus becomes stale faster than bread that is frozen or that which is kept at room temperature.

All-purpose flour is a blend of different wheat grains. Bleached flour has been whitened to create a more uniform flour. Self-rising flour contains added salt and leavening in proper proportions. *Enriched flour* has the nutrients thiamine, riboflavin, and niacin of the vitamin B complex, and sometimes iron, returned to it. This enrichment process also applies to other "enriched" products, such as breakfast cereals and macaroni.

Rice

Whole brown rice contains a generous supply of B vitamins, plus calcium, phosphorus, and iron. *Wild rice* contains twice as much protein, four times as much phosphorus, eight times as much thiamine, and twenty times as much riboflavin as white rice. *White rice*, dehulled polished rice, has no significant amount of B vitamins but may also be enriched, as are flour and cereals. *Converted rice* has undergone a process similar to milling and it has a somewhat higher vitamin content than white rice.

Whole Grains

The structure of a whole grain may be separated into three different parts (see illustration). The *germ* is the heart of the grain, which sprouts when the seed is planted. It is especially rich in the B vitamins, vitamin E, protein, unsaturated fat, minerals (especially iron), and carbohydrates. The *endosperm* constitutes the largest part of the grain. It is composed chiefly of carbohydrates in the form of starch, with some incomplete protein and traces of vitamins and minerals. The *bran* portion of the grain is the covering. It is composed chiefly of the carbohydrate cellulose, with traces of B vitamins, minerals (especially iron), and incomplete proteins.

While the entire grain is edible, the bran and germ are often removed during milling in order to reduce the

TOTAL NUTRIENTS IN THE KERNEL OF WHEAT[1]

Germ is 2½% of Kernel	Bran is 14% of Kernel	Endosperm is 83% of Kernel
Of the whole kernel the germ contains:	Of the whole kernel the bran contains:	Of the whole kernel the endosperm contains:
64% Thiamine	73% Pyridoxine	70-75% Protein
26% Riboflavin	50% Pantothenic Acid	43% Pantothenic Acid
21% Pyridoxine	42% Riboflavin	32% Riboflavin
8% Protein	33% Thiamine	12% Niacin
7% Pantothenic Acid	19% Protein	6% Pyridoxine
2% Niacin		3% Thiamine

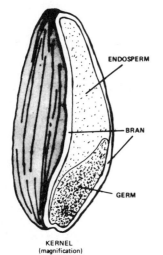

ENDOSPERM

BRAN

GERM

KERNEL
(magnification)

Other Nutrients Found in the Whole Wheat Grain are:

Calcium	Chlorine
Iron	Sodium
Phosphorus	Silicon
Magnesium	Boron
Potassium	Barium
Manganese	Silver
Copper	Inositol
Sulphur	Folic Acid
Iodine	Choline
Fluorine	Vitamin E

And other trace materials

chance of rancidity and to improve the storage quality of the grain. At the same time, important nutrients such as the B vitamins, vitamin E, and iron are lost. In order to enrich flour, bread, and cereal products, thiamine, riboflavin, and iron are added during processing.

LEGUMES

Legumes are plants that have edible seeds within a pod. They include peas, beans, lentils, and peanuts. Legumes are a rich source of incomplete protein, iron, thiamine, riboflavin, and niacin. When sprouted, they provide an excellent source of vitamin C.

Legumes are a hearty and versatile food. Because of their high but incomplete protein content, legumes can be used as a meat substitute when used with other complementary protein foods.

Dried legumes should be stored in tightly covered containers in a cool, dry place. They should be cooked

in liquid to soften their cellulose fiber and to restore flavor and moisture that is lost in the drying process. If one adds baking soda when cooking legumes to speed up the softening of the cellulose, the thiamine content of the legumes will be destroyed.

Soybeans

Generous supplies of soybean products may serve as the major protein source in a meatless diet. However, the balance of essential amino acids in soybeans is not the same as that in meats; therefore more grams of this protein are required to supply the essential amino acids adequately. In addition, soybeans contain vitamins and minerals in a natural relationship that is similar to the human body's needs.

Soy flour, oil, and milk are used in a variety of home-cooked and commerical products. Soy flour has a creamy yellow color and a slightly nutty taste. It is a rich source of protein, the vitamin B complex, calcium, phosphorus, potassium, magnesium, and iron. Soybean

[1] *The Art of Nutritious Cooking* (Bismarck, N.Dak.: Nutrition Search, 1974), p. 15.

oil contains large amounts of linoleic acid, an unsaturated fatty acid essential to the human body. Soybean oil is stable against oxidation and flavor deterioration because of its lecithin and vitamin E content. Soy milk is often recommended for persons who are allergic to cow's milk. Soy milk is low in fat, carbohydrates, calcium, phosphorus, and riboflavin but rich in iron, thiamine, and niacin.

Some forms of soy protein are made into commercial imitation-meat items. Pressed soybean cakes, the product resulting from grinding the soybean residue after the soybeans have been processed for oil, can be added to a variety of cooked dishes. Sprouted soybeans contain increased amounts of vitamin C.

MEATS

"Meat" commonly refers to the flesh of animals; it is the most important source of first-class protein in the modern diet. In addition to protein, beef, lamb, and pork are good sources of the B-complex vitamins (especially thiamine and riboflavin), phosphorus, iron, sulfur, potassium, and copper. Poultry, also a good source of protein, contains the B-complex vitamins (especially niacin), iron, and phosphorus.

The quality of beef, lamb, and pork is designated by the cut—Prime, Choice, or Good—when purchased over the counter. The meat's flavor, tenderness, and ease of cooking vary with the grade and do not affect its nutritional value. In general, lean cuts with less fat are preferable. Prime and Choice cuts of meat are often not the highest in protein content because the animals were "fattened" before slaughter and the lean contains marbling, or fat granules, to increase tenderness. Good grades, therefore, may be more lean and contain more protein per pound. Luncheon meats, frankfurters, and sausages are usually high in fats.

Variety, or organ, meats are usually richer in vitamins and minerals than muscle meats. Variety meats include the liver, tongue, kidneys, heart, brains, and sweetbreads (glands of calves or lambs). Liver is a very rich source of complete protein and B vitamins, especially riboflavin, niacin, and B_{12}. It is also a good source of vitamins A, C, and D; iron; phosphorus; and copper. Because of the high iron and vitamin B_{12} content, liver can aid the body in combating iron-deficiency anemia and pernicious anemia.

Both raw and cooked meat should be refrigerated at a temperature of $30°$ to $32°F$. In order to be at their best flavor and nutritive value, meats should be used within two or three days after purchase. Ground meats and variety meats should be used within 24 hours to prevent spoilage. Meat should not be soaked in water because this leads to loss of water-soluble nutrients. Nearly all meats freeze well and maintain their quality if wrapped and stored properly, although meat that is frozen for more than six months may show freezer burn (drying) and changes in texture. Meats should be frozen quickly and kept at temperatures of $-10°F$ or lower to retard deterioration.

It is preferable that meats be cooked without adding fats or water; broiling and baking at moderate temperatures are recommended. Juices obtained during cooking contain valuable nutrients and should be served with the meat. Pork, or any raw product containing pork, should be cooked thoroughly to kill any trichinosis organisms that may be present. The temperature at the center of a pork roast should be at least $160°$ to $185°F$.

Poultry that is inspected for quality is graded A, B, or C, A being the top quality. White poultry meat is especially rich in niacin and is easier to digest than dark meat, since it contains less fat and connective tissue. Dark meat, however, is superior to white meat as a source of thiamine and riboflavin.

Chilled raw poultry may be kept one or two days in the coldest part of the refrigerator. Stuffing from cooked poultry should be removed and stored separately in a covered container. The body cavity or skin of chickens and turkeys may contain a bacteria that causes food poisoning. In order to prevent a large bacterial growth due to moisture, one should store these birds with loose wrapping so that the surface of the bird will be slightly dry. It is also recommended that poultry be frozen without stuffing and stuffed immediately prior to cooking. Poultry should be thawed completely to enable thorough cooking. Poultry should be cooked thoroughly; the temperature at the center should be about $190°F$.

MILK AND MILK PRODUCTS

Milk and milk products are excellent sources of calcium, complete protein, and riboflavin. Milk also contains phosphorus, thiamine, and vitamins B_6 and B_{12}, but it contains little iron or vitamin C. A glass of milk contains about 300 milligrams of calcium; three glasses of milk daily supply the needed amount of calcium for adults; children and adolescents need four or five glasses per day.

Milk is available in several forms. Most milk is pasteurized to kill bacteria and thereby to prevent the spread of milkborne diseases. The pasteurization process involves heating the milk to a high temperature and cooling it rapidly. Homogenized milk is that which has its fat content finely dispersed throughout, and because of this, it is more easily digested than nonhomogenized milk.

Whole milk usually contains about 3.5 percent fat. Skim milk is whole milk from which the fat is removed. Two percent milk contains two percent fat, which gives it more body and flavor than skim milk. Fortified milk has one or more nutrients, commonly vitamins A and D, added. Nonfat dry milk and fluid skim milk, unless fortified, contain no significant amounts of vitamin A or D because these fat-soluble vitamins are removed with the fat; but they are rich in protein, calcium, and vitamin B_2.

People who are allergic to milk may substitute buttermilk, goat's milk, yogurt, and possibly soy milk, although soy milk lacks much of the value of cow's milk because it is low in calcium and phosphorus.

Buttermilk may be obtained from the residue of the butter-making process, or it may be cultured. Most commercial buttermilk is made by the latter process, in which a harmless bacteria is added to skim milk or churned buttermilk.

Evaporated milk is whole milk with one-half of its water content removed. Condensed milk has water removed and sugar added. Dried milk results from the removal of 95 to 98 percent water from whole milk; nonfat dry milk is skim milk with the water removed.

Butter

Butter is made from milk products, contains vitamins A and D, and is high in fat content. Butter should be kept in the refrigerator and left in its original wrapper until ready for use, to retain its flavor and consistency.

Cheese

Cheese is made by separating most of the curd, or milk solids, from the whey or water part of the milk. Its texture and flavor vary with ripening (aging). Most cheeses contain protein, milk, fat, calcium, phosphorus, vitamin A, and riboflavin. The best way to store cheese is by leaving it in its original wrapper in the refrigerator. If the wrapper is torn, protect the surface from drying out by covering exposed surface with waxed paper, foil, or plastic. Cheeses with a strong odor should be kept in a container with a tight cover.

Yogurt

Milk that has been fermented by a mixture of bacteria and yeasts forms a custardlike product called yogurt. The milk is defatted and soured with *Lactobacillus acidophilus* and other bacteria that are necessary for health of the intestine. Yogurt aids digestion and controls the action of the intestine in favorably stimulating the kidneys.

Yogurt contains the B-complex vitamins and has a higher percentage of vitamins A and D than does the milk it was made from; it is also high in protein.

The beneficial bacteria in yogurt make it a natural antibiotic. Yogurt has been found to be beneficial in treating high cholesterol level, arthritis, constipation, diarrhea, gallstones, halitosis, hepatitis, kidney disorders, and skin diseases.

Yogurt made at home is preferable to commercial yogurt because many of the preservatives added to yogurt found in grocery stores tend to nullify its therapeutic effects.

NUTS

Nuts are the dry fruits or seeds of some kinds of plants, usually of trees. Some readily available nuts are pecans, filberts, Brazil nuts, walnuts, almonds, and cashews. The soft inside part of the nut is the meat, or kernel, and the outer covering is the shell. Nuts are a concentrated food source of proteins, unsaturated fats, the B-complex vitamins, vitamin E, calcium, iron, potassium, magnesium, phosphorus, and copper.

Nuts may be eaten fresh, roasted, boiled, or in the form of flour or butter. Nuts may interfere with digestion unless they are chewed well or chopped into fine particles. When nuts are purchased in the shell, attention should be paid to the firmness of the seal, since partially cracked nuts soon become dry and rancid.

Nuts that are shelled should be stored preferably in the refrigerator, in airtight containers, to preserve their freshness and to prevent oxidation and rancidity of their fat content.

OILS

The term "oil" generally refers to fats in a liquid state. Vegetable oils, such as corn, cottonseed, safflower, soybean, olive, and sunflower, are widely used in cooking. These oils are important in the diet because of their content of unsaturated fatty acids, especially linoleic acid, which is necessary for growth and maintenance of the cells.

Oils may be removed from seeds, such as the safflower, or from beans, such as the soybean, by heat extraction or by pressing. Oils removed by pressing are referred to as "cold-pressed" and retain their vitamin A and E content better than those extracted by heat.

Margarine is a popular butter substitute made from solidified vegetable oils. Margarine contains 87 percent fat along with some salt and flavoring compounds to make it resemble butter in taste. Margarine is fortified with vitamin A, which makes it nutritionally comparable to butter, although margarine is sometimes preferred to butter because it has a higher unsaturated fatty acid content while butter has a higher saturated fatty acid content.

Oils, margarine, and all other fats should be kept refrigerated. They should also be well covered to prevent the absorption of odors from other foods.

SEASONINGS, HERBS, SPICES, AND EXTRACTS

Seasonings, herbs, spices, and extracts are usually derived from foods. They normally have little nutritive value because they are consumed in minute amounts. However, they give variety to the flavor of foods, stimulate the appetite, and encourage the flow of digestive juices. Seasonings, herbs, spices, and extracts are usually derived from the bark, roots, fruits, berries, or leaves of plants, shrubs, or trees.

Salt, or sodium chloride, is the most commonly used seasoning as well as an essential body mineral. Most people, however, consume many times too much salt, the body needs only a small amount, about two or three grams per day. An excess of table salt may cause mineral imbalances in the body because the sodium in it upsets the potassium and calcium levels in the body. Salt may be plain or iodized; salt used in the home should be iodized salt.

Salt substitutes are often used by people who must restrict their intake of sodium. Unrefined salt from evaporated seawater contains many trace minerals, is an especially good source of iodine, and may be found in a refined form.

Pepper ranks next to salt as a common seasoning. Pepper is available in two forms, black and white. Both forms are obtained from the dried berries of the same tropical vine, but they differ in the manner of processing.

Herbs and spices lose their true bouquet and flavor after six months of shelf life. They should be stored in tightly covered containers away from heat and light so that they will not become dry and stale.

Liquid extracts, including vanilla, almond, and fruit extracts (such as lemon and orange), should be stored in a cool, dry place so as not to develop off-flavors or aromas. They must be tightly capped to prevent evaporation.

SEEDS

Seeds are the ripened ovules of plants. The most important nutritive elements of seeds are the B-complex vitamins; vitamins A, D, and E; unsaturated fats; proteins; phosphorus; calcium; and a trace of fluorine.

Edible seeds such as pumpkin seeds, sesame seeds, and sunflower seeds are rich in protein; the B complex; vitamins A, D, and E; phosphorus; calcium; iron; fluorine; iodine; potassium; magnesium; zinc; and unsaturated fatty acids. Sesame seeds are high in calcium content. Sunflower seeds contain up to 50 percent protein.

Seeds have a variety of uses and may be eaten raw, dried, roasted, or cooked. Pumpkin, sesame, and sunflower seeds are popular snack foods, and others, such as caraway, dill, poppy, and anise, are used as seasonings. Seeds can be especially nutritious additions to soups, salads, casseroles, and baked goods. Sunflower-seed oil may be extracted for use in cooking and baking.

Unhulled seeds have a long shelf life, provided they are kept in a cool, dry place in a tightly covered container. Hulled seeds should be refrigerated immediately and used promptly because oxidation of their fat content may make them rancid.

SWEETENERS

Sugars and other concentrated sweets furnish quick energy to the body in readily digestible form. Cane and beet sugars, jellies, jams, candy, syrup, molasses, and honey are concentrated sources of sugar. Fruits are a natural source of sugar and furnish bulk in the diet.

Sugar is a major carbohydrate source but is completely devoid of protein, vitamins, and minerals and is not considered nutritious. Refined white sugar, in granulated or powdered form, and brown sugar are made from either sugar cane or sugar beet. White sugar contains no vitamins or minerals. The B vitamins needed for its assimilation must be obtained from other sources, either foods or supplements. Sugar leads to an imbalance in the calcium-phosphorus relationship. Sugar may also be a contributing factor in the development of overweight, diabetes, arthritis, tooth decay, pyorrhea, asthma, mental illness, nervous disorders, and low blood sugar. Natural sources of sugar, such as fruits, usually contain adequate supplies of vitamins essential for digestion and metabolism. Brown sugar has a slightly higher nutritive value than white sugar.

Artificial Sweeteners

Certain sugar-substitute sweetening agents may be employed by diabetics or persons who must reduce their caloric intake. Saccharine and sorbitol are sugar substitutes that have little energy, or caloric, value.

Carob

Carob is a natural sweetener rich in B vitamins and minerals with a flavor similar to that of chocolate. It is often used as a substitute for chocolate or cocoa, especially by people who are allergic to chocolate or who wish to avoid the caffeine it contains. Carob also contains a fair amount of protein, sugar, and some calcium and phosphorus. It is available in tablet, powder, syrup, and wafer forms.

Chocolate and Cocoa

Chocolate, cocoa, and foods flavored with these substances from the cocoa bean are usually prepared with large amounts of sugar that add carbohydrates to the diet while adding no significant amounts of vitamins and minerals. Chocolate and cocoa contain two stimulants, caffeine and theobromine, which speed up the heartbeat and stimulate the central nervous system. Chocolate also contains oxalic acid, an excess of which could interfere with calcium absorption. Cocoa is lower in fat than chocolate and therefore will keep for longer periods of time. It is slightly higher in nutritive value than chocolate.

Honey

Honey is one of Nature's finest energy-giving foods, consisting of carbohydrates in the most easily digestible form. Honey varies in texture, flavor, and color, depending upon place of origin and the flowers from which the nectar was gathered. Because honey is almost twice as sweet as cane or beet sugar, smaller amounts of it are needed for sweetening purposes. Honey contains large amounts of carbohydrates in the form of sugars, small amounts of minerals, and traces of the B-complex vitamins and vitamins C, D, and E.

Molasses

Molasses is a thick, sticky syrup, light to dark brown in color, with a strong, distinctive flavor. Blackstrap molasses is the residue left after the last possible extraction of sugar from the cane or beet (see "Blackstrap Molasses," p. 180). Ordinary molasses is a good mineral and vitamin source, rich in iron, calcium, copper, magnesium, phosphorus, pantothenic acid, inositol, vitamin E, and the B vitamins.

VEGETABLES

Vegetables are composed primarily of carbohydrates and water and contain very little protein. Vegetables also provide vitamins, minerals, and bulk to the diet and contribute appetite appeal through color, texture, and flavor. In general, light-green vegetables provide vitamins, minerals, and a large amount of the carbohydrate cellulose, necessary to provide bulk in the diet. Yellow and dark-green vegetables are excellent sources of vitamin A. Vegetable leaves are usually rich in calcium, iron, magnesium, vitamin C, and many of the B vitamins. The greener the leaf, the richer it will be in nutrients. Potatoes are relatively high in protein and are excellent sources of vitamin A, vitamin C, niacin, thiamine, and riboflavin as well as iron and calcium. A medium-size potato contains about 90 calories.

Vegetables are commonly available in fresh, frozen, canned, or dried forms. Fresh raw vegetables generally contain more vitamins and minerals than the processed products, although quick-freezing causes almost no nutrient loss. Properly canned vegetables usually contain as many vitamins and minerals as home-cooked fresh vegetables, but dried vegetables show a considerably greater loss of nutrients.

Before being eaten or cooked, fresh vegetables should be thoroughly washed so that chemical sprays and dirt are removed. The vegetable skins should be left on or pared as thinly as possible, so that the vitamins and minerals are preserved. Cooking time should be kept to a minimum when vegetables are boiled in water so that nutrients are conserved and flavor is retained. Baked vegetables will have a higher concentration of nutrients than boiled vegetables.

VEGETABLE JUICES

Fresh vegetable juices are an excellent source of minerals and vitamins. Juices from dark-green and yellow vegetables are especially high in vitamin A. People who want a change from raw or cooked vegetables may find juices appealing and easy to digest. Vegetable juices may also be the preferred form for persons suffering from disorders of the digestive system.

BEVERAGES

Beverages such as alcohol, coffee, cola, and tea add little nutritive value to the diet, except for water. However, milk drinks and fruit and vegetable juices contribute fair amounts of protein, fat, vitamins, and minerals to the diet.

ALCOHOLIC BEVERAGES

Alcoholic beverages may be those produced by fermentation only, such as ale, beer and most wines, and those that are distilled, such as whiskey. Alcoholic beverages supply little to the diet except calories. (See "Alcoholism," p. 109.)

CARBONATED BEVERAGES

Carbonated beverages are high in sugar content and have no nutritional value whatsoever. In order to hold the sugar in suspension and keep it from crystallizing, all soft drinks contain acid, usually orthophosphoric or citric, which eats away tooth enamel and can impair the appetite and the stomach. Certain soft drinks, especially cola, contain large amounts of caffeine, which stimulates the metabolism and leads to depletion of valuable nutrients in the body.

COFFEE

Coffee is produced from the coffee bean. It contains no nutrients but does contain caffeine. Coffee quickens the respiration process, strengthens the pulse, raises the blood pressure, stimulates the kidneys, excites the functions of the brain, and temporarily relieves fatigue or depression. If consumed in excess, coffee can cause increased nervous symptoms, aggravate heart and artery disorders, and irritate the lining of the stomach. It may also create inositol and biotin deficiencies, prevent iron from being properly utilized, and cause other vitamins to be pumped through and out of the body before they can be properly absorbed.

Coffee substitutes are powdered vegetable preparations that are used as coffee alternatives. They usually have barley or chicory-root bases and contain no caffeine.

TEA

Tea is similar to coffee in that it contains caffeine; it contains tannin, or tannic acid, and essential oils as well. The caffeine is the stimulating element; the tannin gives it its color and body; the oils give it flavor and aroma.

Tannin in its concentrated form has had harmful effects on the mucous membrane of the mouth and the digestive tract, but it is generally believed that tannin does not occur in significant enough amounts in tea to be harmful. Tea actually has little nutritive value with the exception of its fluoride content. Herbal teas are preferred to commercial teas because of their therapeutic value, depending upon the herbs used in brewing the tea.

SUPPLEMENTARY FOODS

Supplementary foods may be useful for individuals who wish to increase the nutritional value of their meals. Supplements may be in the form of tablets, liquids, powders, syrups, capsules, granules, or bars; various forms may have differing nutrient characteristics. *Any information concerning ailments is not meant to be prescriptive, but merely represents research findings.*

ALFALFA

Alfalfa is a leguminous plant that is particularly rich in vitamin K and calcium and contains significant amounts of nearly every other vitamin and mineral. The seeds, sprouts, and leaves of the plant are edible but are also available in the form of tablets, powder, or tea.

BLACKSTRAP MOLASSES

Blackstrap molasses is a truly rich source of minerals and vitamins. As the last possible extraction of the cane in refining sugar, it is the richest in nutrients of the sugar-related products. It contains more calcium than milk, more iron than many eggs, and more potassium than any food, and it is an excellent source of B vitamins. It is also rich in copper, magnesium, phosphorus, pantothenic acid, inositol, and vitamin E. One tablespoon of blackstrap molasses contains 3 milligrams of iron and over 100 milligrams of calcium. It is also a good source of natural sugar. Recommended daily dosage is one tablespoon dissolved in one cup lukewarm water or milk, one-half that amount is recommended for children. Molasses may be used as a sugar substitute in cereals and may be eaten instead of jam or jelly. Varicose veins, arthritis, ulcers, dermatitis, hair damage, eczema, psoriasis, angina pectoris, constipation, colitis, anemia, and nervous conditions may respond to supplementing the diet with this mineral-rich molasses.

BONE MEAL

Bone meal is a flourlike substance consisting of the finely ground bones of cattle. As a good supplemental source of calcium, bone meal is especially recommended for anyone whose milk intake must be limited. It also contains phosphorus and the trace minerals copper, manganese, nickel, and fluorine, which are essential for the complete nutrition of teeth and bones. Bone meal can usually be given safely in any dose. The recommended intake of bone meal is three tablets or an equivalent amount per day.

BREWER'S YEAST

Brewer's yeast is a nonleavening yeast that can be added to all foods to increase their nutritional value. Brewer's yeast is one of the best sources of B vitamins and minerals. It contains 16 amino acids, 14 minerals, and 17 vitamins. Brewer's yeast is high in phosphorus in relation to calcium; therefore, 8 ounces of skim milk or four tablespoons of dry powdered milk should be taken with every tablespoon of yeast. The recommended supplemental allowance of brewer's yeast is one tablespoon daily.

Wheat germ and brewer's yeast taken daily may be helpful in preventing heart trouble. Brewer's yeast may protect against toxicity of large does of vitamin D. It is used to prevent constipation and is a good source of enzyme-producing agents.

Brewer's yeast is available in powder, flake, and tablet forms.

DESICCATED LIVER

Desiccated liver is concentrated beef liver, in powder or tablet form, which has been dried in a vacuum at a low temperature so that most of the original nutrient value of liver is conserved. Desiccated-liver tablets, rich in vitamin A, vitamin C, vitamin D, iron, calcium, phosphorus, and copper, are recommended to supplement the diet if liver is not eaten once or twice a week. Desiccated liver may be combined with soups, baked goods, and other foods.

LECITHIN

Lecithin is a natural constituent of every cell of the human body and helps to emulsify cholesterol in the body. Lecithin is available both naturally in egg yolk, soybeans, and corn and as a supplement in capsule, liquid, and granule forms. Lecithin is high in phosphorus and unites with iron, iodine, and calcium to give power and vigor to the brain and aid in the digestion and absorption of fats. Lecithin also consists of ordinary fat, unsaturated fatty acids, and choline.

Lecithin may break up cholesterol and allow it to pass through arterial walls, helping to prevent atherosclerosis. It has also been found to increase immunity against virus infections and to prevent the formation of gallstones. Even distribution of body weight is also aided by lecithin. Lecithin plays an important part in maintaining a healthy nervous system and is found naturally in the myelin sheath, a fatty protective covering for the nerves. Lecithin also helps to cleanse the liver and purify the kidneys.

The National Research Council has not yet established a Recommended Dietary Allowance for lecithin, although it has been suggested that it should be taken daily. There are no known toxic levels for lecithin.

ROSE HIPS AND ACEROLA CHERRIES

Rose hips are the urn-shaped seeds at the base of rose blossoms. They are excellent sources of vitamin A, the B complex, vitamin E, vitamin K, and the bioflavonoids. They can be used either fresh or dried and can be made into tea, jam, syrup, or soup. Another small fruit, the acerola cherry, is a rich natural source of vitamin C and is frequently used together with rose hips to make organic vitamin C supplements. Rose hips and acerola cherries are available as a supplement in the forms of powder, syrup, tablets, and capsules.

SEAWEED

Seaweed is a vegetable from the ocean which is rich in minerals. Sea plants have an advantage over land crops because they grow in seawater, in which the minerals are constantly being renewed. Seaweed is rich in all necessary minerals. There are several varieties of seaweed, including kelp, nari, and Irish moss, all of which are salty in flavor. Kelp is one of the best natural sources of iodine; it is also rich in B-complex vitamins; vitamins D, E, and K; calcium; and magnesium. It is often used as a salt substitute and is available in dried, powdered, and tablet forms. Dulse is dark red in color and is rich in iodine. It can be used fresh in salads, but it should be soaked several times in water first. Seaweed is beneficial in maintaining the health of the mucous membranes and in treating arthritis, constipation, nervous disorders, rheumatism, colds, and skin irritations.

WHEAT GERM

Wheat germ is the heart of the kernel of wheat. It is an excellent source of protein (24 grams per one-half cup), B-complex vitamins, vitamin E, and iron. It also contains copper, magnesium, manganese, calcium, and phosphorus. It is high in phosphorus in relation to calcium, so 8 ounces of skim milk or 4 tablespoons of dry milk powder should be taken with every tablespoon of wheat germ. Wheat germ contains a vegetable oil and therefore should be tightly covered and refrigerated. Wheat-germ oil is extracted from wheat germ; it is a supplemental food high in unsaturated fatty acids and is one of the richest known sources of vitamin E.

SOME RICH SOURCES OF NUTRIENTS

CARBOHYDRATES
Whole grains
Sugar, syrup, and honey
Fruits
Vegetables

FATS
Butter and margarine
Vegetable oils
Fats in meats
Whole milk and milk products
Nuts and seeds

PROTEIN
Meats, fish, and poultry
Soybean products
Eggs
Milk and milk products
Whole grains

WATER
Beverages
Fruits
Vegetables

VITAMIN A
Liver
Eggs
Yellow fruits and vegetables
Dark-green fruits and vegetables
Whole milk and milk products
Fish-liver oil*

VITAMIN B₁
Brewer's yeast
Whole grains
Blackstrap molasses
Brown rice
Organ meats
Meats, fish, and poultry

Egg yolks
Legumes
Nuts

VITAMIN B₂
Brewer's yeast
Whole grains
Blackstrap molasses
Organ meats
Egg yolks
Legumes
Nuts

VITAMIN B₆
Meats
Whole grains
Organ meats
Brewer's yeast
Blackstrap molasses
Wheat germ
Legumes
Green leafy vegetables
Desiccated liver*

VITAMIN B₁₂
Organ meats
Fish and pork
Eggs
Cheese
Milk and milk products

VITAMIN B₁₃
Root vegetables
Liquid whey

BIOTIN
Egg yolks
Liver
Unpolished rice
Brewer's yeast
Whole grains
Sardines
Legumes

CHOLINE
Egg yolks
Organ meats
Brewer's yeast
Wheat germ
Soybeans
Fish
Legumes
Lecithin*

FOLIC ACID
Dark-green leafy vegetables
Organ meats
Brewer's yeast
Root vegetables
Whole grains
Oysters
Salmon
Milk

INOSITOL
Whole grains
Citrus fruits
Brewer's yeast
Molasses
Meat
Milk
Nuts
Vegetables
Lecithin*

LAETRILE
Whole kernels of apricots, apples, cherries, peaches, and plums

NIACIN
Lean meats
Poultry and fish
Brewer's yeast
Peanuts

Milk and milk products
Rice bran
Desiccated liver*

PARA-AMINOBENZOIC ACID
Organ meats
Wheat germ
Yogurt
Molasses
Green leafy vegetables

PANGAMIC ACID
Brewer's yeast
Rare steaks
Brown rice
Sunflower, pumpkin, and sesame seeds

PANTOTHENIC ACID
Organ meats
Brewer's yeast
Egg yolks
Legumes
Whole grains
Wheat germ
Salmon

VITAMIN C
Citrus fruits
Rose hips
Acerola cherries
Alfalfa seeds, sprouted
Cantaloupe
Strawberries
Broccoli
Tomatoes
Green peppers

VITAMIN D
Salmon
Sardines
Herring
Vitamin D–fortified milk and milk products

*Denotes the supplemental form.

Egg yolks
Organ meats
Fish-liver oils*
Bone meal*

VITAMIN E
Cold-pressed oils
Eggs
Wheat germ
Organ meats
Molasses
Sweet potatoes
Leafy vegetables
Desiccated liver*

VITAMIN F
Vegetable oils
Butter
Sunflower seeds

VITAMIN K
Green leafy vegetables
Egg yolks
Safflower oil
Blackstrap molasses
Cauliflower
Soybeans

BIOFLAVONOIDS
Citrus fruits
Fruits
Black currants
Buckwheat

CALCIUM
Milk and milk products
Green leafy vegetables
Shellfish
Molasses
Bone meal*
Dolomite*

CHLORINE
Table salt

Seafood
Meats
Ripe olives
Rye flour
Dulse*

CHROMIUM
Corn oil
Clams
Whole-grain cereals
Brewer's yeast

COBALT
Organ meats
Oysters
Clams
Poultry
Milk
Green leafy vegetables
Fruits

COPPER
Organ meats
Seafood
Nuts
Legumes
Molasses
Raisins
Bone meal*

FLUORIDE
Tea
Seafood
Fluoridated water
Bone meal*

IRON
Organ meats and meats
Eggs
Fish and poultry
Blackstrap molasses
Cherry juice
Green leafy vegetables

Dried fruits
Desiccated liver*

MAGNESIUM
Seafood
Whole grains
Dark-green vegetables
Molasses
Nuts
Bone meal*

MANGANESE
Whole grains
Green leafy vegetables
Legumes
Nuts
Pineapples
Egg yolks

MOLYBDENUM
Legumes
Whole-grain cereals
Milk
Liver
Dark-green vegetables

PHOSPHORUS
Fish, meats, and poultry
Eggs
Legumes
Milk and milk products
Nuts
Whole-grain cereals
Bone meal*

POTASSIUM
Lean meats
Whole grains
Vegetables
Dried fruits
Legumes
Sunflower seeds

SELENIUM
Tuna
Herring
Brewer's yeast
Wheat germ and bran
Broccoli
Whole grains

SODIUM
Seafood
Table salt
Baking power and baking soda
Celery
Processed foods
Milk products
Kelp*

SULFUR
Fish
Eggs
Meats
Cabbage
Brussel sprouts

VANADIUM
Fish

ZINC
Sunflower seeds
Seafood
Organ meats
Mushrooms
Brewer's yeast
Soybean

*Denotes the supplemental form.

Table of Food Composition

The foods in this table have been divided according to food groups and similar types of foods that do not belong to any one group. The chart runs alphabetically according to food groups, with the items in each group also being alphabetized. The first group analyzed is the Beverages, the second Breads, Cereals, Grains, and Grain Products, and so on. If you are unable to locate a particular food in a group, this does not necessarily mean it has not been included. Check the Index in the back of the book, looking for the number in bold type.

Food values have been calculated so as to permit easy computation. All figures are for edible portions only; no bones, seeds, peels (when not usually eaten), etc., are included. These figures are, of necessity, averages of different food samples. Where values of a particular nutrient from different food samples differ too greatly to get a meaningful average, a dash has been used. Both the dash (—) and the trace (t) nutrient values are calculated as zero in evaluations of foods.

For vitamins E and K as well as several of the B vitamins, very little information concerning presence in food is available. The blank spaces on the chart do not mean an absence of a particular nutrient but that meaningful analysis of the food for that nutrient is lacking. Only the zero confirms the absence of a nutrient. The iodine value has not been included for vegetables or fruits because the iodine content of these foods totally depends on the soil in which they are grown. This means that along the coastline the values will be significant while inland they will be nonexistent.

Vitamin E values have been given in milligrams. To approximate the value in IUs, multiply milligrams by 1.5. For example, if 3 milligrams of vitamin E is present, multiply 3 by 1.5, which makes 4.5 IU of vitamin E.

See page 220 for the abbreviations and symbols used in the chart.

CONTENTS: TABLE OF FOOD COMPOSITION

Code No.	Food Item	Measure	Weight g	Calories	Protein g	Fats g	Carbohy-drates g	Water g	Calcium mg	Iodine mg	Iron mg	Magne-sium mg	Phospho-rus mg	Potas-sium mg
	BEVERAGES													
	Alcoholic													
0010	Beer	1 cup	240	101	1.4	0	10.8	221.0	10.0		t	t	72.0	60
	Cordials:													
0020	Anisette	1 cordial	20	74			7.0							
0030	Apricot brandy	1 cordial	20	64			6.0							
0040	Benedictine	1 cordial	20	69			6.6							
0050	Creme de menthe	1 cordial	20	67			6.0							
0060	Curacao	1 cordial	20	54			6.0							
0070	Daiquiri	3 oz	100	122	0.1		5.2		4.0		0.10		3.0	
0080	Gin (86 proof) (also rum, vodka, whiskey, and scotch)	1 oz	28	70	0	0	t	17.9	0		0		0	1
0090	Highball	8 oz	240	166										
0100	Manhattan	3 1/2 oz	100	164	t		7.9		1.0		t		1.0	
0110	Martini	3 1/2 oz	100	140	0.1		0.3		5.0		0.10		1.0	
0120	Old Fashioned	4 oz	100	179			3.5							
0130	Tom Collins	10 oz	300	180	0.3		9.0		6.0		t		6.0	
	Wines													
0140	Sweet (18.8% alcohol)	1 cup	240	329	2.4	0	33.6	184.0	19.0					180
0150	Dry (12.2% alcohol)	1 cup	240	204	0.2	0	9.6	205.0	22.0		0.96	24.0	24.0	221
0160	Champagne	1 cup	240	168	0.4		3.0							
	Carbonated and others													
0170	Club soda	1 cup	230	0	0	0	0	230.0						t
0180	Cola drinks	1 cup	230	88	0		22.0	207.0						
0190	Diet drinks	1 cup	230	0	0	0		230.0	12.4					
0200	Eggnog, all milk	1 cup	310	291	14.6	15.0	24.7		314.0		1.50		328.0	326
0210	Fruit-flavored drinks	1 cup	230	106	0	0	26.0	202.0						0
0220	Ginger ale	1 cup	230	72	0	0	18.0	207.0						
0230	Root beer	1 cup	230	96	0	0	24.0	205.0						
0240	Coffee	1 cup	230	2	0.3	0.1	0.8	226.0	4.6		0.23	15.4	5.0	83
0250	Tea	1 cup	230	4	0.1	t	0.9	229.0	5.0		0.20	t	4.0	58
	BREADS, CEREALS, GRAINS, AND GRAIN PRODUCTS													
0270	Barley, pearled & uncooked	1 cup	224	782	18.0	2.2	173.0	248.0	36.0		4.50	81.0	423.0	358
0280	Biscuits, enr flour, 2 1/2" diam	1 med	38	138	3.0	6.5	17.0	10.4	46.0		0.19		67.0	44
0290	Bran flakes, 40%	1 cup	40	143	3.8	0.4	30.8	1.2	21.0		14	97.0	143.0	171
	Bread													
0313	Corn, whole-ground meal	1 svg	50	104	3.7	3.6	14.0	27.0	60.0		0.55		106.0	79
0326	Cracked wheat	1 slice	23	61	2.0	0.1	13.0	8.0	20.0		0.25	8.0	29	31
0327	Cracked wheat, toasted	1 slice	19	60	2.0	0.1	13.0	4.3	20.0		0.20	8.0	29.0	30
0339	French, enr flour	1 slice	20	58	1.8	0.6	11.1	6.0	9.0		0.40	4.0	17.0	18
0365	Italian, enr flour	1 slice	20	55	1.8	0.2	11.3	6.4	3.0		0.40		15.0	15
0401	Pumpernickel	1 slice	32	79	2.9	4.0	17.0	7.8	27.0		0.80	23.0	73.0	145
0414	Raisin	1 slice	23	60	1.5	0.6	12.0	8.2	16.0		0.30	6.0	20.0	54
0415	Raisin, toasted	1 slice	19	60	1.5	0.6	12.0	4.2	16.0		0.30	6.0	20.0	53
0440	Rye	1 slice	23	56	2.1	0.3	12.0	8.2	17.0		0.37	10.0	34.0	33
0441	Rye, toasted	1 slice	20	56	2.1	0.3	12.0	5.0	17.0		0.40	10.0	34.0	34
0453	White, enr	1 slice	23	62	2.0	0.7	12.0	8.2	19.0		0.58	5.0	22.0	24
0454	White, toasted	1 slice	20	62	2.0	0.7	12.0	5.0	20.0		0.58	5.0	23.0	24
0466	Whole wheat	1 slice	23	55	2.1	0.6	11.0	8.4	19.0		0.53	18.0	58.0	59
0467	Whole wheat, toasted	1 slice	19	55	2.4	0.6	11.0	5.6	22.0		0.50	18.0	52.0	62
0479	Bread stuffing, uncooked[1]	1 cup	230	478	10.0	29.0	44.0	140.0	92.0		2.30		152.0	133
0481	Bread crumbs, dry	1 cup	88	345	11.0	4.0	65.0	5.7	107.0		3.20		124.0	134
0492	Buns, soft, enr flour (hamburger, hot dog)	1 avg	30	89	2.5	1.7	16.0	9.4	22.0		0.60	11.0	26.0	28
0503	Corn flakes	1 cup	25	93	2.0	0.2	21.0	1.6	4.0		1.32	4.0	7.9	23
0513	Corn-grits, cooked	1 cup	242	123	2.9	0.2	27.0	210.0	2.4		0.50	7.0	24.0	27
0531	Corn meal—yellow, cooked	1 cup	240	115	2.6	0.5	25.0	210.0	2.0		0.50	16.0	34.0	38

[1] Made with egg, water, and fat
[2] Value for yellow variety; white has only a trace.

Sodium mg	Copper mg	Vitamin A IU	(Thiamine) B1 mg	(Riboflavin) B2 mg	Vitamin B6 mg	Vitamin B12 mcg	Biotin mcg	Choline mg	Folic Acid mg	Inositol g	Niacin mg	Pantothenic Acid mg	Vitamin C mg	Vitamin D IU	Vitamin E mg	Vitamin K mg
17.0			t	0.07	0.140	0					1.44	0.90	0			
		0	14.00	1.00							t		8.00	0		
0.3		0	0	0							0		0			
		35	0.030	0.02							t		0			
		t	t	t							t		0			
											t		21.0	0		
10.0			0.020	0.05							0.48					
5.0			t	0.02	0.144	0					0.24	0.07				
59.1		0	0	0							0		0			
		0	0	0							0		0			
26.0		0	0	0							0		0			
156.0		940	0.140	0.56							0.30		3.00	31.0		
18.0		0	0	0							0		0			
		0	0	0							0		0			
18.0		0	0	0							0		0			
2.3	0.01	0	0.010	0.01	t	0					0.90	0.01	0	0		0.090
1.6	0.01	0	0	0.04							0.10		1.00			
6.7		0	0.270	0.11	0.470	0			0.340		6.94	1.13	0			
238.0		t	0.020	0.04							0.19		t			
251.0	0.24	1,877	0.460	0.56	0.850				0.040		4.70	0.35	14.10	187.0		
314.0		75	0.070	0.10							0.30		0.50			
122.0		t	0.030	0.02	0.020	0			0.010		0.30	0.14	t			
120.0		t	0.020	0.02							0.30		t			
116.0		t	0.020	0.02	0.010	0			0.002		0.10	0.08	t			
117.0		0	0.060	0.05							0.50	0.16	0			
182.0		0	0.070	0.04	0.050	0										
84.0		t	0.010	0.02							0.20		t			
84.0		t	0.010	0.02							0.20		t			
128.0	0.04	0	0.040	0.02	0.023	0			0.004		0.32	0.10	0			
130.0		0	0.030	0.02	0	0			0		0.30		0			
117.0	0.04	t	0.060	0.05	0.020	t	0.2		0.003	t	0.55	0.10	t		0.23	
118.0	0.03	t	0.050	0.05	0						0.56					
122.0	0.04	t	0.070	0.02	0.080	0	0.4		0.010	0.01	0.64	0.18	t		0.1	
119.0		t	0.040	0.02					0.010	0.01	0.60		t			
159.0		966	0.120	0.21							1.84		t			
648.0	0.18	t	0.190	0.26							3.10		t			
152.0		t	0.080	0.05							0.70		t			
242.0	0.03	1,173	0.290	0.35	0.550				0.002		2.90	0.05	8.80	10.2		
496.0	4.60	145	0.070	0.06	0.100[2]	0	1.7		0.010	0.01	0.48	0.97	0			
264.0	0.48	144	0.050	0.02				24.0	0.020		0.24	1.70	0			2.80

Code No.	Food Item	Measure	Weight g	Calories	Protein g	Fats g	Carbohydrates g	Water g	Calcium mg	Iodine mg	Iron mg	Magnesium mg	Phosphorus mg	Potassium mg
0544	Cornstarch	1 tbsp	8	29	t	t	7.0	0.1	0		0	0.2	0	t
0557	Cracked-wheat cereal, cooked	1 cup	42	138	4.4	0.9	30.0		18.0		1.50			
	Crackers													
0570	Graham	1 med	7	28	0.6	0.7	5.1	0.4	2.8		0.11	1.3	10.0	27
0583	Rye	1 med	3	13	0.2	0.7	1.5	0.2	1.6		0.01		11.6	18
	Snack, standard, round	1 med	3	17	0.2	0.9	2.0				0.10			
0609	Soda, 2 1/2" square	1 square	6	26	0.5	0.8	4.2	0.2	1.3		0.09	1.7	5.3	7
0622	Cream of wheat, cooked	1 cup	200	134	4.5	0.4	28.0	175.0	99.0		9.00		124.0	
0635	Danish pastry	1 small	35	148	2.6	23.5	16.0	8.0	17.0		0.30	8.0	38.0	39
0648	Farina, instant, cooked	1 cup	238	131	4.1	0.2	26.0	204.0	183.0		15.00	9.5	143.0	31
	Flour													
0661	Buckwheat, light	1 cup	110	382	7.0	1.3	86.0	13.2	12.0		1.10	53.0	97.0	352
0674	Cake	1 cup	100	364	7.5	0.8	79.4	12.0	17.0		0.50	26.0	73.0	95
0678	Carob (St. John's bread)	1 tbsp	9	16	0.4	0.1	7.3	1.0	32.0				9.0	
0685	Chestnut	1 cup	110	398	6.7	4.1	84.0	12.5	55.0		3.50		180.0	932
0690	Potato	1 cup	110	386	8.8	0.9	86.0	8.4	36.0		19.00		196.0	1,747
0700	Rye, medium	1 cup	110	385	13.0	1.9	79.0	12.0	30.0		2.90	80.0	288.0	223
0710	Soy, full-fat	1 cup	110	418	45.0	13.3	36.0	9.0	264.0		9.90	322.0	715.0	1,952
0720	Wheat, all-purpose enr	1 cup	110	394	12.0	1.1	84.0	13.0	18.0		3.20	28.0	96.0	105
0730	Wheat, whole	1 cup	120	410	15.0	2.4	82.0	14.0	49.0		4.00	136.0	446.0	444
0743	French toast	1 slice	65	183	5.5	12.0	14.0		77.0		0.90	16.0	94.0	
0756	Macaroni, cooked, unenr/salt	1 cup	140	155	5.3	0.6	32.0	101.0	11.0		0.56	25.0	70.0	85
0769	Macaroni w/cheese, cooked	1 cup	220	468	19.0	24.0	44.0	128.0	398.0		2.00		354.0	264
0782	Melba toast, unsalted	1 slice	4	15	0.5	123.0	2.7							
	Muffins													
0795	Plain, enr flour	1 med	48	139	3.7	4.9	20.0	18.0	50.0		0.80	13.0	73.0	60
0808	Blueberry	1 med	40	112	2.9	3.7	16.8	15.6	34.0		0.60	10.0	53.0	46
0821	Noodles, cooked, unenr/salt	1 cup	160	200	6.6	2.4	37.0	113.0	16.0		0.96		94.0	70
0834	Noodles, chow mein	1 cup	28	137	3.7	6.6	16.0	0.3						
0847	Oat flakes	1 cup	43	147	7.7	1.9	29.0		148.0		15.00		58.0	129
0860	Oatmeal or rolled oats, cooked	1 cup	236	130	4.7	2.4	23.0	204.0	21.0		1.42	49.0	138.0	144
	Pancakes													
0873	Buckwheat, 4" diam	1 med	45	90	3.1	4.1	10.7	29.0	99.0		0.60	22.0	152.0	110
0886	Wheat, 4" diam	1 med	45	104	3.2	3.2	15.3	22.5	45.0		0.60	11.0	63.0	55
	Pizza													
0899	Cheese, 14" diam	1/8	75	177	9.0	6.2	21.0	36.0	166.0		0.75		146.0	98
0912	Sausage, 14" diam	1/8	100	232	7.8	9.0	30.0	51.0	17.0		1.20		92.0	168
0925	Popcorn, w/oil and salt	1 cup	14	66	1.4	3.1	8.3	0.4	1.1		0.31		30.0	
0938	Pretzel	1 med	6	23	0.6	0.3	4.5	0.3	1.3		0.09		7.9	8
0951	Puffed rice	1 cup	14	56	0.8	0.5	13.0	0.5	2.8		0.25		13.0	14
0964	Puffed wheat	1 cup	12	43	1.6	0.2	9.5	0.3	3.0		0.50		40.0	12
0977	Raisin bran	1 cup	57	184	4.3	0.8	22.0	5.0	23.0		20.00	100.0	165.0	230
	Rice													
0990	Brown, cooked	1 cup	150	178	3.8	0.9	37.0	105.0	18.0		0.80	45.0	110.0	105
1003	Brown, raw	1 cup	190	744	14.3	3.6	161.0	23.0	67.0	t	3.30	182.0	460.0	214
1029	Instant	1 cup	148	161	3.3	t	35.8	108.0	4.0		1.20		28.0	t
1042	Parboiled, cooked	1 cup	150	155	3.2	0.2	35.0	110.0	29.0		1.20		85.0	65
1055	Parboiled, dry	1 cup	187	669	14.0	0.6	152.0	19.0	112.0		5.40	48.0	374.0	281
1068	White, cooked	1 cup	150	158	3.0	0.2	36.0	109.0	15.0		1.40	12.0	42.0	42
1081	White, raw	1 cup	191	675	13.0	0.8	154.0	23.0	46.0		5.54	55.0	180.0	176
1094	Wild, raw	1 cup	191	696	27.0	1.3	144.0	16.0	36.0		8.02	246.0	648.0	420
1107	Rice flakes	1 cup	30	111	1.8	0.1	26.0	1.0	8.7		0.48		40.0	54
1120	Rice pilaf	1 cup	188	192	4.2	0.6	38.1	138.0	30.4		1.43	16.0	71.0	96
1130	Rice polish or bran	1 cup	100	266	12.0	13.0	54.3	9.8	69.0		16.00		1,106.0	714
1140	Rice w/tomato and meat	1 cup	250	218	4.5	4.2	41.0	196.0	35.0		1.50		98.0	578
	Rolls													
1150	Breakfast, sweet	1 lg	50	158	4.2	4.5	25.0	16.0	43.0		0.40	16.0	54.0	62
1160	Dinner, enr flour	1 med	38	113	3.1	2.1	20.0	9.7	28.0		0.72	14.0	32.0	36
1170	Whole wheat	1 med	40	103	4.0	1.1	19.5	12.8	42.0		0.96	46.0	112.0	117
1180	Rusk	1 avg	23	96	3.2	2.0	16.0	1.1	4.6		0.30		27.0	37
1190	Shredded-wheat biscuit	1 avg	28	99	3.8	0.6	21.0	1.9	12.0		0.98	40.0	109.0	97

Sodium mg	Copper mg	Vitamin A IU	(Thiamine) B₁ mg	(Riboflavin) B₂ mg	Vitamin B₆ mg	Vitamin B₁₂ mcg	Biotin mcg	Choline mg	Folic Acid mg	Inositol g	Niacin mg	Pantothenic Acid mg	Vitamin C mg	Vitamin D IU	Vitamin E mg	Vitamin K mg
t		0	0.000	0.00							0.00		0.0	0.0		
0.4		0	0.180	0.05							1.50		0.0	0.0		
47.0	0.01	0	0.003	0.02							0.11		0.0			
26.5	0.01	0	0.010	0.01							0.04		0.0			
		0											0.0			
66.0	t	0	0.001	t							0.06		0.0			
—		0	0.110	0.07							0.85		0.0	0.0		
128.0		108	0.020	0.05							0.30		t			
447.0		0	0.170	0.10	0.050	0.0					1.20		0.0	0.0		
1.0	0.77	0	0.090	0.04							0.44		0.0			
2.0		0	0.030	0.03	0.045	0.0				t	0.70	0.32	0.0			
12.0			0.250	0.41							1.10					
37.0		t	0.460	0.15							3.74		21.00			
1.1	0.46	0	0.330	0.13					0.020		2.75		0.0			
1.1		121	0.970	0.34	0.720		77.0	246.0	0.470	0.23	2.50	1.90	0.0			
2.2	0.21	0	0.480	0.29	0.170	0.0	1.1	57.2	0.009	0.05	3.58	0.55	0.0			
3.6	0.52	0	0.660	0.14	1.120	0.0	10.8		0.050	0.13	5.16	1.30	0.0		3.00	0.004
		555	0.090	0.16							0.50		t			
—	0.03	0	0.010	0.01							0.42		0.0			
1,195.0	0.09	946	0.220	0.44							1.98		t			
212.0		48	0.080	0.11							0.67		t			
253.0		88	0.060	0.08							0.50		0.40			
400.0		112	0.050	0.03							0.64					
300.0		2,018	0.500	0.60							5.00		15.00			
515.0	1.18	0	0.190	0.05	0.080	0.0			0.078		0.24		0.0	0.0	4.90	0.177
209.0		104	0.050	0.07							0.30		t			
191.0		54	0.080	0.10							0.60		t			
527.0		473	0.050	0.15							0.75		6.00			
729.0		560	0.090	0.12							1.50		9.00			
271.0	0.05			0.01	0.030	0.0					0.24		0.0			
101.0	0.01	0	0.001	t	0.001	t					0.04	0.03	0.0		0.01	
0.3	0.05	0	0.060	0.01	0.010	0.0					0.62	0.05	0.0	0.0		
1.0	0.08	0	0.070	0.03	0.020	0.0					0.90		0.0	0.0		
256.0		2,666	0.660	0.80	0.120						6.60		20.00	266.0		
423.0		0	0.140	0.03	0.930		18.0	168.0	0.030	0.18	21.00	2.30	0.0			
19.0		0	0.710	0.10							9.78		0.0		4.56	
404.0		0	0.190								1.50		0.0			
538.0		0	0.160	0.01							1.80		0.0			
17.0		0	0.820	0.06	0.187		18.7	183.0	0.040	0.05	6.55	2.56	0.0			
561.0		0	0.160						0.020		1.50		0.0		0.27	
10.0		0	0.840		0.070		9.6	113.0	0.030	0.02	6.69	1.20	0.0			
13.0		0	0.860	1.20							12.00		0.0			
296.0		0	0.110	0.02	0.040	0.0		t			1.62	0.10		0.0	0.01	
931.0		16	0.150	0.48							1.37		0.60			
t		0	2.260	0.25	2.500		60.0	170.0	0.150	0.50	28.00	2.80	0.0			
790.0		1,650	0.100	0.08							1.75		38.00			
195.0		35	0.040	0.08							0.40		t			
192.0		t	0.110	0.07							0.84		t			
226.0		t	0.140	0.05							1.20		t			
57.0	0.05	53	0.020	0.05							0.25		t			
0.8	0.05	0	0.060	0.03	0.070	0.0			0.020		1.23	0.20	0.0	0.0		

Code No.	Food Item	Measure	Weight g	Calories	Protein g	Fats g	Carbohy-drates g	Water g	Calcium mg	Iodine mg	Iron mg	Magne-sium mg	Phospho-rus mg	Potas-sium mg
	Spaghetti													
1200	w/Meat sauce	1 cup	250	335	19.0	12.0	38.0	175.0	125.0		3.75		238.0	670
1210	w/Tomatoes and cheese	1 cup	250	260	8.7	8.7	37.0	193.0	80.0		2.25		135.0	408
1220	Tortilla, yellow corn	6″ diam cake	30	63	1.5	0.6	13.5	60.0			0.90	32.0	42.0	
1230	Waffles	1 avg	75	206	7.0	7.3	28.0	31.0	85.0		1.28	19.0	130.0	109
1235	Wheat bran	1 oz	29	62	4.6	1.3	17.9	3.3	34.5		4.30	142.0	325.0	370
1240	Wheat germ	1 tbsp	6	24	1.8	0.7	2.7	0.7	4.0		0.50	19.0	67.0	50
1250	Wheat-germ cereal, toasted	1 cup	65	254	20.0	7.5	27.0	2.7	31.0		5.80		705.0	616
1260	Wheat-meal cereal, cooked	1 cup	360	154	6.5	1.0	30.0	315.0	25.0		1.80		190.0	170
1270	Wheat, unground (bulgar), cooked	1 cup	250	420	16.0	1.7	85.0	140.0	50.0		3.25		500.0	218
1280	Wheat flakes	1 cup	21	105	2.6	0.6	23.0	0.6	9.0		2.00		75.0	45
1290	Zweiback	1 avg	23	97	2.5	2.0	17.0	1.1	3.0		0.14		16.0	35
	CONDIMENTS, DRESSINGS, AND SAUCES													
1300	Bacon, imitation bits	1 tsp	1.6	7	0.6	0.3	0.4							
1310	Barbecue sauce	1 tbsp	14	15	0.2	9.7	1.1	11.3	2.9		0.11		2.8	24
1320	Catsup, tomato	1 tbsp	17	19	0.3	0.1	4.3	11.7	3.7		0.14	4.0	8.5	62
1330	Cheese sauce	1 tbsp	19	33	1.5	2.4	1.2		44.0		0.05		32.5	
1340	Chili sauce, tomato	1 tbsp	17	17	0.4	t	4.1	11.3	3.3		0.13		8.7	62
1350	Curry powder	1 tsp	2	4	0.2	0.2	0.5		13.0		1.50	5.7	5.0	37
1360	Hollandaise sauce	1 tbsp	21	48	1.0	4.1	1.6		22.0		0.18		28.0	
1370	Horseradish, prepared	1 tsp	5	2	0.1	t	0.5	4.4	3.0		0.05		1.6	14
1380	Mustard, prepared, brown	1 tbsp	12	11	0.7	0.8	0.5	9.4	14.9		0.24	5.8	16.1	16
1390	Pepper, seasoned	1 tsp	2.9	7	0.3	0.2	1.0							
1400	Relish, pickle, sweet	1 tbsp	13	18	0.1	0.1	4.4	8.2	2.6		0.10		1.8	
	Salad dressing													
1410	Blue cheese and Roquefort	1 tbsp	15	76	0.7	7.7	1.1	4.8	12.0		0.03		11.0	6
1412	Blue cheese and Roquefort, low-calorie	1 tbsp	15	20	0.4	1.0	0.6	12.6	9.6		0.02		7.1	
1430	Caesar	1 tbsp	15	73	0.3	8.0	0.6							
1440	French	1 tbsp	15	62	0.1	5.6	2.6	5.8	1.6		0.06	1.5	2.1	12
1442	French, low-calorie	1 tbsp	15	14	0.1	0.6	2.3	11.6	1.7		0.06		2.1	12
1450	Green Goddess	1 tbsp	15	72	0.1	7.4	0.8							
1460	Italian	1 tbsp	15	83	t	8.8	1.0	4.1	1.5		0.03		0.6	2
1470	Mayonnaise	1 tbsp	14	101	0.1	11.2	0.3	2.1	3.0		0.10	0.3	4.0	5
1480	Russian	1 tbsp	15	74	0.2	7.6	1.1	5.2	2.8		0.09		5.6	24
1500	Thousand Island	1 tbsp	15	75	0.1	7.2	2.3	4.8	1.6		0.09		2.6	17
1502	Thousand Island, low-calorie	1 tbsp	15	27	0.1	2.1	2.3	10.0	1.6		0.09		2.6	17
	Salt													
1510	Celery	1 tsp	5	2	0.2	0.1	0.1							
1520	Garlic	1 tsp	6	4	0.1	0.1	0.7					1.1		
1530	Iodized	1 tsp	5	0	0.0	0.0	0.0	t	12.0	1.0	0.01	6.0		t
1540	Onion	1 tsp	5	5	0.1	0.1	1.0							
1550	Seasoned	1 tsp	4	3	t	t	0.7							
1560	Sandwich spread	1 tbsp	17	64	0.1	6.0	2.5	7.7	2.6		0.12		3.4	16
1570	Soy sauce	1 tbsp	15	8	0.8	0.2	1.5	9.4	12.3		0.72		14.6	55
	Spaghetti sauce													
1580	Meatless	1 tbsp	17	12	0.3	0.3	1.8		5.3		0.11			
1590	w/Meat	1 tbsp	17	16	0.7	0.8	1.3		5.3		0.30		8.5	
1600	w/Mushrooms	1 tbsp	16	14	0.2	0.7	1.5		0.2		0.20		5.0	
1610	w/Mushrooms and meat	1 tbsp	17	14	0.5	0.5	1.7		5.1		0.11			
1620	Steak sauce (tomato type)	1 tbsp	17	16	0.3	0.1	3.5		5.0		0.20			
1630	Tartar sauce	1 tbsp	14	74	0.2	8.1	0.6	4.8	2.5		0.13		4.5	11
	Tomato paste, see no. 8950													
	Tomato puree, see no. 8960													
	Vinegar													
1640	Cider	1 tbsp	15	3	t	0.0	0.9	14.0	0.9		0.09		1.4	15
1650	Distilled	1 tbsp	15	2	0.0	0.0	0.1	14.0	—		—	0.1		2
1660	White sauce, medium	1 tsp	17	27	0.7	2.1	1.5	12.5	20.0		0.03		15.8	24
1670	Worcestershire sauce	1 tsp	5	4	0.1	0.0	0.9		5.0		0.30		3.0	

Sodium mg	Copper mg	Vitamin A IU	(Thiamine) B_1 mg	(Riboflavin) B_2 mg	Vitamin B_6 mg	Vitamin B_{12} mcg	Biotin mcg	Choline mg	Folic Acid mg	Inositol g	Niacin mg	Pantothenic Acid mg	Vitamin C mg	Vitamin D IU	Vitamin E mg	Vitamin K mg
1,018.0		1,600	0.250	0.30							4.00		23.00			
955.0		1,075	0.250	0.18							2.25		13.00			
2.3		6	0.040	0.02	0.050	0.0					0.30		0.00			
358.0		248	0.130	0.19							0.98		t			
2.6		0	0.210	0.10	0.440				0.029		0.06	0.70	0.00			0.020
0.2	0.14	0	0.160	0.04	0.060	0.0		24.4	0.010	0.05	0.25	0.10	0.00		1.80	0.002
1.3		72	1.070	0.64							3.50		6.50			
760.0		0	0.210	0.07							2.16		0.00			
1,498.0		0	0.130	0.08							6.00		0.00			0.090
—	0.07	1,333	0.330	0.40	0.600				0.047		3.30	0.67	10.00	—		
58.0		9	0.010	0.02							0.21		0.00			
40.0																
114.0		50	0.001	t							0.04		0.70			
177.0	0.10	238	0.020	0.01							0.27		2.55			
		103	0.050	0.04							0.05		t			
223.0		233	0.020	0.01							0.27		2.70			
9.0																
		208	0.010	0.03							0.05		0.25			
4.8	0.01															
150.0	0.05															
4.0	0.02															
93.0	0.07															
164.0		32	0.002	0.02							0.02		0.30			
166.0		26	t	0.01							0.01		0.30			
236.0																
206.0		—													1.30	
118.0		—													0.20	
140.0															1.54	
314.0	0.11	t	t	t							t		t		1.80	
84.0	0.03	39	0.003	0.01												
130.0		104	0.010	0.01	0.010						0.09		0.90		1.34	
105.0		48	0.003	0.01							0.03		0.45		1.50	
105.0		48	0.003	0.01							0.03		0.45		0.33	
1,430.0																
1,850.0																
1,938.0	0.02	0	0.0	0.0							0.0		0.0			
1,620.0																
1,230.0																
106.0		48	0.002	0.01							t		1.02			
1,099.0		0	0.003	0.04							0.06		0.0			
96.0																
122.0		252	0.010	0.01							0.20					
124.0		302	0.010	0.01							0.15					
103.0																
265.0																
99.0		99	0.001	0.01							t		1.00			
0.1													0.0			
0.1	0.01															
64.4		78	0.010	0.03							0.03		t			

Code No.	Food Item	Measure	Weight g	Calories	Protein g	Fats g	Carbohy-drates g	Water g	Calcium mg	Iodine mg	Iron mg	Magne-sium mg	Phospho-rus mg	Potas-sium mg
	DAIRY PRODUCTS													
	Butter, see no. 7140													
	Cheese													
1680	Blue or Roquefort	1 svg	28	103	6.0	8.5	0.6	11.0	88.0		0.14		95.0	
1690	Cheddar, American	1 piece	17	68	4.3	5.5	0.4	6.0	128.0		0.17	7.6	81.0	14
1691	Cheddar, American, grated	1 tbsp	7	28	1.7	2.2	0.1	2.6	53.0		0.07	3.2	33.0	6
1700	Brick	1 svg	28	103	6.2	8.5	0.5	11.5	204.0		0.30	3.2	127.0	
1710	Camembert (domestic)	1 svg	28	84	4.9	6.9	0.5	14.6	29.0		0.10		52.0	
1715	Colby	1 oz	28	110	6.0	9.0	1.0						52.0	31
1720	Cottage, large or small curd, creamed	1 cup	225	235	31.0	9.5	6.5	176.0	212.0		0.68		342.0	191
1721	Cottage, uncreamed (dry)	1 cup	260	223	44.2	0.8	7.0	205.0	234.0		1.04		455.0	187
1730	Cream	1 cup	224	838	18.0	82.0	4.7	114.0	139.0		0.45		213.0	166
1731	Cream	1 tbsp	14	53	1.1	5.3	0.3	7.1	8.5		0.05		12.0	11
1740	Edam	1 oz	28	87	7.7	5.7	1.1		225.0		0.20	12.0	136.0	
1750	Gruyere	1 oz	28	115	8.1	8.9	0.5		308.0		0.30	12.0	230.0	
1760	Limberger	1 oz	28	69	5.9	7.8	0.6	13.0	165.0		0.20		110.0	
1770	Parmesan	1 oz	28	110	10.0	7.3	0.8	8.4	320.0		0.10	13.0	219.0	42
1780	Pasteurized, processed (American)	1 oz	28	103	6.5	8.4	0.53	1.1	195.0		0.25	13.0	216.0	22
1790	Pasteurized, processed, pimento (American)	1 oz	28	107	6.5	8.5	0.5	11.2						
1800	Swiss (domestic)	1 oz	28	99	7.8	7.9	0.5	11.2	259.0		0.25	12.0	158.0	29
1810	Cheese fondue	1 lb	453	1,200	66.0	82.0	45.0	246.0	1,436.0		5.38		1,331.0	747
1820	Cheese souffle	1 lb	453	988	45.0	77.5	28.0	294.0	910.0		4.50		883.0	548
1830	Cheese spread (American)	1 oz	28	81	4.5	6.0	2.3	14.0	158.0		0.20	13.0	245.0	67
	Cream													
1840	Fluid: light or half and half	1 cup	240	322	7.7	28.0	11.1	191.0	259.0	t	26.4	204.0	310
1841	Fluid: light or half and half	1 tbsp	15	20	0.5	1.8	0.7	12.0	16.2	t	1.6	13.0	19
1850	Heavy or whipping	1 cup	238	861	5.2	90.0	7.4	135.0	179.0	t	20.0	140.0	212
1860	Sour or cultured	1 oz	30	57	0.8	5.4	1.0		31.0		3.0	23.0	17
	Whipped, artificial, see no. 3110													
1870	Custard, baked	1 cup	248	285	13.0	14.0	28.0	191.0	278.0		0.99		290.0	362
	Eggnog, see no. 0200													
	Egg													
1880	Boiled, poached, or raw	1 med	50	79	6.5	5.7	0.4	37.0	27.0		1.15	5.0	103.0	65
1885	Fried	1 med	50	108	6.2	8.6	0.4	34.0	30.0		1.20	5.0	111.0	70
1890	Scrambled or omelet	1 med	64	116	7.6	8.3	1.5	46.0	51.0		1.10	7.0	121.0	93
1895	White	1 med	31	16	3.4	t	0.3	27.0	3.0		0.03	3.0	5.0	43
1900	Yolk[3]	1 med	17	58	2.7	5.2	0.1	8.7	24.0		0.94	3.0	97.0	17
	Ice cream													
1910	All flavors, commercial	1 cup	188	389	7.5	24.0	39.0	117.0	231.0		0.19	15.0	186.0	211
1920	Bar, frozen	1 med	60	167	2.1	11.0	15.0		70.0			8.0	52.0	
	Cone, see nos. 2740 and 2745													
1930	Soda, chocolate (vanilla ice cream)	1 reg		225	2.7	8.3	46.0		75.0		0.70		93.0	
1932	Soda, vanilla	1 reg		261	2.3	7.1	48.7		69.0		0.10			
1940	Ice milk, commercial	1 cup	190	289	9.1	9.7	43.0	127.0	296.0		0.19	13.0	236.0	317
	Milk, cow's													
1950	Buttermilk	1 cup	246	90	8.9	0.2	13.0	223.0	298.0	t	36.0	234.0	344
1960	Canned, evaporated	1 cup	252	348	18.0	20.0	24.0	186.0	635.0		0.25	63.0	517.0	764
1970	Chocolate drink, skim milk	1 cup	290	220	9.6	6.7	32.0	240.0	313.0		0.58		263.0	411
1974	Hot cocoa	1 cup	252	244	9.6	12.0	27.0	199.0	298.0		1.01		285.0	365
1980	Skim, dry, instant	1 cup	64	228	23.0	0.4	33.0	2.6	828.0		0.38	92.0	643.0	1,104
1981	Skim, dry, instant, reconstituted	1 cup	245	76	7.7	0.1	11.0	223.0	276.0		0.13	31.0	214.0	368
1985	Skim, dry, regular	1 cup	126	453	45.0	1.0	66.0	3.8	1,648.0		0.76	180.0	1,280.0	2,199
1990	Skim, liquid (fortified)	1 cup	246	89	8.9	0.2	13.0	223.0	298.0	t	35.0	234.0	357
2000	Whole, dry	1 cup	103	516	27.0	28.0	39.0	2.1	936.0		0.52	101.0	729.0	1,370
2002	Whole, liquid (fortified)	1 cup	244	159	8.5	8.8	12.0	213.0	287.0	t	37.0	226.0	346
2005	Milk, goat's, fresh	1 cup	244	163	7.7	9.8	11.0	213.0	315.0		0.03	41.0	259.0	439
	Milk, half and half, see nos. 1840 and 1841													

[3]Contains a small amount of egg white.
[4]Values for reconstituted food.

Sodium mg	Copper mg	Vitamin A IU	(Thiamine) B1 mg	(Riboflavin) B2 mg	Vitamin B6 mg	Vitamin B12 mcg	Biotin mcg	Choline mg	Folic Acid mg	Inositol g	Niacin mg	Pantothenic Acid mg	Vitamin C mg	Vitamin D IU	Vitamin E mg	Vitamin K mg
		347	0.010	0.17							0.34		0			
119.0	0.02	223	0.010	0.08	0.010	0.17	0.6	8.2	0.003	t	0.02	0.09	0			
49.0	0.01	92	0.001	0.03	0.005	0.07	0.2	3.4	0.001	t	0.01	0.04	0			
		347		0.13							0.03		0			
		283	0.010	0.21							0.20					
515.0	0.05	380	0.070	0.56	0.090	2.25			0.070		0.23	0.50	0			
754.0		26	0.080	0.65							0.26		0			
560.0	0.09	3,450	0.050	0.54	0.120	0.49					0.22	0.60	0			
35.0	0.01	215	0.003	0.03	0.010	0.03					0.01	0.04	0			
	0.01	510	0.011	0.14							0.10		0			
		560	0.002	0.14							0.10		0			
		320	0.020	0.14							0.10		0			
205.0	0.10	300	0.010	0.20	0.030						0.10	0.15	0			
318.0	0.02	342	0.006	0.12	0.020	0.20	1.3		0.003		t	0.13	0			
199.0	0.03	319	0.003	0.11	0.020	0.50					0.03	0.10	0			
2,455.0		3,986	0.270	1.52							0.90		t			
1,649.0		3,624	0.230	1.09							0.90		t			
455.0		240	0.003	0.15							0.03		0			
110.0		1,152	0.070	0.38	0.080	0.60					0.24	0.77	2.40			
6.9		72	0.010	0.02	0.010	0.04					0.01	0.12	0.15			
76.0		3,665	0.050	0.26	0.070	0.50					t		2.40			
12.0		230	010	0.04	0.030											
196.0		868	0.100	0.47							0.25		t			
61.0	0.05	590	0.060	0.15	0.060	1.00	11.3	252.0	0.003	0.02	0.05	0.80	0	24.0	0.23	0.006
169.0	0.03	710	0.050	0.15							0.10		0	27.0		
164.0	0.03	691	0.050	0.18							0.10		0	31.0		
47.0	0.02	0	t	0.08	0.070	0.31	2.2	0.6	t		0.03	0.04	0	0.0		
8.8	0.05	578	0.040	0.08	0.050	1.02	8.8	253.0	0.002		0.02	0.72	0	27.0		
75.0	0.06	978	0.080	0.36							0.19	0.55	0.19		0.11	
28.0		209	0.020	0.01							0.10					
		297	0.030	0.13							0.20		1.00	0.0		
		295	0.024	0.11							0.10		1.00	0.0		
129.0		399	0.100	0.42							0.19		1.90			
320.0	0.01	t	0.100	0.44	0.090	0.54			0.030		0.25	0.80	2.50			
118.0	0.33	806	0.100	0.86	0.130	0.40	11.3[4]	38.0[4]	0.003		0.50	1.60	2.50			
133.0		232	0.120	0.46							0.30		0.29	5.3		
129.0		603	0.100	0.45							0.50		2.52	5.0		
337.0	0.31	19	0.220	1.14	0.240	2.10					0.58	2.30	4.50			
112.0	0.10	6.3	0.070	0.38	0.800	0.68					0.19	0.77	1.50			
670.0	0.01	38	0.440	2.30	0.690						1.13		8.82			
118.0	0.01	998	0.100	0.44	0.100	1.00			t		0.25	0.90	2.50	100.0		
417.0	0.19	1,164	0.300	1.50							0.72	2.50	6.20			
122.0	–	354	0.070	0.42	0.090	0.98		36.6	0.002	0.03	0.24	0.75	2.44	100.0	0.10	0.007
83.0	0.11	390	0.100	0.27	0.110	0.20					0.70	0.78	2.44			

Code No.	Food Item	Measure	Weight g	Calories	Protein g	Fats g	Carbohydrates g	Water g	Calcium mg	Iodine mg	Iron mg	Magnesium mg	Phosphorus mg	Potassium mg
2010	Milk, human (U.S. samples)	1 oz	30	23	0.3	1.2	2.8	26.0	10.0		0.03	1.0	4.0	15
	Milk pudding, vanilla, see no. 3030													
2020	Yogurt, partially skim	1 cup	250	125	8.5	4.3	13.0	223.0	300.0		t		235.0	358
	DESSERTS AND SWEETS													
2030	Apple, brown Betty	1 svg	100	151	1.6	3.5	28.0	65.0	18.0		0.60	6.7	22.0	100
2040	Apple butter, canned	1 tbsp	20	37	0.1	0.2	9.1	10.0	3.0		0.10		9.0	50
2050	Banana bread	1 slice	49	134	2.4	3.9	23.0		8.0		4.00	30.0		
	Brownie, see no. 2460													
	Cake[5]													
2060	Angel food	1 slice	40	108	2.8	0.1	24.0	13.0	3.6		0.08	18.8	8.8	35
	Boston cream pie, see no. 2830													
2070	Chocolate malt, w/chocolate icing	1 slice	50	173	1.7	4.4	33.3		32.0		0.35		83.0	40
2080	Coffee, w/egg (enr flour[6])	1 slice	50	161	3.2	4.8	26.0	15.0	31.0		0.80		87.0	55
	Devil's food, no icing	1 slice	45	165	2.2	7.7	23.4	11.0	33.0		0.40		62.0	63
2100	Devil's food, cupcake, w/boiled white icing	1 avg	50	184	1.9	7.3	31.0	10.7	30.0		0.35		53.0	55
2110	Devil's food, cupcake, w/chocolate icing	1 avg	50	184	2.1	8.2	28.0	11.0	35.0		0.50		66.0	77
2120	Fruit, dark	1 slice	30	114	1.4	4.6	17.0	5.4	22.0		0.78		40.0	149
2130	Gingerbread, w/enr flour	1 slice	55	174	2.1	5.9	28.0	17.0	37.0		1.30		38.0	250
	Shortcake, see no. 2080 or 2140													
2140	Sponge, no icing	1 slice	40	118	3.0	2.3	22.0	13.0	12.0		0.48		44.8	35
2150	White, no icing	1 slice	40	150	1.8	6.4	22.0	9.7	25.0		0.08		36.0	30
2160	Yellow, no icing	1 slice	40	145	1.8	5.1	23.0	9.4	28.0		0.16		45.0	31
	Cake icing													
2170	Caramel	1 svg	10	36	0.1	0.7	7.6	1.4	10.0		0.20		6.0	5
2180	Chocolate	1 svg	10	38	0.3	1.4	6.7	1.4	6.0		0.10		11.0	20
2190	Coconut	1 svg	10	36	0.2	0.8	7.5	1.5	1.0		0.10		3.0	17
2200	White, boiled	1 svg	10	32	0.1	0	8.0	1.8	0.2		t		0.2	2
2210	White, uncooked	1 svg	10	38	0.1	0.7	8.2	1.1	2.0		t		0.2	2
2220	Candied citron	1 lb	453	1,424	0.9	1.4	364.0	81.5	376.0		3.60		109.0	544
	Candy													
2230	Caramel, plain or chocolate	1 piece	5	20	0.2	0.5	3.8	0.4	7.4		0.07		6.1	10
2240	Caramel, plain or chocolate, w/nuts	1 piece	5	21	0.2	0.8	3.5	0.4	0.7		0.08		7.0	12
	Chocolate cream													
2250	Coconut filling	1 piece	15	66	0.4	2.6	10.0	1.0	7.2		0.17		12.0	25
2260	Fudge filling	1 piece	15	65	0.6	2.4	11.0	.9	15.0		0.20		17.0	29
2270	Vanilla filling	1 piece	15	65	0.6	2.6	11.0	1.1	19.0		0.09		17.0	27
2280	Fudge, chocolate	1" piece	45	180	1.2	5.5	34.0	3.7	35.0		0.45		38.0	66
2290	Fudge, chocolate, w/nuts	1" piece	45	192	1.8	7.8	31.0	3.5	36.0		0.54		51.0	80
2300	Fudge, vanilla	1" piece	45	179	1.4	5.0	34.0	4.5	50.0		0.23		37.0	57
2310	Fudge, vanilla, w/nuts	1" piece	45	191	1.9	7.9	32.0	4.3	50.0		0.40		51.0	51
2320	Gumdrop	1 piece	10	33	t	0.1	8.5	1.2	0.6		0.05		t	t
2330	Hard	1 oz	28	108	0	0.3	27.0	0.4	5.9		0.53	t	2.0	1
2340	Jelly beans	1 oz	28	102	t	0.1	26.0	2.0	3.4		0.30		1.1	t
2350	Lollipop	1 med	27	102	0	0	27.0		0		0		0	
2360	Marshmallow	1 lg	6	19	0.1	t	4.7	1.0	1.1		0.10		0.4	t
2370	Milk chocolate bar	2 oz	56	291	4.3	18.0	32.0	0.5	128.0		0.62	32.0	130.0	53
2380	Milk chocolate bar, w/almonds	2 oz	56	298	5.2	20.0	290.0	0.8	128.0		0.90		152.0	248
2390	Mint patty	1 med	11	43	0.3	1.6	7.9							
2400	Peanut brittle	1 piece	25	110	2.1	4.0	18.2	0.5	10.0		0.50		31.0	38
2410	Cherry, maraschino	1 med	7	8	t	t	2.0	4.6	1.0		t			
2420	Chewing gum	1 stick	3	9	2.5			0.1						
2430	Chocolate syrup, thin type	1 tbsp	20	49	0.5	0.4	11.0	6.0	3.4		0.32	12.6	18.0	56

[5]Unenriched flour used for all cakes unless otherwise stated.
[6]Values per 100 g for unenriched flour: iron, 6 mg; B_1, 0.05 mg; B_2, 0.11 mg; niacin, 0.6 mg.

Sodium mg	Copper mg	Vitamin A IU	(Thiamine) B_1 mg	(Riboflavin) B_2 mg	Vitamin B_6 mg	Vitamin B_{12} mcg	Biotin mcg	Choline mg	Folic Acid mg	Inositol g	Niacin mg	Pantothenic Acid mg	Vitamin C mg	Vitamin D IU	Vitamin E mg	Vitamin K mg
5.0	0.02	72	0.003	0.12	0.003	0.01					t	0.07	2.00			
128.0		175	0.100	0.45	0.012	0.28					0.25	0.78	2.50			
153.0		100	0.060	0.04							0.40		1.00			
0.4	0.07	0	0.002	t							0.04		0.40	0		
		273	0.060	0.06							0.50		0	3		
113.0		0	0.004	0.06							0.08		0			
159.0		80	0.020	0.04							0.10		t			
22.0		80	0.900	0.80							0.70		t			
132.0		68	0.010	0.05							0.10		t			
117.0		60	0.010	0.04							0.10		t			
118.0		80	0.010	0.05							0.10	0.1	t			
47.0	0.03	36	0.040	0.04							0.24		t			
130.0		50	0.070	0.06							0.50		0			
67.0		180	0.020	0.06							0.08		t			
129.0		12	0.010	0.03	0.020						0.08		t			
103.0		60	0.010	0.03							0.08		t			
8.0		28	0.001	0.01							t		t			
6.0		21	0.002	0.01							0.02		t			
12.0		0	0.001	t							0.02		t			
14.0		0	t	t							t		0			
5.0		27	t	t							t		t			
1,315.0																
11.0		t	0.002	0.01							0.01		t			
10.0		1	0.010	0.01							0.01		t			
30.0		0	0.003	0.01							0.03		0			
34.0		t	0.010	0.02							0.03		0			
27.0		t	0.010	0.01							0.02		t			
86.0		t	0.010	0.04							0.09		t			
77.0		t	0.020	0.04							0.14		t			
94.0		t	0.010	0.06							0.05		t			
84.0		t	0.020	0.06							0.05		t			
3.5		0	0	t							t		0			
9.0	t	0	0	0							0		0			
3.4		0	0	t							0		0			
		0	0	0							0				0	
2.3		0	0	t							t		0			
151.0		215	0.030	0.19							0.17		0.80	50.0	0.60	
45.0		129	0.050	0.23							0.45		t			
7.8		7	0.022	0.01							1.20		0			
		35	0.003	t							t		t			
		0	0	0							0		0			
10.0	0.09	t	0.010	0.04							0.08		0			

Code No.	Food Item	Measure	Weight g	Calories	Protein g	Fats g	Carbohydrates g	Water g	Calcium mg	Iodine mg	Iron mg	Magnesium mg	Phosphorus mg	Potassium mg
	Cookies													
2440	Animal-shaped	1 med	2	9	0.1	0.2	1.6	0.1	1.0		0.01		2.3	2
2450	Assorted	1 med	8	38	0.4	1.6	5.5	0.2	3.0	12.0	0.06		13.0	5
2460	Brownie, w/nuts	1 piece	50	243	3.3	16.0	25.0	5.0	21.0		1.00		74.0	95
2470	Butter, thin	1 avg	6	27	0.4	1.0	4.2	0.3	7.6		0.03		5.6	4
2480	Chocolate	1 med	11	49	0.8	1.7	7.7	0.4	5.7		0.12		14.0	14
2490	Chocolate chip	1 med	9	46	0.5	2.7	5.3	0.3	3.1		0.20		8.9	11
2500	Coconut bar	1 avg	13	64	0.8	3.2	8.1	0.5	9.4		0.20		16.0	30
2510	Date nut	1 med	16	76	0.8	3.5	10.0							
2520	Fig bar	1 avg	14	50	0.5	0.8	10.0	2.0	11.0		0.14		8.4	28
2530	Gingersnap	1 avg	5	21	0.3	0.4	4.0	0.2	3.7		0.12		2.4	23
2540	Ladyfinger	1 avg	6	21	0.5	0.5	3.9	1.2	2.5		0.10		9.8	4
2550	Macaroon	1 sm	10	48	0.5	2.3	6.6	t	2.7		0.09		8.9	46
2560	Marshmallow	1 lg	16	65	0.6	2.1	11.6	1.6	3.4		0.08		9.1	15
2570	Molasses	1 med	8	34	0.5	0.8	6.1	0.3	4.1		0.17		6.6	11
2580	Oatmeal, w/raisin	1 lg	20	90	1.2	3.1	14.3	0.6	4.2		0.58		20.0	74
2590	Peanut	1 lg	14	66	1.4	2.7	9.0	0.3	5.9		0.13		16.2	25
2600	Raisin	1 avg	12	46	0.5	0.6	9.7	1.0	8.5		0.25		19.0	33
2610	Sandwich	1 avg	8	40	0.4	1.8	5.4	0.2	2.1		0.06		19.0	3
2620	Shortbread, plain	1 avg	8	39	0.6	1.8	5.4	0.2	0.6					
2630	Shortbread, striped	1 avg	10	50	4.1	2.4	6.5							
2640	Sugar, soft	1 lg	8	36	0.5	1.3	5.4	0.6	6.2		0.11		8.2	6
2650	Vanilla wafer	1 avg	5	23	0.3	0.8	3.7	0.1	2.1		0.02		3.1	4
2660	Cream puffs and eclairs, w/custard filling	1 avg	107	249	7.0	14.9	22.0	62.0	87.0		0.75		122.0	129
	Custard, see no. 1870													
	Doughnut													
2670	Cake	1 avg	33	129	1.5	6.1	17.0	7.8	13.0		0.46[7]	7.0	63.0	30
2680	Raised or yeast	1 avg	33	136	2.1	8.8	12.0	9.4	13.0		0.50[7]	7.0	25.0	26
2690	Raised, jelly-filled	1 avg	65	226	3.4	8.8	30.0		28.0		0.80	16.0	42.0	
	Gelatin													
2700	Fruit-flavored	1 cup	239	141	3.6	0	34.0	201.0	0		0		0	
2710	Fruit-flavored, w/fruit	1 square	188	126	2.4	0.2	31.0	154.0						
2720	Vegetable, lettuce, and salad dressing	1 square	164	115	2.2	5.7	15.0		24.0		0.50		27.0	
2730	Honey, strained or extracted	1 tbsp	21	64	0.1		16.0	3.6	1.0		0.11	0.6	1.3	11
	Ice cream, see nos. 1910–1932													
	Ice cream bar, see no. 1920													
2740	Ice cream cone, plain	1 med	12	45	1.2	0.3	9.3	1.1	19.0		0.10		24.0	29
2745	Ice cream cone, w/1/2 cup ice cream	1 avg	80	188	4.0	7.5	24.0		108.0		1.80	5.2	102.0	152
	Ice milk, see no. 1940													
2750	Ices (water, snow cone), all flavors	1 cup	150	117	0.6	t	48.9	100.0	t		t		t	4
2760	Jams, marmalades, preserves, all flavors	1 tbsp	20	54	0.1	t	14.0	5.8	4.0		0.20	1.0	1.8	18
2770	Jellies, all flavors	1 tbsp	20	55	t	t	14.0	5.8	4.2		0.30	1.0	1.4	15
	Molasses													
2780	Blackstrap or third extraction	1 tbsp	20	43	—	—	11.0	4.8	137.0		3.22	51.6	17.0	585
2785	Light, first extraction	1 tbsp	20	50		—	12.5	4.8	33.0		0.86	9.2	9.0	183
	Pie[8]													
2790	Apple, 9" diam	1 piece	135	346	3.0	15.0	50.0	64.0	11.0		0.41		30.0	108
2800	Banana cream	1 piece	135	298	6.1	13.0	39.0	73.0	89.0		0.68		111.0	274
2810	Blackberry	1 piece	113	275	2.9	12.0	39.0	58.0	22.0		0.57		29.0	113
2820	Blueberry	1 piece	110	266	2.6	12.0	37.0	56.0	12.0		0.66		25.0	72
2830	Boston cream	1 piece	107	323	5.4	10.0	53.0	37.0	72.0		0.54		108.0	95
2840	Butterscotch	1 piece	130	347	5.7	14.0	49.0	59.0	98.0		1.20		105.0	124
2850	Cherry	1 piece	135	352	3.5	15.0	51.0	63.0	19.0		0.41		34.0	142
2860	Coconut custard	1 piece	130	303	7.8	16.0	32.0	72.0	122.0		0.91		151.0	212
2870	Custard	1 piece	130	278	7.9	14.0	30.0	76.0	125.0		0.78		147.0	178

[7]Values per 100 g for unenriched flour: iron, 0.5 mg; B_1, 0.03 mg; B_2, 0.06 mg; niacin, 0.3 mg.

[8]All piecrust made with unenriched flour. If made with enriched flour, increase value per 1,000 g by the following amounts: iron, 0.3 mg; B_1, 0.03 mg; B_2, 0.03 mg; niacin, 0.3 mg per crust.

Sodium mg	Copper mg	Vitamin A IU	(Thiamine) B_1 mg	(Riboflavin) B_2 mg	Vitamin B_6 mg	Vitamin B_{12} mcg	Biotin mcg	Choline mg	Folic Acid mg	Inositol g	Niacin mg	Pantothenic Acid mg	Vitamin C mg	Vitamin D IU	Vitamin E mg	Vitamin K mg
6.1		3	0.001	t							0.01		t			
29.0		6	0.002	0.01							0.03		t			
126.0		100	0.100	0.06							0.35		t			
25.0		39	0.002	0.01							0.02		0			
15.0		18	0.004	0.01							0.06		t			
31.0		10	0.010	0.01							0.08		t			
19.0		21	0.010	0.01							0.05		0			
35.0		15	0.010	0.01							0.04		t			
29.0		3	0.002	t							0.02		t			
4.3		39	0.004	0.01							0.01		0			
3.4		0	0.004	0.02							0.06		0			
33.0		42	0.003	0.01							0.03		t			
31.0		6	0.003	0.01							0.06		0			
32.0	0.02	10	0.020	0.02							0.10		t			
24.0		28	0.010	0.01							0.39		t			
6.2		25	0.010	0.01							0.07		t			
39.0		0	0.003	t							0.04		0			
4.8		6	0.003	t							0.04		0			
25.0	0.01	9	0.010	0.01							0.10		t			
13.0	0.01	6	0.001	0.01							0.02		0			
89.0		375	0.040	0.18							0.11		t			
165.0		26	0.050[7]	0.05[7]							0.40[7]	0.13	t			
77.0		20	0.050[7]	0.06							0.43		0			
		121	0.12	0.10							0.90		t			
122.0		0	0	0							0		0			
64.0													5.60			
		1,977	0.04	0.06							0.30		8.00			
1.1	0.04	0	t	0.01	0.004	0			0.001		0.06	0.04	0.21	0		
28.0		t	0.01	0.02							0.10		t			
69.0		302	0.04	0.17							0.20		t			
t		0	t	t							t		1.50			
2.4	0.06	2	t	0.01	0.010	0					0.04		0.40[9]			
3.4	0.02	2	t	0.01	0.010	0					0.04		0.80[9]			
19.0		—	0.02	0.04	0.050		1.8	17.2	0.002	0.03	0.40	0.09		0		
3.0	0.30	—	0.01	0.01	0.040	0			0.002		0.04	0.07	0			
406.0	0.08	41	0.03	0.03	0						0.54	0.15	1.35	3.4		
262.0	0.08	338	0.05	0.18							0.41		1.35			
303.0		102	0.02	0.02							0.34		4.52			
295.0		33	0.02	0.02							0.33		3.30			
199.0		225	0.03	0.12							0.21		t			
278.0		338	0.04	0.13							0.26		t			
410.0		594	0.03	0.03							0.68		t			
312.0		299	0.08	0.25							0.39		0			
373.0		299	0.07	0.21							0.39	1.20	0			

[9]Higher values per 100 g were found for the following jams or jellies: gooseberry, 10 mg; red cherry or strawberry, 15 mg; guava, 40 mg; black currant, 45 mg; rose hip or acerola, 330 mg.

Code No.	Food Item	Measure	Weight g	Calories	Protein g	Fats g	Carbohy-drates g	Water g	Calcium mg	Iodine mg	Iron mg	Magne-sium mg	Phospho-rus mg	Potas-sium mg
	Pie (Cont.)													
2880	Meringue, chocolate	1 piece	120	302	5.8	14.0	38.0	58.0	83.0		0.84		118.0	167
2890	Meringue, lemon	1 piece	120	306	4.4	12.0	45.0	57.0	17.0		0.60		59.0	60
2900	Mince	1 piece	135	366	3.4	16.0	52.0	58.0	38.0		1.35		51.0	240
2910	Peach	1 piece	132	337	3.3	14.0	50.0	63.0	13.2		0.60		38.0	197
2920	Pecan	1 piece	113	472	5.8	26.0	58.0	22.0	53.0		3.20		116.0	139
2930	Pumpkin	1 piece	130	274	5.2	15.0	30.0	77.0	66.0		0.65		90.0	208
2940	Raisin	1 piece	140	378	3.6	15.0	57.0	60.0	25.0		1.26		56.0	269
2950	Rhubarb	1 piece	130	329	3.2	14.0	4.7	62.0	83.0		0.90		34.0	207
2960	Strawberry	1 piece	170	337	3.2	13.0	52.0	99.0	27.0		1.20		43.0	204
2970	Piecrust, baked, w/enr flour	9″ shell	135	675	8.2	45.2	59.1	20.0	19.0		7.0		67.0	67
2980	Pop bar, twin, frozen	1 bar	128	95	t	t	24.0							
	Popover, fruit-filled, see no. 3100													
	Pudding													
2990	Milk, bread, w/raisin	1 cup	250	468	14.0	15.0	70.0	147.0	273.0		2.75		285.0	538
3000	Milk, chocolate	1 cup	248	367	7.7	12.0	64.0	163.0	238.0		1.24		243.0	424
3010	Milk, rice, w/raisin	1 cup	250	365	9.0	7.7	65.0	165.0	245.0		1.00		235.0	442
3020	Milk, tapioca	1 cup	250	335	13.0	13.0	42.0	180.0	263.0		1		273.0	338
3030	Milk, vanilla	1 cup	248	275	8.7	9.7	39.0	188.0	290.0		t		226.0	342
3040	Sherbert, orange	1 cup	185	237	1.7	2.1	59.0	124.0	30.0		t		24.0	41
	Syrup													
	Chocolate, see no. 2430													
3050	Maple	1 tbsp	20	50	0	0	13.0	6.6	21.0		0.24		1.6	35
3060	Sorghum	1 tbsp	20	52	—	—	13.6	4.6	34.0		2.50		5.0	120
3070	Table blend, corn	1 tbsp	20	58	0	0	15.0	4.8	9.2		0.82		3.2	1
3075	Table blend, maple or cane	1 tbsp	20	50	0	0	13.0	6.6	3.2		0.80		0.2	5
	Shortbread, see no. 2620													
	Sugar													
3080	Beet or cane, granulated	1 cup	200	770	0	0	199.0	1.0	10.0		0.20	1.0	2.0	6
3085	Beet or cane, granulated	1 tbsp	12	46	0	0	12.0	0.1	0.6		0.01	t	0.1	t
3090	Brown	1 tbsp	14	52	0	0	13.0	0.3	11.0		0.40	8.7	5.0	32
3092	Brown, firmly packed	1 cup	220	821	0	0	213.0	4.6	187.0		7.50	136.0	42.0	757
3095	Powdered	1 tbsp	12	46	0	0	12.0	0.1	0		0.01		0	t
3100	Turnover, fruit-filled	1 avg	50	112	4.4	4.6	13.0	27.0	48.0		0.80[10]	12.0	70.0	75
3110	Whipped topping	1 tbsp	5	13	0.2	9.0	1.0	13.0						
	FISH AND SEAFOODS													
3120	Anchovy, canned	3 fillet	12	21	2.3	1.2	t	7.0	20.0				25.0	
3125	Anchovy paste	1 tsp	7	14	1.4	0.8	0.3							
3140	Bass, fried	1 lb	453	756	96.0	38.0	30.0	275.0						
3150	Bluefish, baked or boiled, w/butter	1 lb	453	720	118.0	24.0	0	308.0	131.0		3.20		1,300.0	
3160	Clams, steamed or canned	1 lb	453	224	36.0	3.2	13.0	349.0	248.0		19.00		618.0	631
3170	Cod, broiled	1 lb	453	740	131.0	24.0	0	293.0	143.0		4.60		1,260.0	1,872
3180	Codfish cake, fried, w/potato and egg	1 cake	50	86	7.4	4.0	4.7	33.0						
3190	Crab, deviled	1 lb	453	852	516.0	42.6	60.0	287.0	213.0		5.40		620.0	752
3200	Crab Imperial[11]	1 svg	240	352	35.0	18.2	9.4		144.0		2.20		398.0	314
3210	Crabmeat, cooked or canned	1 lb	453	398	78.0	8.6	2.3	355.0	194.0		3.60	153.0	789.0	498
3220	Fishstick, frozen, breaded, fried	1 stick	22	38	3.6	2.0	1.4	14.5	2.4		0.09		37.0	
3230	Flounder, baked	1 lb	453	894	138.0	38.0	0	263.0	106.0		6.44	138.0	1,582.0	2,700
3240	Frog's legs, fried	1 lb	453	1,230	77.0	86.0	37.0		84.0		6.00		693.0	
3250	Haddock, fried	1 lb	453	717	88.0	29.0	26.0	300.0	180.0		5.41		1,114.0	1,570
3260	Haddock, plate dinner	1 reg	340	328	28.6	14.3	21.4		65.0		1.70		316.0	
3270	Halibut, broiled	1 lb	453	752	116.0	32.0	0	302.0	74.0		3.68		1,141.0	2,415
3280	Herring, kippered	1 sm	100	205	22.0	13.0	0	61.0	66.0		1.40		254.0	
3290	Herring, pickled	1 lb	453	976	91.0	68.0	0	269.0		6.0				
3300	Kelp	1 cup	220	—	16.5	2.4	88.4	48.0	2,405.0	3.0	0.22	1,670.0	528.0	11,601
3310	Lobster, steamed	1 med	200	179	37.0	3.0	0.6	154.0	130.0		1.60	44.0	384.0	360
3320	Lobster Newburg	1 svg	100	194	18.5	10.6	5.1	64.0	87.0		0.90		192.0	171

[10]When made with enriched flour, values per 100 g are iron, 0.9 mg; B$_1$, 0.05 mg; B$_2$, 2 mg; niacin, 0.3 mg.

[11]Prepared with butter, flour, milk, onion, green pepper, eggs, and lemon juice.

Sodium mg	Copper mg	Vitamin A IU	(Thiamine) B₁ mg	(Riboflavin) B₂ mg	Vitamin B₆ mg	Vitamin B₁₂ mcg	Biotin mcg	Choline mg	Folic Acid mg	Inositol g	Niacin mg	Panto- thenic Acid mg	Vitamin C mg	Vitamin D IU	Vitamin E mg	Vitamin K mg
307.0		228	0.04	0.14							0.24		t			
338.0		204	0.04	0.10							0.24		3.60			
605.0	0.12	t	0.10	0.05							0.54		1.35			
354.0		964	0.03	0.05							0.90		3.96			
250.0		181	0.18	0.08							0.34		t			
278.0		3,211	0.04	0.13							0.65	0.67	t			
399.0		t	0.04	0.04							0.42		1.40			
351.0	0.13	65	0.03	0.05							0.39		3.90			
330.0		68	0.03	0.07							0.68		43.00			
825.0		0	0.040	0.04							7.00		0			
503.0	0.20	750	0.150	0.48							0.25		2.50			
139.0		372	0.050	0.35							0.25		t			
178.0	0.08	275	0.080	0.35							0.50		t			
390.0	0.10	725	0.100	0.45							0.25		2.50			
161.0	0.12	397	0.070	0.40							0.25		2.50			
18.5		111	0.020	0.06							t		3.70			
2.0		0									0		0			
4.0				0.02							0.02			0		
14.0		0	0	0							t		0	0		
0.4		0	0	0							0		0	0		
2.0	0.04	0	0	0							0			0		
0.1	t	0	0	0							0			0		
3.4	t	0	0.001	t							0.03		—	0		
66.0	0.04	0	0.020	0.07							0.44		—	0		
0.1	t	0	0	0							0			0		
110.0		165	0.070	0.12							0.50		t			
		6	0.010													
	2.80															
471.0	4.53	227	0.500	0.45							8.60					
			0.050	0.50	0.380				0.010		4.50	2.70				
506.0	3.6	828	0.370	0.51							14.00					
3,928.0			0.360	0.50							6.80		27.00			
1,747.0			0.140	0.29							2.60		12.00			
3,850.0	1.22	9,830	0.720	0.36	1.600	0.05			0.018		13.00	2.70	9.02			
		0	0.010	0.02							0.35					
1,090.0	3.31		0.320	0.37							0.12		9.20			
		0	0.510	1.05							5.40					
798.0	0.86		0.180	0.32							14.00		9.02		1.80	
1,319.0		313	0.270	0.24							5.70					
616.0	3.20	3,128	0.230	0.32	1.900		3.6				38.00	1.20				
		30		0.28							3.30					
6,615.0	t			0.73							12.54					
420.0	3.40	551	0.200	0.14		1.00					1.40	3.00	0			
229.0			0.070	0.11												

Code No.	Food Item	Measure	Weight g	Calories	Protein g	Fats g	Carbohydrates g	Water g	Calcium mg	Iodine mg	Iron mg	Magnesium mg	Phosphorus mg	Potassium mg
3330	Lobster Thermidor	1 med	415	405	28.5	26.6	14.8		190.0		1.90		451.0	
3340	Mackerel, canned	1 lb	453	798	87.0	50.0	0	298.0	834.0		9.50		1,236.0	
	Oysters													
3350	Cooked or fried	1 cup	240	561	21.0	33.0	45.0	131.0	365.0		19.00		578.0	487
3360	Raw[12]	1 cup	240	152	25.0	5.3	15.4	190.0	204.0	58.0	17.30		367.0	
3370	Oyster stew, w/milk	1 cup	230	223	12.0	15.0	10.0	189.0	262.0		4.40		255.0	306
	Perch													
3380	Ocean, fried	1 lb	453	1,021	87.0	61.0	31.0	267.0	152.0		5.98		1,040.0	1,306
3390	Yellow, broiled	1 lb	453	389	87.0	4.0	0	359.0			2.70		808.0	1,030
3400	White, fried	1 lb	453	752	74.0	37.0	0		53.0		4.12		779.0	
3410	Pike, blue and northern, broiled	1 lb	452	403	82.0	4.9	0	360.0						
3420	Pike, walleye, broiled	1 lb	453	392	86.0	5.4	0	355.0			1.80		959.0	1,429
3430	Red snapper, broiled	1 lb	453	421	89.7	40.8	0	356.0	72.5		3.60		969.0	1,463
	Salmon													
3440	Pink, canned	1 lb	453	639	93.0	27.0	0	147.0	888.0	6.0	3.60	136.0	1,296.0	1,635
3450	Baked or broiled	1 lb	453	824	122.0	33.0	0	287.0			5.40		1,867.0	1,998
3460	Smoked	1 lb	453	797	97.9	43.0	0	267.0	64.0				1,110.0	
3470	Sockeye (red), w/bones cooked	1 lb	453	746	92.0	42.0	0	304.0	1,168.0	6.0	5.40	131.0	1,550.0	1,551
3480	Loaf, w/rice	1 svg	100	122	12.0	4.5	7.3	74.4						
3490	Sardines, canned in oil w/bone	1 lb	453	1,408	93.0	110.0	2.7	229.0	1,234.0		16.00		1,957.0	2,526
3500	Scallops, breaded, fried	1 lb	453	875	83.0	39.9	48.0	272.0						
	Seaweed, see nos. 3300 and 7955													
3520	Shad, baked	1 lb	453	879	105.0	51.0	0	289.0	108.0		2.70		1,412.0	1,700
	Shrimp													
3540	Cooked or french fried	1 lb	453	989	92.0	49.0	45.0	285.0	325.0		9.02	230.0	861.0	1,033
3550	Canned, dry-packed	1 lb	453	525	110.0	5.0	3.2	319.0	520.0		14.00	271.0	119.0	553
3570	Smelts, raw	4 or 5 med	100	98	18.6	2.1	0	79.0			0.40		272.0	
3590	Swordfish, broiled	1 lb	453	764	129.0	28.0	0	293.0	124.0		5.98		1,265.0	
3610	Trout, broiled	1 lb	453	883	97.0	51.6	0	300.0						
	Tuna													
3630	Canned in oil, drained	1 lb	453	853	130.0	37.0	0	275.0	36.2		8.57	300.0	1,055.0	1,340
3640	Salad	1 cup	250	425	36.5	26.3	8.7	175.0	50.0		3.30		355.0	
3660	Casserole, w/noodles	1 svg	200	280	17.8	11.8	25.0							
3680	Turtle, canned	1 lb	453	480	106.0	3.2	0	340.0		3.0				
	FOOD SUBSTITUTES													
	Cream substitute													
3800	Liquid	1 tbsp	14	24	0.1	1.7	1.8	72.0						
	Powdered	1 tsp	3	15	0.3	0.8	1.8	t	2.0		0.01			
4000	Orange crystals, w/water	1 cup	240	110	1.4	0.5	26.0	211.0	24.0		0.53		38.4	502
	Whipped cream substitute, see no. 3110													
	FRUITS AND JUICES													
	Acerola cherries, see no. 7950													
5300	Apple cider, sweet	1 cup	249	124	0.2	0	34.4		15.0		1.20	1.0	25.0	249
5330	Apple juice, fresh or canned	1 cup	250	118	0.2	t	30.0	217.0	15.0		1.50	10.0	23.0	253
	Apples													
5360	Raw, whole	1 med	130	76	0.3	0.8	17.0	110.0	9.0		0.39	10.4	13.0	143
	Sauce, see nos. 5400 and 5410													
5400	Stewed, canned, sweetened	1 cup	300	273	0.6	0.3	71.4	227.0	12.0		1.50	15.0	15.0	195
5420	Stewed, canned, unsweetened	1 cup	240	100	0.5	0.5	23.0	221.0	10.0		1.20	12.5	12.0	187
	Apricots													
5420	Canned in syrup	1 cup	250	215	1.5	0.2	53.0	193.0	28.0		0.75	17.5	38.0	585
5430	Dried, uncooked	1 cup	150	390	7.5	0.7	89.0	38.0	101.0		8.50	93.0	162.0	1,468
5440	Raw	1 med	38	19	0.4	0.1	4.1	28.0	6.5		0.19	4.6	8.7	107
5450	Nectar	1 cup	250	143	0.7	0.2	34.0	226.0	23.0		0.50		30.0	378
5460	Avocado	1 lg	216	361	4.5	33.0	12.0	160.0	22.0		1.30	97.0	91.0	1,305
5470	Banana, raw	1 med	150	128	1.6	0.3	30.0	114.0	12.0		1.10	49.5	39.0	555
5480	Blackberries, raw	1 cup	144	84	1.7	1.3	17.0	127.0	46.0		1.30	45.0	27.0	245
5490	Blueberries, canned in syrup	1 cup	250	252	1.0	0.5	61.0	183.0	23.0		1.50	15.0	20.0	138

[12] Western or Pacific.
[13] An average of 906 to 1,450.

Sodium mg	Copper mg	Vitamin A IU	(Thiamine) B1 mg	(Riboflavin) B2 mg	Vitamin B6 mg	Vitamin B12 mcg	Biotin mcg	Choline mg	Folic Acid mg	Inositol g	Niacin mg	Pantothenic Acid mg	Vitamin C mg	Vitamin D IU	Vitamin E mg	Vitamin K mg
		984	0.150	0.51							4.80		0			
	7.00	1,939	0.270	0.95	1.22		81.0		0.030		26.00	2.10				
495.0	59.00	1,056	0.410	0.70							7.68					
	59.00		0.290			2.2					3.12	1.20	72.00			
780.0		782	0.140	0.41							2.10					
707.0		0	0.450	0.51	1.040						8.28	1.60	0			
305.0	8.50		0.270	0.76							7.60					
		0	0.280	0.34							18.80		0			
	3.85															
229.0	3.85		1.120	0.72							10.00					
304.0	3.44		0.770	0.09												
1,753.0	0.32	317	0.140	0.63	1.400		23.0				36.20	2.50	0			
523.0		722	0.720	0.27							44.00					
2,354.0	0.34	1,037	0.180	0.72	2.000		68.0		0.002	0.08	33.00	2.62	0	1,422.0		
2,300.0	0.18	632	0.070	0.56	1.300		108.0		0.020		15.00	2.70		1,350		
356.0	3.50	135	0.590	1.17							39.00				27.20	
839.0			0.180	0.36							12.00				2.70	
	0.77	271	0.050	0.14	0.500				0.009		8.20	0.95				
			0.010	0.12							0.14					
		9,430	0.180	0.23							50.00					
	0.47		0.360	0.90							38.00					
3,580.0		361	0.230	0.54	1.900		13.6		0.91					1,178.0[13]		
		725	0.100	0.28							12.50			2.50		
19.0		5	0	0							t		t			
17.0		29	0.002	0.01												
2.4		480	0.200	0.07							0.96		106.00			
10.0	0.32	90	0.050	0.07							t		2.00			
2.5	0.02		0.030	0.05	0.040	0	1.2	1.5	0.001	0.06	0.25	0.05	2.50			
1.0	0.02	117	0.040	0.03	0.039	0	1.6		0.003	0.04	0.13	0.14	5.20		0.40	
6.0	1.05	120	0.060	0.03							t		3.00			
4.8	0.02	96	0.050	0.02	0.040						t	0.21	2.40			
2.5	0.13	4,350	0.050	0.05	0.135				0.015		1	0.23	10.00			
39.0	0.56	16,350	0.020	0.24	0.250	0			0.010		4.95		18.00			
0.4	0.04	1,026	0.010	0.02	0.023	0			0.001		0.23	0.08	0.38			
t		2,375	0.030	0.03							0.50		7.50			
8.6		626	0.240	0.43	0.907	0	11.9		0.060		3.46	2.30	31.00			
1.5	0.23	285	0.080	0.09	0.765	0	6.0		0.010		1.05	0.39	15.00		0.33	0.003
1.4	0.23	288	0.040	0.06	0.075	0			0.021		0.60	0.36	30.00			
2.5	0.28	100	0.030	0.03	0.120				0.013		0.50	0.22	15.00			

Code No.	Food Item	Measure	Weight g	Calories	Protein g	Fats g	Carbohy-drates g	Water g	Calcium mg	Iodine mg	Iron mg	Magne-sium mg	Phospho-rus mg	Potas-sium mg
5500	Blueberries, raw	1 cup	140	87	1.0	0.7	19.0	116.0	21.0		1.40	8.4	18.0	113
5510	Boysenberries, frozen, sweetened	1 cup	150	144	1.2	0.4	36.6	111.0	25.5		0.90	18.0	25.5	157
5520	Cantaloupe, raw	1/4	100	30	0.7	0.1	7.5	91.0	14.0		0.40	16.0	16.0	251
	Cherries													
5530	Sour, canned, pitted, in syrup	1 cup	257	111	2.1	0.5	56.7	190.0	39.0		0.77		33.0	334
5540	Sour, raw	1 cup	200	116	2.4	0.6	28.6	167.0	44.0		0.80	28.0	38.0	218
5550	Sweet, canned w/syrup	1 cup	200	178	0.2	0.4	42.0	156.0	28.0		0.60	18.0	24.0	248
5560	Sweet, raw	1 cup	200	140	2.6	0.6	32.0	167.0	44.0		0.80	22.5	38.0	382
	Cider, sweet, see no. 5300													
	Cranberries													
5570	Cocktail juice	1 cup	250	163	2.5	2.5	40.0	208.0	13.0		0.75	5.0	7.5	25
5580	Sauce	1 cup	277	404	0.3	0.5	100.0	172.0	17.0		0.55	5.5	11.0	83
5590	Raw	1 cup	100	460	0.4	0.7	10.8	88.0	14.0		0.50		10.0	2
5600	Cranberry-orange relish uncooked	1 cup	250	445	1.0	1.0	114.0	134.0	47.5		1.00		20.0	180
	Dates													
5610	Dried	1 med	10	27	0.2	t	6.3	2.3	5.9		0.30	5.8	6.3	65
5620	Dried, pitted	1 cup	178	488	3.9	0.9	120.0	40.0	105.0		5.34	103.0	112.0	1,153
5630	Elderberries, raw	1 cup	457	329	11.9	2.3	75.0	365.0	174.0		7.30		127.0	1,371
	Figs													
5640	Dried	1 lg	21	58	0.9	0.3	13.0	4.8	26.0		0.63	14.9	16.0	134
5650	Raw	1 med	38	30	0.5	0.1	6.8	18.0	13.0		0.23	7.6	8.4	74
5660	Stewed or canned w/syrup	1 med	38	32	0.2	0.1	7.6	29.0	4.9		0.15		4.9	57
5670	Fruit cocktail, canned in heavy syrup	1 cup	256	195	1.0	0.3	47.0	204.0	23.0		1.02	17.9	31.0	412
5680	Gooseberries	1 cup	150	59	1.2	0.3	14.6	133.0	27.0		0.75	13.5	22.5	233
	Grapefruit													
5690	Canned sections	1 cup	250	175	1.5	0.2	42.0	203.0	33.0		0.75	28.8	35.0	338
5700	Raw, red flesh, 5" diam	1 med	260	108	1.3	0.3	25.0	230.0	46.0		1.14	31.2	46.0	385
5710	Juice, canned, sweetened	1 cup	250	175	1.2	0.2	32.0	217.0	20.0		1.00		35.0	405
5720	Juice, canned, unsweetened	1 cup	250	75	1.2	2.5	17.0	223.0	20.0		0.88		35.0	383
5730	w/Orange juice, canned, sweetened	1 cup	250	125	1.2	0.2	30.0	217.0	25.0		0.75		38.0	460
5740	w/Orange juice, canned, unsweetened	1 cup	250	108	1.5	0.5	25.0	222.0	25.0		0.75	22.5	38.0	460
	Grapes													
5750	American Concord	1 cup	153	106	2.0	1.5	21.0	125.0	24.0		0.61	19.9	18.0	242
5760	European, Muscot, or Tokay	1 cup	160	107	1.0	0.5	25.0	130.0	19.0		0.64	9.6	32.0	277
5770	Green, seedless	1 cup	200	102	1.0	0.2	27.2	171.0	16.0		0.60		26.0	220
5780	Juice	1 cup	250	165	0.5	t	41.0	189.0	28.0		0.75	30.0	30.0	290
	Lemon													
5790	Juice, fresh	1 tbsp	15	4	0.1	t	1.2	55.0	1.0		0.03	4.5	2.0	85
5800	Slice, raw, w/peel	1/10 lemon	10	2	0.1	t	0.9	8.0	2.6		0.06		1.6	14
	Lemonade													
5810	Frozen concentrate	1 tbsp	16	31	t	t	8.0	8.0	0.6		0.03	0.8	0.9	11
5820	Diluted concentrate	1 cup	250	110	0.2	t	27.0	221.0	2.5		t	2.5	2.5	40
5830	Lime juice, fresh	1 tbsp	15	4	0.1	t	1.3	46.0	1.0		0.03		2.0	16
	Limeade													
5840	Frozen concentrate	1 tbsp	16	29	t	t	7.7	8.0	0.8		0.02		0.9	9
5850	Diluted concentrate	1 cup	250	103	t	t	26.0	222.0	2.5		t	2.5	2.5	33
5860	Mandarin oranges, canned in light syrup	1 cup	250	125	1.3	0.5	30.0	213.0	45.0		0.50	36.0	35.0	445
	Muskmelon, see no. 5520													
5870	Nectarine, raw	1 med	87	50	0.5	t	12.0	71.0	3.1		0.39	11.3	19.0	229
	Olive													
5880	Green, pickled	1 lg	7	9	0.1	0.9	0.1	5.5	4.3		0.11	1.54	1.2	4
5890	Ripe, canned	1 lg	7	13	0.1	1.4	0.2	5.0	7.4		0.12		1.2	2
	Orange													
5895	Fresh	1 med	180	88	1.8	0.4	20.0	154.0	74.0		0.72	19.8	36.0	360
5900	Juice, canned, sweetened	1 cup	250	130	1.7	0.5	30.0	216.0	25.0		0.10		45.0	498
5910	Juice, canned, unsweetened	1 cup	250	120	2.0	0.5	29.0	219.0	25.0		0.10	27.5	45.0	498

[14]Values for orange-fleshed varieties.

Sodium mg	Copper mg	Vitamin A IU	(Thiamine) B1 mg	(Riboflavin) B2 mg	Vitamin B6 mg	Vitamin B12 mcg	Biotin mcg	Choline mg	Folic Acid mg	Inositol g	Niacin mg	Pantothenic Acid mg	Vitamin C mg	Vitamin D IU	Vitamin E mg	Vitamin K mg
1.0	0.21	140	0.040	0.08	0.094	0			0.011		0.70	0.22	20.00			
1.5		210	0.030	0.15							0.90		12.00			
12.0	0.05	3,400[14]	0.040	0.03	0.086	0	0.3		0.007	0.12	0.60	0.25	33.00		0.14	
5.1		1,748	0.080	0.05	0.110						0.51	0.30	13.00			
4.0	0.24	2,000	0.100	0.12	0.170				0.012		0.80	0.14	20.00			
2.0		1,300	0.060	0.04	0.060	0			0.010		0.40	0.24	10.00			
4.0	0.24	220	0.100	0.12	0.064	0			0.012		0.80	0.52	20.00			
2.5		t	0.030	0.03							t		40.00			
2.8		55	0.030	0.03	0.060	0					t		5.54			
82.0	0.09	40	0.030	0.02	0.040						0.10	0.22	11.00			
2.5		175	0.075	0.05							0.25		450.00			
0.1	0.02	5	0.016	0.01	0.015	0					0.20	0.08	0			
1.8	0.39	89	0.260	0.28	0.270	0			0.043		3.90	1.39	0			
		2,742	0.320	0.27							2.29	164.00				
7.1	0.04	17	0.020	0.02	0.037	0			0.007		0.15	0.09	0			
0.8	0.03	30	0.020	0.02	0.043	0			0.010		0.15 1	0.11	0.76			
0.8		11	0.010	0.01	0						0.08	0.03	0.38			
13.0	0.08	358	0.050	0.03	0.085	0					1.02		5.12			
1.5	0.12	435											49.50			
2.5	1.00	25	0.080	0.05	0.050	0					0.50	0.30	80.00			
2.9	0.12	1,144	0.160	0.06	0.090	0	78.0		0.010	0.47	0.57	0.07	105.00		0.58	
2.5	0.03	25	0.080	0.05	0.030	0	2.0		0.010	0.25	0.50	0.43	77.50		0.10	
6.2		25	0.080	0.05	0.033		2.0		0.010	0.25	0.50	0.43	80.00			
2.5		250	0.130	0.05							0.50		85.00			
2.5		250	0.130	0.05							0.50		85.00			
4.6	0.05	153	0.080	0.05	0.120	0			0.010		0.46	0.11	6.12			
4.8	0.10	160	0.080	0.05							0.48		6.40			
8.0	0.26	140	0.080	0.02							0.40		4.00			
5.0	0.02		0.100	0.05	0.050		0.8		0.008		0.50	0.10	t			
0.1	0.01	3	0.010	t	0.030				t		0.01	0.06	7.00			
0.2	0.02	2	0.004	t							0.01		5.30			
0.3	t	3	0.003	t							0.05		4.68			
t	0.03	t	t	0.03	0.013	0					0.25	0.03	18.00			
0.1		2	0.003	t							0.01		3.00			
t		t	0.002	t							0.02		1.86			
t		t	t	t							t		5.00			
2.5		1,050	0.150	0.05							0.25		55.00			
4.7	0.07	1,287	t	t	0.015	0			0.017				10.00			
168.0		21	0	0		0							t			
53.0		4.9	t	t	0.001	0			t			t				
1.8	0.14	360	0.180	0.05	0.108	0	t		0.010	0.38	0.72	0.45	90.00		0.43	0.002
2.5		500	0.180	0.05	0.088	0	2.0		0.005	0.35	0.75	0.37	100.00			
2.5		500	0.180	0.05	0.088	0	2.0		0.005	0.35	0.75	0.37	100.00			

Code No.	Food Item	Measure	Weight g	Calories	Protein g	Fats g	Carbohydrates g	Water g	Calcium mg	Iodine mg	Iron mg	Magnesium mg	Phosphorus mg	Potassium mg
	Orange (Cont.)													
5920	Juice, concentrate, diluted	1 oz	19	13	0.2	t	3.1	25.0	2.6		0.03	2.78	4.6	54
5930	Juice, concentrate, frozen	1 tbsp	16	25	0.4	t	5.9	9.0	5.2		0.06		8.6	103
5940	Juice, fresh													
	w/Apricot juice	1 cup	249	125	1.0	t	32.0	87.0	2.0		0.20			
	w/Grapefruit juice, see nos. 5730 and 5740													
5960	Papaya, raw	1 lg	400	156	2.4	0.4	40.0	355.0	80.0		1.20		64.0	936
	Peach													
5970	Canned in syrup	1 cup	257	201	1.0	0.3	50.0	203.0	10.0		0.77	15.42	31.0	334
5980	Fresh	1 med	114	43	0.7	0.1	10.0	102.0	10.0		0.57	11.4	22.0	234
	Pears													
5990	Canned, sweetened	1 cup	250	194	0.5	0.5	47.0	203.0	13.0		0.51	13.0	18.0	214
6000	Dried, cooked, unsweetened	1/3 cup	100	126	1.5	0.8	31.7	65.0	16.0		0.60		23.0	269
6010	Fresh	1 med	182	111	1.3	0.7	27.8	151.0	15.0		0.60	12.7	20.0	237
6020	Persimmon, Japanese, raw	1 med	125	96	0.9	0.5	22.0	98.0	7.5		0.38	10.0	33.0	218
	Pineapple													
6030	Canned, sliced, in syrup	1 slice	122	90	0.4	0.1	22.0	98.0	13.0		0.37	9.8	6.1	117
6040	Canned, crushed, in syrup	1 cup	260	192	0.8	0.3	47.0	197.0	29.0		0.78		13.0	250
6050	Raw	1 cup	140	73	0.5	0.3	17.0	119.0	24.0		0.70	17.0	11.0	204
6060	Juice, canned	1 cup	250	138	1.0	0.2	32.4	214.0	38.0		0.75	28.8	23.0	373
	Plum													
6070	Canned in syrup	1 cup	256	213	1.0	0.3	52.0	198.0	23.0		2.30	12.5	26.0	364
6080	Fresh, 2" Damson	1 med	60	29	0.3	t	6.7	49.0	7.2		0.30	5.4	11.0	102
	Prunes													
6090	Cooked, sweetened	1 cup	270	464	2.2	0.5	112.0	143.0	52.0		4.05		81.0	707
6100	Cooked, unsweetened	1 cup	270	321	2.7	0.8	76.0	179.0	65.0		4.86	59.0	100.0	883
6110	Dried, raw	1 lg	10	26	0.2	0.1	6.2	2.8	5.1		0.39	0.4	7.9	69
6120	Juice, canned, unsweetened	1 cup	240	185	1.0	0.2	45.0	192.0	34.0		9.84	24.0	48.0	564
	Pumpkin, see no. 8790													
6130	Raisins, dried	1 cup	160	462	4.0	0.3	111.0	29.0	99.0		5.60	56.0	162.0	1,221
	Raspberries													
6140	Red, frozen, sweetened	1 cup	200	196	1.4	0.4	47.0	121.0	26.0		1.20		34.0	200
6150	Red, raw	1 cup	133	76	1.6	0.7	16.0	112.0	29.0		1.20	26.6	29.0	223
6160	Rhubarb, cooked, sweetened	1 cup	270	381	1.3	0.3	93.0	170.0	211.0		1.62	35.0	41.0	548
	Strawberries													
6170	Frozen, sliced, sweetened	1 cup	227	247	1.1	0.4	60.0	162.0	32.0		1.59	20.4	39.0	254
6180	Raw	1 cup	149	55	1.0	0.7	11.0	134.0	31.0		1.49	17.9	31.0	244
6190	Tangerine, raw	1 lg	114	52	0.9	0.2	12.0	101.0	46.0		0.46		21.0	144
	Watermelon													
6200	4" x 8" piece	1 wedge	925	241	4.6	1.8	52.0	857.0	65.0		4.63	84.2	93.0	925
6210	Balls or cubes	1 cup	210	56	1.0	0.4	12.0	195.0	15.0		1.15	19.1	23.0	223
	MEATS, POULTRY, AND GAME													
	Beef													
6230	Chuck, pot roasted	1 lb	453	1,481	117.0	108.0	0	224.0	50.0		15.00	131.0	634.0	1,676
6240	Chili con carne, w/beans	1/2 cup	115	167	8.6	7.0	12.2	83.0	37.0		2.00		145.0	268
6250	Chili con carne, w/no beans	1/2 cup	115	230	11.8	17.0	6.7	77.0	43.7		1.60		175.0	
6260	Corned	1 lb	453	1,685	104.0	138.0	0	199.0	41.0		13.00		421.0	680
6270	Corned beef hash, canned	1/2 cup	115	208	10.1	13.0	12.3	78.0	15.0		2.30		77.0	230
6280	Dried or chipped, uncooked	3 oz	85	173	29.1	5.4	0	41.0	17.0		4.30		343.0	170
6290	Dried or chipped, creamed	1/2 cup	120	185	9.8	12.0	t	86.0	126.0		0.96		168.0	184
6300	Hamburger, regular, cooked	4 oz	85	190	20.6	17.2	0	46.0	9.4		2.70	18.0	165.0	383
6310	Hamburger, lean, cooked	4 oz	86	188	23.5	9.7	0	52.0	10.3		3.00	18.0	198.0	480
6320	Hash, canned[15]	1 cup	225	290	21.7	9.9	28.7		28.0		2.90		1.0	
6330	Heart, braised[16]	1 lb	453	1,685	117.0	131.0	0.4	201.0	49.8		25.00	82.0	766.0	
6340	Kidney, braised	1 lb	453	1,142	149.0	54.0	3.6	24.0	82.0		59.00		1,105.00	1,468
6350	Liver, fried	1 lb	453	1,052	120.0	48.0	24.0	254.0	49.0		35.64	82.0	1,909.0	1,721
6390	Pot pie, 4 1/2" diam	1 avg	227	558	23.0	33.0	42.7	125.0	32.0		4.09		161.0	361
6370	Rump roast, oven roasted	1 lb	453	1,571	107.0	124.0	0	218.0	45.3		14.00	82.0	892.0	1,670

[15] 75 g beef and 150 g potatoes per 225 g.
[16] Losses of B vitamins are high in braised and stewed meats.
[17] Values vary widely from 100 to 100,000 IU per 100 g.

Sodium mg	Copper mg	Vitamin A IU	(Thiamine) B$_1$ mg	(Riboflavin) B$_2$ mg	Vitamin B$_6$ mg	Vitamin B$_{12}$ mcg	Biotin mcg	Choline mg	Folic Acid mg	Inositol g	Niacin mg	Pantothenic Acid mg	Vitamin C mg	Vitamin D IU	Vitamin E mg	Vitamin K mg
0.3	t	57.1	0.025	t	0.008	0					0.09	0.05	12.80			
0.3		111	0.047	0.01							0.19		25.00			
2.5	0.20	500	0.230	0.08	0.100	0	0.8	30.0	0.005	0.30	1.00	47.50	125.00		0.10	
		1,440	0.050	0.02							0.50		10.00			
12.0	0.04	7,000	0.160	0.16		0					1.20	0.87	224.00			
5.1	0.13	1,105	0.030	0.05	0.050	0	0.6		0.003		1.54	0.13	7.71			
1.1	0.10	1,516	0.020	0.06	0.027	0			0.004		1.14	0.19	7.98			0.009
2.5	1.00	t	0.030	0.05	0.036	0					0.25	0.06	2.55			
3.0		30	t	0.08							0.30		2.00			
3.6	0.02	36	0.040	0.08	0.034	0	t				0.18	0.13	7.28			
7.5		3,388	0.040	0.03							0.13		13.80			
1.2	0.12	61	0.100	0.02	0.090	0			0.001		0.22	t	8.54			
2.6		130	0.210	0.05							0.52		18.00			
1.4	0.10	98	1.300	0.04	0.120	0			0.008		0.28	0.22	24.00			
2.5	0.01	125	0.130	0.05	0.240	0			0.025		0.50	2.50	23.00			
2.6		3,098	0.050	0.05	0.070	0			0.260		1.04	0.18	5.12			
0.6		150	0.040	0.02	0.030	0					0.30	0.11	3.60			
8.1	0.50	1,620	0.080	0.16							1.62		2.70			
11.0	0.68	2,025	0.080	0.16	1.620											
.8	0.03	160	0.010	0.02	0.020	0			0.001		0.16	0.05	0.30			
4.8	0.05	—	0.020	0.02							0.96		4.80			
43.0	0.40	32	0.180	0.13	0.380	0	7.2		0.020	0.19	0.80	0.07	1.60			0.010
2.0		140	0.040	0.12	0.060	0			0.008		1.20	0.43	42.00			
1.3	0.24	173	0.040	0.12	0.080	0			0.007		1.20	0.32	33.00			
5.4		216	0.050	0.14	0.070	0			0.010		81.00	0.19	16.00			
2.3		68	0.050	0.14	0.100	0	t		0.020	0.27	1.14	0.31	120.00		0.48	0.030
1.5	1.00	89	0.050	0.10	0.080	0	6.0		0.013		0.89	0.05	88.00		0.19	0.020
2.3	0.11	479	0.070	0.02	0.076	0			0.008		0.11	0.23	35.00			
9.2	0.37	5,458	0.280	0.28	0.630	0	33.1		0.009	0.59	1.85	2.80	65.00			
2.1	0.08	1,230	0.060	0.06	0.140	0	11.3		0.002	0.13	0.47	6.30	17.00			
271.0	0.45	181	0.230	0.90	2.000				0.070		18.10	2.80	0		0.60	
611.0		69	0.030	0.08	0.120						1.50	0.16	0	0		
498.0		173	0.020	0.14							2.50			0		
7,882.0		0	0.090	0.80		0.01					6.80		0	0		
621.0		t	0.010	0.10	0.090						2.40		0	0		
3,660.0		0	0.060	0.27							3.20		0	0		
859.0		432	0.070	0.23							0.70		t	2.0		
40.0	0.05	34	0.080	0.18	0.390				0.010		4.60	0.37	0	0	0.31	0.030
41.0	0.05	17	0.080	0.20					0.010		5.20		0	0	0.32	0.030
40.0		30	0.150	0.22	0.170						4.60		21.00	0		
	1.30	136	1.300	3.10					0.140		25.80	10.20	27.00	0		
1,147.0	1.13	5.209	2.300	21.80					0.260		48.00	15.40	0	0		
834.0	9.50	241,902[17]	1.200	18.90	3.800		450.0	2,310.0	1.330	0.23	74.70	34.90	122.00	154.0	2.90	0.420
645.0		1,861	0.250	0.27							4.54		6.81			
271.0		227	0.270	0.81	1.970	8.20	15.4	371.0		0.52	19.50	2.80	0	0	0.59	

Code No.	Food Item	Measure	Weight g	Calories	Protein g	Fats g	Carbohy-drates g	Water g	Calcium mg	Iodine mg	Iron mg	Magne-sium mg	Phospho-rus mg	Potas-sium mg
	Beef (Cont.)													
6380	Round steak, lean cut	1 lb	453	856	141.0	27.6	0	277.0	58.9		16.80	111.0	1,214.0	2,193
6390	Short ribs, cooked	1 lb	453	1,092	128.0	61.0	0	259.0	54.0		16.00	91.0	116.0	1,922
6400	Sirloin, T-bone, Porterhouse, or Rib steak, broiled	1 lb	453	1,848	101.0	157.0	0	199.0	45.3		13.10	95.0	843.0	18
6410	Stew, vegetable	1 lb	453	403	29.0	19.0	28.0	373.0	54.0		5.40		339.0	1,133
6420	Tongue, cooked	1 lb	453	1,105	97.4	22.5	1.8	275.0	32.0		10.00	72.0	530.0	742
6430	Brains, cooked (all kinds)	1 lb	453	566	47.0	39.0	3.6	357.0	45.3		10.90		1,413.0	922
	Calf													
6440	Liver, fried	1 lb	453	1,182	134.0	59.8	18.0	233.0	59.0		64.00	178.0	2,432.0	2,052
6450	Sweetbread (pancreas), braised	1 lb	453	760	148.0	14.0	0	284.0						
	Chicken													
6460	Broiled, no skin	1 lb	453	616	108.0	17.0	0	321.0	91.1		4.90	72.0	770.0	1,241
6470	Fried, breast	1 lb	453	920	147.0	29.0	6.8	265.0	54.0		7.70		1,250.0	
6480	Fried, leg	1 lb	453	1,065	148.0	46.0	4.5	249.0	68.0		10.40		1,069.0	
6490	Fried, thigh	1 lb	453	1,074	132.0	51.0	11.3	253.0	58.9		10.40		1,069.0	
6500	Liver, simmered	1 lb	453	747	120.0	19.9	14.0	294.0	49.8		38.50		720.0	684
6510	Roasted	1 lb	453	1,314	114.0	92.0	0	242.0	99.7		9.50		1,070.0	
6520	A la king	1 lb	453	865	51.0	63.0	23.0	309.0	23.6		4.50		661.0	747
6530	w/noodles	1 lb	453	694	42.0	35.0	48.0	321.0	50.0		4.10		467.0	281
6540	Chow mein	1 lb	453	462	56.0	18.0	18.0	353.0	104.0		4.50		530.0	857
6550	Fricassee	1 lb	453	729	69.0	42.0	14.5	321.0	27.0		4.00		512.0	634
6560	Pot pie, 4 1/2″ diam	1 avg	227	533	22.9	30.6	42.0	128.0	68.0		2.90		227.0	336
6570	Duck, domestic, cooked	1 lb	453	1,477	72.5	130.0	0	245.0	45.3		7.25		797.0	1,291
6580	Goose, roasted	1 lb	453	1,929	107.0	166.0	0	177.0	45.3		9.50		1,087.0	1,903
6590	Gravy, meat	1 tbsp	18	41	0.3	3.5	2.0		t		0.10		2.0	
	Hot dog, see no. 7430													
	Lamb													
6600	Chopped, broiled	1 lb	453	1,843	91.0	161.0	0	194.0	40.0		5.00	100.0	708.0	1,313
6610	Leg, roasted	1 lb	453	1,264	145.0	85.6	0	244.0	50.0		7.70	95.0		1,313
6620	Liver, fried	1 lb	453	1,182	146.0	56.0	12.7	228.0	72.0		81.00	104.0	2,591.0	1,499
6630	Shoulder, cooked	1 lb	453	1,531	98.0	123.0	0	225.0	45.3		5.40	100.0	779.0	1,314
	Meat loaf, see no. 7480													
6640	Pate de fois gras	1 tbsp	20	84	2.7	7.6	0.9	7.4						
6650	Pheasant, raw	1 lb	453	684	110.0	23.0	0	133.0	63.0		16.80		1,186.0	
	Pork													
6660	Bacon, broiled or fried, crisp, drained	1 lb	453	2,767	137.0	236.0	14.5	36.7	63.0		14.90	133.0	1,015.0	1,069
6670	Bacon, Canadian, cooked, drained	1 lb	453	1,255	125.0	79.3	1.4	226.0	86.1		18.50	109.0	988.0	1,957
6680	Ham croquettes	1 lb	453	1,137	73.8	68.0	53.0	244.0	313.0		9.50		723.0	376
6690	Chops, roasted	1 lb	453	1,690	102.0	139.0	0	204.0	45.3		13.00	122.0	1,051.0	2,573
6700	Chop suey	1 lb	453	543	47.0	30.1	23.0	344.0	109.0		8.60	67.0	448.0	770
6710	Ham, cured, roasted	1 lb	453	1,309	95.0	100.0	0	243.0	40.0		11.80	90.6	779.0	1,504
6720	Liver, fried	1 lb	453	1,091	135.0	52.1	11.3	245.0	67.0		132.00	109.0	2,442.0	1,789
6730	Pigs' feet, pickled	1 lb	453	901	75.8	67.0	0	304.0						
6740	Roast	1 lb	453	1,690	102.0	137.0	0	205.0	45.3		13.10	131.0	1,051.0	1,040
6750	Spareribs, cooked	1 lb	453	1,992	94.0	176.0	0	180.0	40.0		11.80		548.0	
6760	Rabbit, baked	1 lb	453	978	133.0	45.8	0	271.0	95.0	0.3	6.70		1,173.0	1,667
	Sausage, see nos. 7500–7630													
6770	Tongue, all kinds, pickled	1 lb	453	1,210	87.0	91.9	1.4	256.0						
	Turkey													
6780	Pot pie, 4 1/2″ diam	1 avg	227	538	23.6	30.6	42.0	128.0	61.3		3.18		229.0	449
6790	Roasted, dark meat	1 lb	453	920	136.0	38.0	0	274.0	36.0[19]	0.4[19]	6.70	77.0	1,137.0	1,802
6800	Roasted, light meat	1 lb	453	797	149.0	17.7	0	280.0			5.40	127.0	1,137.0	1,861
	Veal													
6810	Cutlet, broiled	1 lb	453	1,060	120.0	60.7	0	267.0	50.0			81.5	1,019.0	2,387
6820	Roast rump	1 lb	453	1,064	126.0	58.0	0	266.0	54.0		15.80	90.6	684.0	2,270
6830	Venison (deer), raw	1 lb	453	571	95.0	18.0	0	335.0	45.3		22.70	150.0	1,128.0	—

[18]Values vary widely from 100 to 10,000 IU per 100 g.
[19]Value for light and dark meats combined.

Sodium mg	Copper mg	Vitamin A IU	(Thiamine) B1 mg	(Riboflavin) B2 mg	Vitamin B6 mg	Vitamin B12 mcg	Biotin mcg	Choline mg	Folic Acid mg	Inositol g	Niacin mg	Pantothenic Acid mg	Vitamin C mg	Vitamin D IU	Vitamin E mg	Vitamin K mg
203.0	0.36	45.3	0.360	1.09	1.970	8.20	11.8	3.1	0.050	0.05	27.00	2.80	0	0	0.59	
252.0		91	0.310	0.95							23.00		0	0		
240.0	0.54	272	0.270	0.81	1.970	8.20	11.8	308.0	0.050	0.01	20.80	2.80	2.40	59.0	0.59	
167.0	0.09	4,439	0.270	0.31		2.90					8.60		31.70	0		
276.0	0.32		0.230	1.30							19.00		0	0		
566.0	0.95	0	1.000	1.20	7.20						20.00	12.70	82.00	0		
535.0	0.36	148,131[17]	1.100	18.90	3.000	2.70					74.70	36.00	168.00	63.0		
	0.36		0.270	0.72	13.000											
299.0	1.80	408	0.230	0.87	3.100	2.00	45.3		0.010	0.23	39.80	3.60			1.70	
	0.63	408	0.230	1.00							66.50		0			
	1.00	634	0.310	1.80							32.00					
	0.99	91	0.270	2.20							30.80		0			
276.0	1.20	55,719[18]	0.770	12.20							53.00		72.50	91.0		0.030
	1.20	4,348	0.310	0.99	0.590		51.0		0.010	0.22	33.50	3.60	0			
1,404.0		2,084	0.180	0.77							9.90		23.00			
1,132.0		815	0.090	0.31							8.20		t			
1,300.0		498	0.140	0.40							7.70		18.00			
698.0		317	0.090	0.31							10.90		0	317.0		
581.0		3,019	0.250	0.25							4.10		0.45			
371.0	1.85	t	0.860								30.00		0	0		
390.0	13.60	0	0.360	1.08							36.70					
		0	0.010	0.01							t		—	0		
317.0	1.10	0	0.540	0.95	1.200	9.70		344.0	1.4		20.80	2.50	0	0	0.72	
317.0	0.27	0	0.670	1.20	1.200	9.70	26.7	380.0	1.4	0.26	24.80	2.50	0	0	0.72	
385.0	7.20	337,485	2.200	23.00			570.0		1.300		113.00	32.10	163.00	81.5		
317.0		0	0.590	1.04	1.200	9.70			1.4		21.30	2.50	0	0	0.72	
			0.020	0.06							0.50		0	—		
4,625.0	2.40	0	2.300	1.50	0.570	3.17	34.0	362.0		0.19	23.60	1.50	0	0	2.40	0.200
11,574.0		0	4.170	0.77							22.70		0	0		
1,549.0		1,118	1.270	1.00							11.30		t			
272.0	1.40	0	2.300	1.04	2.170		23.6	349.0	0.010	0.20	22.00	1.99	0	0	3.20	
1,907.0		1,087	0.500	0.67							9.06		58.90			
3,252.0	4.00	0	2.130	8.15	2.030	3.20	22.7	550.0	0.010	0.14	1.63	3.60	0	0	7.20	0.070
503.0	5.16	67,497	1.540	19.80	2.9000	145.00	453.0	2,500.0	1.000		101.00	29.00	100.00	199.0		0.550
240		0	2.300	1.04			15.8				22.20		—	0		
		0	1.950	0.95							1.54		0	0		
186.0			0.230	0.32							51.20		0			
620.0		3,019	0.250	0.30							5.70		4.54			
448.0	0.90[19]		0.180	1.04					0.040[19]		0.90	4.90		0		
371.0			0.230	0.63					0.040[19]		50.00	4.90		0		
245.0	1.13	0	0.320	1.13							24.50	0.84	0	0		
362.0		0	0.400	1.31							29.00		0	0	0.23	
—		0	1.040	2.17							28.50		—			

Code No.	Food Item	Measure	Weight g	Calories	Protein g	Fats g	Carbohy-drates g	Water g	Calcium mg	Iodine mg	Iron mg	Magne-sium mg	Phospho-rus mg	Potas-sium mg
	Plate dinners, frozen													
6840	Beef roast[20]	1 avg	336	356	44.0	10.7	20.5	247.0	33.6		5.40		255.0	820
6850	Chicken, fried[21]	1 avg	336	581	43.0	29.0	38.0	222.0	138.0		4.03		487.0	376
6860	Meat loaf[22]	1 avg	336	440	27.0	22.5	32.9	248.0	64.0		4.70		393.0	386
6870	Swiss steak	1 avg	284	251	23.3	9.4	18.5		76.0		4.30		173.0	
6880	Turkey, sliced[23]	1 avg	236	376	28.2	10.1	42.7	251.0	87.4		3.70		292.0	591
	NUTS, NUT PRODUCTS, AND SEEDS													
	Almonds													
6900	Dried	1 cup	140	765	26.0	76.0	26.0	6.6	328.0		6.58	378.0	706.0	1,082
6910	Roasted and salted	1 cup	140	878	26.0	81.0	26.0	1.0	329.0		6.58	378.0	706.0	1,082
6920	Brazil nuts, unsalted	1 cup	300	1,962	42.0	201.0	32.7	14.0	558.0		10.00	675.0	2,088.0	2,145
6930	Butternuts	5 avg	15	96	3.6	9.2	1.3	0.6			1.00			
6940	Cashews, unsalted	1 cup	100	569	15.0	45.0	26.0	5.2	39.0		3.80	274.0	373.0	464
6950	Chestnuts, fresh	1 cup	200	382	5.8	3.0	84.2	105.0	54.0		3.40	82.0	176.0	908
	Coconut													
6960	Fresh	1 cup	100	346	3.5	35.3	9.4	51.0	13.0		1.70	46.0	95.0	256
6965	Shredded, moist, sweetened	1 cup	62	344	2.2	23.0	32.0	2.1	10.0		1.24	47.7	69.0	219
6980	Hazelnuts (filberts)	11 avg	15	97	1.6	9.5	3.0	0.9	38.0		0.50	27.6	48.0	71
6990	Hickory nuts	15 sm	15	101	2.1	10.1	2.0	0.5			0.40	24.0	54.0	
7000	Mixed nuts, shelled	1 cup	200	1,252	32.0	110.0	35.0		186.0		6.64		906.0	1,120
	Peanut butter													
7010	Commercial	1 tbsp	15	88	3.8	7.0	2.8	0.3	8.6		0.29	26.0	57.0	94
	Natural	1 tbsp	15	85	3.9	6.7	2.4	0.3	9.0		0.30	26.0	61.0	101
	Peanuts													
7020	Roasted, w/skin	1 cup	240	1,397	60.0	107.0	48.0	4.3	173.0		5.28	420.0	976.0	1,683
	Roasted, salted	1 cup	240	1,418	62.0	110.0	45.0	3.8	180.0		4.80	420.0	963.0	1,616
7040	Pecans, raw halves	1 cup	104	715	10.0	74.0	15.2	3.5	76.0		2.50	148.0	301.0	627
7050	Pistachio nuts	1 cup	100	594	19.0	54.0	19.0	5.3	131.0		7.30	158.0	500.0	972
7060	Pumpkin and squash kernels	1 cup	230	1,271	67.0	107.0	35.0	10.0	117.0		26.00		2,631.0	
7070	Sesame seeds, dry, decorticated	1 cup	230	1,339	42.0	123.0	41.0	13.0	253.0		5.50	416.0	1,361.0	
7080	Sunflower seeds, dry	1 cup	100	560	24.0	43.0	19.0	4.8	120.0		7.10	38.0	837.0	920
	Walnuts													
7090	Black	1 cup	100	628	21.0	59.6	15.1	3.1	t		6.00	190.0	570.0	460
	English, raw	1 cup	100	651	15.0	59.0	15.0	3.5	99.0		3.10	131.0	380.0	450
	OILS, FATS, AND SHORTENINGS													
7130	Bacon fat	1 tbsp	14	126	0	14.0								39
7140	Butter, salted	1 tbsp	14	100	0.1	11.2	0.1	2.2	2.8	0.46	0	1.9	2.0	3
7150	Chicken fat	1 tbsp	14	126	0	14.0	0							
	Cod-liver oil, see no. 7960													
7160	Hydrogenated cooking fat, fortified	1/2 cup	113	814	0.7	91.5	0.5		23.0				18.0	
7170	Lard	1 tbsp	14	126	0	220.0		0	0	1.0	0	0	0	0
7180	Margarine (fortified)	1 tbsp	14	100	0.1	11.3	0.1	1.0	3.0	1.0	0		2.0	3
	Mayonnaise, see no. 1470													
	Oil													
7200	Corn	1 tbsp	14	126	0	14.0	0	0	0	1.7	0	0	0	0
7210	Cottonseed	1 tbsp	14	126	0	14.0	0	0	0	1.5	0	0	0	0
7220	Olive	1 tbsp	14	124	0	14.0	0	0	0	1.2	0	0	0	0
7230	Peanut	1 tbsp	14	124	0	14.0	0	0	0	1.4	0	0	0	0
7240	Safflower	1 tbsp	14	124	0	14.0	0	0	0	2.0	0	0	0	0
7250	Soybean	1 tbsp	14	124	0	14.0	0	0	0	1.8	0	0	0	0
7260	Wheat germ	1 tbsp	14											

[20]With whole oven-browned potatoes, peas, and corn.
[21]With mashed potatoes, mixed vegetables (carrots, beans, corn, peas).
[22]With tomato sauce, mashed potatoes, and peas.
[23]With mashed potatoes and peas.
[24]Value for salted nuts is 200 mg per 100 g.

Sodium mg	Copper mg	Vitamin A IU	(Thiamine) B1 mg	(Riboflavin) B2 mg	Vitamin B6 mg	Vitamin B12 mcg	Biotin mcg	Choline mg	Folic Acid mg	Inositol g	Niacin mg	Pantothenic Acid mg	Vitamin C mg	Vitamin D IU	Vitamin E mg	Vitamin K mg
870.0		370	0.200	0.34							7.10		17.00			
1,156.0		1,982	0.240	0.60							17.00		13.40			
1,320.0		1,445	0.340	0.47							5.70		13.40			
1,072.0		4,354	0.140	0.31							4.30					
1,340.0		437	0.230	0.30							7.70		13.40			
5.6	1.70	0	0.340	1.29	0.140	0	25.2		0.063		4.90	0.73	t	0		
277.0		0	0.070	1.29	0.133	0	25.2		0.063		4.90	0.81	0			
3.0	4.20	t	3.300	0.36	0.510	0			0.015		4.60	0.69	30.00	0		
	0.18															
15.0[24]		100	0.430	0.25		0					1.80	1.30	—			
12.0	0.12	—	0.440	0.44							0.12					
23.0	0.69	0	0.050	0.02	0.044	0			0.028		0.50	0.20	3.00	0		
11.0	0.34	0	0.030	0.02							0.25		2.50			
0.1	0.20	16	0.069	0.08			2.4		0.010		0.80	0.17	1.10	0		
	0.20	—	0.080	—							0		—	0		
26.0		40	1.200	0.26							8.00		t	0		
91.0	0.09	0	0.020	0.02	0.050		5.8	22.0	0.010	0.03	2.20	0.38	0			
91.0		—	0.020	0.02	0.050	0			0.008		2.40	—	0			
12.0	2.30	t	0.770	0.32	0.700	0	81.0	384.0	0.140	0.43	40.00	5.76	2.40		18.50	
1,003.0	1.00	t	0.770	0.32							40.00		0			
0.3	1.14	135	0.890	0.14	0.190	0	28.0	52.0	0.028		0.94	1.78	2.08	0		
—	1.17	230	0.670	—							1.40		0			
—		161	0.550	0.44							5.50		—			
	3.70		0.410	0.30							12.40		0			
30.0	1.77	50	1.960	0.23							5.40					
3.0		300	0.220	0.11					0.077		0.70		—			
2.0	1.40	30	0.330	0.13	0.730	0	37.0		0.080		0.90		2			
142.0																
138.0	t	462			t	t			0.7				0	13.0	0.14	
		0														
1,115.0		3,730												10.0		
0	t	0	0	0	t	0			0.7		0		0	0		
138.0	0.01	462							0.7				0		7.60	
0		0	0	0					0.7		0		0	1.3	5.00	0.001
0		0	0	0					0.7		0		0		8.50	
0	0.01	0	0	0					0.7		0		0		5.32	
0	t	0	0	0					0.7		0		0		8.50	
0		0	0	0					0.7		0		0		13.00	
0	0.06	0	0	0					0.7		0		0		2.90	
															28.00	

Code No.	Food Item	Measure	Weight g	Calories	Protein g	Fats g	Carbohy-drates g	Water g	Calcium mg	Iodine mg	Iron mg	Magne-sium mg	Phospho-rus mg	Potas-sium mg
	SANDWICHES[25]													
7270	Bacon, lettuce, tomato w/toast	1 avg	148	282	6.8	16.0	29.0		53.0		1.50		89.0	
7280	Chicken salad, no lettuce	1 avg	110	245	14.0	9.0	27.0		50.0		1.50		101.0	
7290	Club—bacon, chicken, tomato	1 avg	315	590	36.0	21.0	42.0		103.0		4.30		394.0	
7300	Cream cheese and jelly	1 avg	119	386	6.6	16.0	50.0		60.0		1.10		74.0	
7310	Egg salad, no lettuce	1 avg	138	279	11.0	13.0	31.0		68.0		2.40		153.0	
7320	Ham salad, no lettuce	1 avg	114	321	11.0	17.0	30.0		45.0		2.00		102.0	
7330	Ham, no lettuce	1 avg	81	281	11.0	15.0	24.0		40.0		1.70		93.0	
7340	Hamburger, 4 oz, beef w/lettuce, catsup	1 lg	192	454	32.0	26.0	21.0		43.0		4.80	42.0	271.0	673
7350	Hamburger, 2 1/2 oz, beef w/catsup	1 avg	122	309	21.0	20.0	20.0		34.0		3.20	30.0	176.0	428
7360	Liverwurst on rye, no lettuce	1 avg	91	251	9.4	12.3	27.0		38.0		2.50			143
7370	Peanut butter	1 avg	83	328	12.0	20.0	30.0		61.0		1.00		177.0	
7380	Roast beef (hot) w/gravy	1 avg	160	421	19.0	25.0	30.0		43.0		2.90		163.0	
7390	Tuna fish	1 avg	105	278	11.0	14.0	26.0		48.0		1.20		135.0	
7400	Turkey, hot or cold	1 lg	156	402	29.0	18.0	28.0		62.0		5.8		370.0	
	SAUSAGE, COLD CUTS, AND LUNCHEON MEATS													
	Frankfurter													
7430	Cooked	1 lb	453	1,377	56.0	123.0	7.2	258.0	23.0		6.8		462.0	983
7440	w/Beans	1 lb	453	653	35.0	32.0	57.0		168.0		8.6		540.0	1,188
	Ham													
7450	Deviled, canned	1 lb	453	1,592	63.0	147.0	0	229.0	36.0		9.5		417.0	
7460	Luncheon meat, broiled	1 lb	453	1,061	86.0	77.0	0	268.0	50.0		12.7		753.0	
7470	Spiced, canned	1 lb	453	1,334	68.0	113.0	5.9	249.0	41.0		10.0	97.0	490.0	1,007
7480	Meat loaf	1 lb	453	907	72.1	59.9	15.0	290.0	41.0		8.2		807.0	
7490	Potted meat	1 lb	453	1,125	79.4	87.0	0	275.0	182.0		6.9		428.0	
	Sausage													
7500	Blood	1 lb	453	1,787	64.0	167.0	1.4	210.0	38.0		9.8		72.5	
7510	Bockwurst	1 lb	453	1,198	51.3	108.0	2.7	280.0						
7520	Bologna	1 lb	453	1,379	54.9	125.0	5.0	255.0	32.0		8.2	40.0	581.0	1,043
7530	Braunschweiger	1 lb	453	1,447	67.1	124.0	10.4	238.0	45.0		26.8		1,111.0	
7540	Brown and serve, cooked	1 lb	453	1,912	75.0	171.0	12.7	181.0						
7550	Cervelat (all types)	1 lb	453	1,393	84.4	111.0	7.3	220.0	50.0		12.7		971.0	
7560	Country style	1 lb	453	1,565	68.5	141.0	0	226.0	41.0		10.4		762.0	
7570	Head cheese	1 lb	453	1,216	70.3	99.8	4.5	266.0	41.0		10.4		785.0	
7580	Liverwurst	1 lb	453	1,393	73.5	116.0	8.2	244.0	41.0		24.5		1,080.0	
7590	Polish	1 lb	453	1,379	71.2	117.0	5.4	243.0	41.0		10.9		798.0	
7600	Pork link or bulk	1 lb	453	2,156	820.0	200.0	t	158.0	32.0		10.9	72.5	734.0	1,219
7610	Salami	1 lb	453	1,411	79.4	116.0	6.4	231.0	45.0		11.8		907.0	
7620	Thuringer	1 lb	453	1,393	84.4	111.0	7.3	220.0	50.0		12.7		971.0	
7630	Vienna, canned	1 lb	453	1,089	63.5	90.0	1.4	285.0	36.0		9.5		694.0	
7640	Tamales w/sauce	1 avg	100	140	4.5	7.0	14.0		20.0		1.2		39.0	
	SOUPS													
	Asparagus													
7660	Cream of, w/water	1 cup	255	70	2.5	1.8	11.0	237.0	28.0		0.8		41.0	128
7665	Cream of, w/milk	1 cup	260	157	7.3	6.2	18.0	225.0	188.0		0.8		166.0	320
7680	Bean and pork, w/water	1 cup	250	168	8.0	5.7	21.0	211.0	63.0		2.2		128.0	395
	Beef													
7690	Consomme, broth or bouillon	1 cup	240	31	5.0	0	2.6	230.0	t		0.5		31.0	130
7700	Bouillon cubes or powder	1 cube	3.4	7	0.7	0.1	0.2	0.1						3
7710	Noodle, w/water	1 cup	250	70	4.0	2.7	7.2	233.0	7.5		1.0		50.0	80
	Celery													
7720	Condensed	1 cup	255	184	3.6	11.0	19.0	216.0	102.0		21.0		76.5	230
7725	Cream of, w/water	1 cup	255	92	1.8	5.4	9.4	233.0	51.0		0.5		38.0	115
7730	Cream of, w/milk	1 cup	260	179	6.8	9.9	16.0	224.0	211.0		0.8		164.0	307
	Chicken													
7740	Consomme, broth or bouillon	1 cup	240	22	3.4	.5	1.9	232.0	12.0		1.20		72.0	

[25]Enriched white bread was used for all sandwiches unless otherwise stated. Butter or margarine was used in the amount of 5 g for each sandwich except the hot sandwiches, in which gravy was used.

Sodium mg	Copper mg	Vitamin A IU	(Thiamine) B_1 mg	(Riboflavin) B_2 mg	Vitamin B_6 mg	Vitamin B_{12} mcg	Biotin mcg	Choline mg	Folic Acid mg	Inositol g	Niacin mg	Pantothenic Acid mg	Vitamin C mg	Vitamin D IU	Vitamin E mg	Vitamin K mg
		870	0.160	0.14							1.60		13.00			
		10	0.140	0.14							3.20		1.00			
		1,705	0.380	0.41							10.00		27.00			
		575	0.120	0.14							1		2.00			
		580	0.160	t							1		2.00			
364.0		270	0.160	0.22							5.00		0.30			
		30	0.280	0.14							2.30		2.00			
		165	0.280	0.14							2.30		2.00			
387.0	0.05	370	0.220	0.33					0.010		7.50		1.80		0.21	0.030
		1,745	0.130	0.38							2.20		0			
		165	0.100	0.08							5.40		0			
		0	0.170	0.21							4.90		0			
		231	0.140	0.11							4.10		1.00			
		45	0.180	0.233							6.80		0			
4,911.0	0.36	0	0.680	0.91	0.590			258.0			11.00	1.90	0	0		
2,445.0		590	0.300	0.26							5.70		t			
		0	0.640	0.45							7.30		0	0		
		0	2.000	0.68							11.80					
5,597.0		0	1.410	0.95	1.100						13.60				0.14	
		324	0.590	1.00							11.30		0	12.9		
2,137.0	0.31		0.120	1.02							5.50		0			
		0											0	0		
5,897.0	0.09	0	0.720	0.98	0.450			272.0			12.00		0	0	0.27	
		29,620	0.780	6.55							37.00		0	75.5		
		0	0.510	1.17							19.20		0	0		
			1.000	0.87							14.00					
		0	0.180	0.45							4.00		0	0		
		28,800	0.910	5.90							25.90		0	75.5		
		0	1.540	0.86							14.10		0	0		
4,340.0		0	3.600	1.50	0.750	0.250		217.0	0.050		16.80	3.10	0	0	0.75	
		0	1.130	1.10							18.60		0	0		
			0.510	1.17							19.20					
4,454.0			0.390	0.58							11.90		0	0		
670.0													0			
1,134.0		520	0.080	0.31							0.78		t			
1,046.0		332	0.050	0.10							0.77					
1,008.0		650	0.130	0.08							1.00			2.50		
782.0	1.90	t	t	0.02							1.20		—			
816.0																
955.0	1.00	50	0.050	0.08							1.00		t			
2,030.0		434	0.026	0.10							1.02			2.60		
1,102.0		416	0.050	0.29							0.78			2.60		
1,015.0		204	0.030	0.05							0.03		t			
722.0	0.02															

Code No.	Food Item	Measure	Weight g	Calories	Protein g	Fats g	Carbohydrates g	Water g	Calcium mg	Iodine mg	Iron mg	Magnesium mg	Phosphorus mg	Potassium mg
	Chicken (Cont.)													
7750	Cream of, condensed	1 cup	255	201	6.1	12.0	17.1	214.0	48.5		1.02		74.0	168
7755	Cream of, w/water	1 cup	255	100	3.0	6.1	8.4	234.0	26.0		0.51		36.0	84
7760	Cream of, w/milk	1 cup	260	190	7.8	11.0	15.0	222.0	182.0		0.52		161.0	276
7770	Gumbo, w/water	1 cup	250	58	3.2	1.5	7.7	235.0	20.0		0.50		25.0	113
7780	Noodle, w/water	1 cup	250	65	3.5	2.0	8.2	133.0	10.0		0.50		38.0	58
7790	Rice, w/water	1 cup	250	50	3.2	1.2	6.0	237.0	7.5		0.25		25.0	103
7800	Chili, beef	1 cup	250	168	7.9	4.7	23.4		28.5		3.30		151.0	
	Clam chowder													
7810	Manhattan, w/water	1 cup	255	84	2.3	2.5	13.0	234.0	36.0		1.02		49.0	191
7820	New England, w/water	1 cup	240	130	4.3	7.7	10.5	214.0	91.2		0.96		82.0	221
7830	Minestrone, w/water	1 cup	250	108	4.8	3.5	15.0	224.0	37.5		1.00		60.0	307
	Mushroom													
7840	Cream of, condensed	1 cup	240	266	4.6	19.0	20.0	190.0	82.0		0.72		103.0	197
7845	Cream of, w/water	1 cup	255	143	2.5	10.0	11.0	228.0	43.0		0.51		54.0	105
7850	Cream of, w/milk	1 cup	260	229	7.3	15.0	17.0	216.0	203.0		0.52		179.0	296
7860	Onion, dry mix	1 oz	28	98	3.9	3.0	15.1	0.8	27.0		0.39		32.0	155
7870	Pea, split	1 cup	250	148	8.7	3.2	21.0	214.0	30.0		1.50		153.0	275
7880	Potato, cream of, w/water	1 cup	260	115	3.6	5.7	12.0	234.0	62.0		1.04		68.0	239
	Tomato													
7890	Cream of, condensed	1 cup	240	173	3.8	5.0	31.0	194.0	26.0		1.44		65.0	451
7895	Cream of, w/water	1 cup	240	86	1.9	2.4	15.0	217.0	14.0		0.72	22.0	34.0	226
7900	Cream of, w/milk	1 cup	245	169	6.4	6.9	22.0	206.0	164.0		0.74		152.0	409
7910	Turkey noodle, w/water	1 cup	250	83	4.5	3.0	8.7	231.0	15.0		0.75		45.0	80
	Vegetable													
7920	Beef, w/water	1 cup	250	80	5.2	2.2	9.7	230.0	13.0		0.75		50.0	165
	Vegetarian, w/water	1 cup	250	80	2.2	2.0	14.0	230.0	20.0		1.00		40.0	175
	SUPPLEMENTARY FOODS													
7950	Acerola cherries	3 1/2 oz	100	28	0.4	0.3	6.8	92.0	12.0		0.20		11.0	83
7955	Agar-agar		100				0.3		16.3	567.0		6.30		22.0	
7958	Bone-meal tablet[26]	6 tablets	5						990.0		2.00	4.0	495.0	
7960	Cod-liver oil	1 tbsp	14							2.5				
7962	Desiccated liver[26]		10		7.0						0.66			
7965	Malt, dried	1 tbsp	28	103	3.7	0.5	22.0	1.5			1.12			
7968	Rose hips drops[26]	1 tbsp	.3											
7970	Soybean milk	1 cup	230	76	7.8	3.4	5.1	213.0	48.0		1.80		110.0	
	Yeast													
8010	Brewer's, debittered, powdered	1 tbsp	10	28	3.9	0.1	3.8	0.5	21.0[27]		1.70	23.0	175.0	189
8020	Torula, calcium-fortified	1 tbsp	8	22	3.1	0.1	3.0	0.5	34.0[28]		1.50	13.2	137.0	164
	VEGETABLES													
	Artichoke													
8050	Cooked	1 sm	100	44	2.8	0.2	9.9	86.5	51.0		1.10		69.0	301
8055	Raw	1 sm	100	44	2.9	0.2	10.6	85.5	51.0		1.30		88.0	430
	Asparagus													
8070	Cooked	1 spear	16	3	0.3	t	0.6	15.0	3.4		0.10	3.2	8.0	29
8075	Raw	1 spear	16	4	0.4	t	0.8	15.0	3.5		1.60		9.9	44
	Beans													
8090	Green, cooked	1 cup	125	31	2.0	0.2	8.9	116.0	62.5		.75	40.0	46.3	189
8100	Lima, green, raw	1 cup	160	197	13.0	0.8	35.4	108.0	83.2		4.50	10.7	227.0	1,040
8105	Lima, dry, cooked	1 cup	192	265	15.7	1.2	49.0	123.0	55.7		6.00	129.0	196.0	1,175
8120	Navy, baked w/pork and													
	tomato sauce	1 cup	268	327	16.0	7.0	51.0	189.0	145.0		4.80	99.0	247.0	353
8130	Red kidney, canned	1 cup	260	234	14.8	1.0	42.6	198.0	75.0		4.68		4.9	686
8140	Yellow or wax, cooked	1 cup	100	22	1.4	0.2	4.6	93.0	50.0		0.60		37.0	151
	Bean sprouts (mung beans)													
8150	Cooked	1 cup	100	28	3.2	0.2	5.2	91.0	17.0		0.90		48.0	156

[26] Values obtained from various products presently on the market.
[27] Values range from 70 to 760 m per 100 g.
[28] Values range from 60 to 1,000 m per 100 g.

CHAPTER TWO

Horse for Sale

That I had never been sold away was a blessing of immeasurable comfort. I had lived my entire life as a school horse here in this valley. Friends had come and gone, yet my comforts remained constant: the Blue Ridge Mountains, the Allegheny Mountains, and the Maury River all surrounding me. These mountains, all blue to me, were home.

I was grateful, too, that I had lived a life of service under the care of a decent-enough owner. I had seen cruel hands on others, and I was deeply aware of my position. Though throughout much of my life I longed for something more—the greatness, perhaps, that my dam foresaw—I was content to have been treated fairly. My fortune changed, however, when my owner's fortune changed overnight.

The day before had ended the same as most days. We were led to our rooms, given our grain, and the barn was closed up for the evening. But the next morning, no one came to feed us. By the time the sun had moved high into the sky, we all were hungry and panicked. We kicked our doors until finally some of the students arrived to feed us and turn us out.

Monique, the proprietor of the stable and my owner, did not show. That was the first day since my birth that I had not seen her. Though I did not love Monique, I depended on her.

The students who came in her place spoke in hushed tones and whispered of the terrible and sudden death of Monique's husband. These whispers also spoke of a debt incurred by the dead man, a debt so enormous that it might force Monique out of her fine brick home and off of several hundred mountainous acres. In the second it took her husband to release his final breath, Monique had been stripped of her status as a wealthy and privileged landowner. There was no recourse left for Monique but to sell everything, including us horses, so that she could return to her native land, a country so far away that she planned never to return to the blue mountains.

Monique priced all of us reasonably. Many of my fieldmates sold quickly, purchased by current or former students who held a sentimental attachment to their favorite school horses. I recognized these buyers and had taught some of them myself, in their youth and mine. Yet I alone remained — the sole horse for sale.

I suppose, if you have never before been any girl's or boy's favorite horse, no heart longs for you.

With good reason, I was apprehensive that I would be sold at auction in Lynchville. Lynchville held no promising future for a horse like me. In fact, Lynchville offered no future at all, only a guarantee that my remaining days would likely be spent in suffering. Kill sales, like the one in Lynchville, employ unspeakably cruel techniques. Among horses, the code of kill buyers is widely understood — they'll do whatever it takes to load a frightened horse who resists his fate en route to slaughter. I have heard that breaking all four legs or cutting out eyes is commonplace. I would as soon have chosen to fend for myself in the blue mountains and taken my chances against bear and coyote than to have loaded willingly for Lynchville.

Monique warned of the distinct possibility of Lynchville as she appealed to our neighbors to extend some small charity to her by taking me in temporarily. The stables around Rockbridge County had known me since I was a colt. This fact alone should have made it easier for me to find a home, for who would so easily turn away a longtime neighbor now in need? As we set out, I was hopeful that my breeding and years of experience were assets enough to offset my obvious liabilities.

Rockbridge County has never seen a shortage of young, healthy horses. When a horse half my years, and of impeccable health, could easily have been purchased at an attractive price, there seemed no economic benefit to using me as a school horse. Though athleticism and endurance run through my Appaloosa blood, though agility and strength flow into my Appaloosa muscles, though courage and loyalty live deep in my Appaloosa bones, my aches and difficulties defy all this.

My prior career as a school horse had been long and diversified. In my youth, I introduced dozens of girls to the artistry of dressage. I carried many a young man through the mechanics of learning to jump. School horses are rarely asked to jump much higher than three feet, for by the time our pupils grow strong and skilled enough to master an intricate course of twelve three-foot jumps, they are well on their way to competing on finer horses than I. Still, for twenty or so faithful years, I had schooled without complaint, nearly every day and often for many hours.

Monique tried desperately to convince each of the barns we visited that I would make a versatile and valuable addition to their stable, capable of teaching hunt seat, dressage, basic equitation, and jumping. We made the rounds to places I had shown before, all managed by trainers I had seen on and off throughout my life in the blue mountains. I concealed my flaws as best I could. We made no less than four trips to local barns, all of which held plenty of school horses and were not in need of another.

For some time now, my powerful hind had hurt on days when it was too hot or too cold. It hurt me to jump, as a school horse must. This pain was not all that hindered me. My other ailment, I did not like to think about, and for years, had tried to deny. Our neighbors had all heard Monique's complaints about my refusal to jump. They were disinclined, each of them, to believe that I could be of value to their riding schools.

I felt certain that Monique would have accepted any offer made. Yet her pleading on my behalf resulted not in a purchase or even an offer. I feared that the Lynchville auction was my destiny. I resigned myself to never again seeing my blue mountains or feeling the Maury River swirl around my feet or hearing its roar after a heavy rainfall.

CHAPTER THREE

Reprieve

Long after Monique's house, barn, and land had sold to new owners, I remained alone, standing in my field. Though the new owners were horse people themselves, their primary interest was in the breeding of fine Thoroughbreds for the track. They brought no horses with them, as they intended to start a breeding farm only after certain improvements had been made to the buildings and land. As I was not only gelded but also of the wrong breed, not to mention my age, lack of pigmentation, and chronic conditions, the new owners declined Monique's offer of me as a gift. They did, however, agree to let me stay on if Monique would make arrangements for my care until a proper home could be found. I do not know what those arrangements might have entailed as no evidence of them ever presented itself to me.

I had been cared for well enough throughout my life. Like most school horses, I relied on structure and routine. Until this time, I had come to expect fresh hay and a rather healthy scoop of grain twice daily—once to be given just after sunrise and once again in the evening. Now I waited and waited for someone to come with hay, grain, and water, but no one arrived.

By nightfall of my first solitary day, I had eaten all of my grain and much of my hay, and drunk a good bit of water. I remained convinced that the morning sun would bring a caretaker with more rations. Morning came and brought with it a dense fog, but no caretaker. I was not alarmed, but assumed that once the fog lifted, provisions would arrive for me. The fog hung so thick that I could not see even the copper vane atop the barn. For the entire day, the mountains were but shadowy layers of themselves, for there was no sun to light up the trees or disperse the clouds.

I could see nothing of Saddle Mountain, which naturally rises and falls in precisely the shape of an English saddle. I strained to see the highest peak, what would be the saddle's cantle, but it was lost to the sky. Even the lower peak, the pommel, was hostage to the grave clouds which had descended upon me. The unseasonable mix of moist pockets of heat and cold sealed in the fog until nearly nightfall. I finished the hay left in the ring and passed the time by searching for one spot in the field that would give me some glimpse at all of Saddle Mountain. For the entire day, I could not see beyond my own feet.

Long after the fog lifted, I waited there at the gate, sure that Monique herself would show up, or an attendant on her behalf. Only once did I see any activity near the barn. I made a dancing fuss of my displeasure at being kept alone and without suitable food for so long. No one responded to my pleas for help. The activity was not intended for me; workmen had come to survey the barn and surrounding property for the new owners, who had not yet arrived. There was nothing left in the hay ring — nor a fleck of grain in my bucket — and I had resorted to licking the muddy water in the tub at the back of my field. Had I foreseen that I would be standing alone in the back of the field for more than one season, even more than one day, naturally I would have conserved my first day's rations.

During this time of uncertainty, I was consoled by the evidence around me that I was still home. Seeing my blue mountains and just knowing, from the sloping tree line, where I could find the Maury River provided my only solace. Though in my solitude I deeply felt the absence of my former life of comfort and routine, I realized that I remained, after all, in the very field in which I was born.

Upon taking full measure of this fact, that everything I had ever known was as near me as ever, I found it unnecessary to stand a moment longer pacing at the gate, filled with indignation and concern about my future. The new day did, indeed, feel new! With the fog chased off, my thoughts were as clear to me as the blue mountains now on display for as far as I could see in the golden light of morning. I must test my resourcefulness on this land I knew so well, or suffer greatly while waiting for a phantom custodian to arrive.

Fortunately, the winter had been milder than average. I judged by the duration of sunlight during the day that winter had surpassed its halfway point. During Monique's prosperity, the field had held twenty horses comfortably, so I knew I could survive for some time on grass. I also knew that should I awaken to find no grass, I could subsist for a short while on the lichen that covered the protruding boulders in my field. I had seen deer graze in this way, on lichen and moss. With no snowfall, except for a light dusting that had occurred nearer the darkest time of winter, my field was, if not lush, at least sporadically green.

While the absence of a snow cover on the ground

gave me grass to graze, it left me without a ready source of water. Because of my extensive experience as a trail mount, access to the Maury River was as familiar as my own skin. On a trail ride of eight or ten miles, I would often lead riders across the Maury River. At certain points, the Maury runs narrow like a brook — narrow enough that, on a good day, I could jump clear across its banks. At least, in my youth I could. I knew every sycamore tree along its banks and each stark-white river birch, too.

I was even more familiar with the fence line than the river. I knew its vulnerabilities and where it was in need of repair. The front fence line, the side best seen from the road, was made of handsomely maintained white-painted wood. The back fence line consisted of cedar posts strung with barbed wire. A cedar-post fence, if properly constructed, makes smart use of wood planks secured diagonally across the barbed wire between every few vertical cedar posts. The purpose of these diagonal posts is to reinforce the barbed wire, keeping it taut and stable down the line.

Though not ideal for the containment of horses, the barbed-wire fence proved a blessing in my quest for water. I knew exactly where the fence line was weak. I trotted to the place in the fence where the cedar reinforcements had long ago rotted away and used this to my advantage, for I was determined to forge a path to the Maury. It took some work, but I managed to widen a hole enough to give me mostly clear access to the unfenced portion of the farm, which in turn opened the Maury River to me. In pushing open the fence, I sustained numerous cuts and gashes, but none were life-threatening. I grazed on new grass and drank freely from the water. It was in this way that I kept myself fed and hydrated during Monique's absence.

Though I missed the regimen of two good meals served daily, and the warmth of my private room in the barn, I also felt satisfied. I survived, in fact quite well. Near the river, I discovered a lush patch of sarsaparilla, growing just for me it seemed. Though, if truth be told, I prefer the taste of peppermint to sarsaparilla, I found that the pain in my hocks and hips eased considerably when I cabbaged this plant routinely from the forest. A dense thicket of old, proud cedar trees in the middle of my field provided suitable cover, protecting me well from rain and even from wind. And though the winter sunlight cannot be considered harsh, there were times I found that the sun proved too strong for my eyes. The respite of the cedar stand gave me needed relief. I even found warmth there after sunset. I have always been partial to cedar trees, perhaps because of their abundance and familiarity to me. During this time, they proved essential.

As soon as I had secured my basic needs of food, fresh water, and very adequate shelter, my thoughts turned to my owner, Monique. Alone with the blue mountains and the Maury River, I reflected on all that had passed between Monique and myself since my birth. I had known her my entire life. Since I could remember, it was her voice that called me in from the field and her hand that filled my grain box. To my knowledge, I had received acceptable medical treatment, when needed, for both prevention and cure. I had remained active and working. My most basic needs were never neglected. I now pondered as I had never done before the questions of why I had so long remained in her care and why we had grown into such adversaries over the course of my life.

In the many years that had passed between us, horses had been born; horses had been put down for illness or injury. Ponies had been bought for pleasure, then sold for not bringing enough pleasure or not quite measuring up. I knew that I had been spared sale because some part of Monique could never part with her last remaining connection to Starry Night, the stunning snowflake Appaloosa who was my dam.

Monique was so entirely devoted to my dam that she wanted to replicate her in me. Her dejection at my albinism never waned from the moment she discovered me nursing from Dam in the field. She realized right away that she had miscalculated. Not only was my appearance abhorrent, but to Monique and others like her, my albinism was evidence that I was a weaker, flawed specimen.

As constant was her love for Dam, Monique was as uniformly constant in her indifference toward me. Because of Dam's great attachment to me and her sense of purpose in raising me, Monique tolerated me, I believe. After my dam's death, which came sooner than it should have, Monique and I did not replace her with each other, for too much resentment had built up between us. We avoided each other, at best.

As I grazed in solitary confinement, with no horses or people to distract me from my thoughts, I realized I had never before considered the possibility that my dam's death had hardened me, too, as much as it had hardened Monique. Standing alone in my field, the very field where Dam and I were torn apart, I found that what I longed for most was the belonging that I had with Dam and the mares of my field when I was a colt—a belonging that I had not found since. Yet it seemed a prayer that I petitioned too late.

Perhaps I would have been content to stay alone in the field until the new owners completed their work and dispensed with me. Or perhaps I would have gambled all and fled to the blue mountains to start over on my own. The thought of innumerable seasons of fallen leaves whirling under me as I cantered higher and higher up the mountainside was luring me to set out for the forest. Granted, though I had only run through the mountains under saddle, I had always been reliable and resourceful on the trail. The terrain of the blue mountains can be challenging, but I had never lost my footing, even down the narrowest, rockiest cliffs. It would have been a different life to be sure, but I had begun to consider the idea of forging a feral, solitary existence in the blue mountains.

The doorway I had made in the fence line stood open and waiting for me to decide. Though I had spent plenty of time trying desperately to remove my halter, for it cut deeply into my face and I wished it to be off completely, I now began to take heart that the halter had, indeed, been left fastened to me. Halters serve but one purpose—to catch and lead a horse. I had first wondered for what purpose Monique had abandoned me; now I wondered for what purpose she had left me haltered.

One afternoon, as I was again evaluating the option of fleeing to the mountains by way of my hard-earned passage through the barbed wire, Monique herself appeared at the gate and called me to her. I trotted to the gate, demonstrating my eagerness to join with her. Curious, and surprised to see her, I greeted her warmly with a light touch to her chest. I detected a new softness to her, perhaps there all along, perhaps made with grief from the loss of her husband. In days prior, I surely would have objected to my conditions and made known to her my displeasure at the halter having been left so tightly bound to my face. I gave Monique no fight as she hooked the lead rope to my halter. I thought of Dam and her devotion to the woman standing before me and decided that I could start over with Monique, and hoped that Monique could, too.

Monique did not speak to me, so I made the first overture. I nickered long and low into her ear. I blew across her neck with the intent to acknowledge everything we had been through together and also my willingness to begin anew. Monique paused. She sighed deeply and looked around the field, the same field that had once held Dam, the mares, and me when I was a colt. I lifted my head to see more clearly. Was Monique remembering Dam, as was I? The blue mountains encircled the two of us, urging our reconciliation, it seemed to me. I blew on Monique again. I pushed my head into her neck, not hard as if I wanted grain this very instant, but softly, to welcome her home to our field.

I believe now, and will always believe, that for an instant, Monique considered forgiving me as I had just, finally, forgiven her. But the relief that mutual forgiveness brings was not to be. She took me by the halter and pulled my cheek to her face.

"Since when have you nuzzled anybody? Much less me?" She then pushed my head away.

I made no further attempt to reconcile. Monique brushed her hand across her eyes and led me out of the field.

She had arrived with a trailer in tow; I dropped my head and consented to load without a struggle. Unsure whether I was going to Lynchville or someplace I had not considered, I looked toward the blue mountains for what I prayed would not be the last time.

CHAPTER FOUR

My New Home

Despite my failure to fulfill her expectations, our lifetime together had entreated Monique to make an act of kindness on my behalf. She had arranged for one last visit to a local barn in an effort to plead my case. The Maury River Stables, owned by Mrs. Isbell Maiden, was the fifth facility we had visited in our mission to find a proper home for me. I knew as we turned into the drive that this place would soon become my home. While Monique approached Mrs. Maiden, I remained in the trailer, watching the two women from the window.

I had always observed Monique to be taller than the average woman; she had no need of a mounting block.

She always held herself with exceptionally straight posture, which she urged all of her students to emulate. She could not have been credited with exceptional posture on that day. Bent over in defeat and having lost an entire life, Monique made a desperate picture of grief. Wearing dark glasses, and with her head wrapped in a scarf that tied under her chin, she spoke quickly and curtly of the gravity of my situation. The scarf and dark glasses were surely added for dramatic effect, but that is solely one horse's opinion.

Unhesitatingly, Mrs. Maiden agreed to house me, albeit temporarily, with the understanding that Monique would work toward finding a suitable, permanent home elsewhere. I committed myself to expressing only gratitude toward Mrs. Maiden. Even this temporary improvement in my situation, one that allowed me to stay in the blue mountains, was beyond my greatest hope.

Monique didn't seem wholly satisfied with the offer. Rather, she acted quite put upon when Mrs. Maiden suggested that compensation be granted for my food and care, even if only for a portion of it. I overheard Mrs. Maiden tell Monique that she herself had been in the position before of having to rebuild her entire life after a great loss.

"That's why I'm helping you," she impressed upon Monique. "I believe in women helping women."

I maintain that her husband's death and the resulting divestiture of her entire stable and riding school had exhausted Monique entirely of all civility.

"You can drop the women helping women bit," she snarled at Mrs. Maiden. "All of your horses are leftovers like him. Why do you think I brought him here? I've never known you to turn away any horse for any reason."

Upon hearing this, I wondered why we had not started out with the Maury River Stables to begin with, but as we were safely arrived and all seemed to be working out in my favor, I did not make a commotion. I did badly want out of the trailer. Still, I did not kick or snort. I listened to the two women negotiating the terms of my acceptance to the Maury River Stables.

If Mrs. Maiden felt intimidated by Monique, as many people had over the years, she did not show it. Mrs. Maiden reaffirmed her position, "That's true; I love all horses. But I can barely keep the barn running month to month. Anything you could do to offset my costs for keeping Chancey while you get straightened out would help."

Monique acquiesced; she wanted to be done with me. She agreed to send funds when she could, but I believe we all understood that funds would not be forthcoming.

I unloaded agreeably when Mrs. Maiden asked for me. Though I was thankful that Monique's last compassionate act brought me to the Maury River Stables, I had hoped for a warmer good-bye or even some small acknowledgment of our many years together. But my owner had no departing words for me. Mrs. Maiden led me toward the barn as Monique started the truck. I turned back to watch her leave, and stood square as she drove off. Mrs. Maiden waited for Monique's truck to disappear before she inspected me thoroughly.

I gathered that I was sorry-looking when I arrived at the Maury River Stables. I did not request, or expect, the kindness Mrs. Maiden showed me right away by designing a plan to return me to good health. In fact, it was not until Mrs. Maiden's inspection that I was made aware that my health had deteriorated as greatly as it evidently had during my isolated days in Monique's field.

I was first placed in a round pen, where I now understand all new horses are kept for an introductory period of sorts. The day was pleasant enough, though the sun was too bright in my eyes, as I could not escape its glare at all in the round pen. My eyes burned in the full gaze of the sun. By contrast, in my old field I could easily find shelter under my cedar stand, a shadow cast near a hay ring, or even shade thrown off by a tractor to protect my fair eyes and pink skin.

Mrs. Maiden called to a young girl for help. The girl came quickly but kept her eyes cast to the ground as she walked. I judged her to be ten years of age and later was proven correct in that judgment. She was tiny then, and with her dark hair cut short above her ears, looked very much at home in worn overalls and dirty boots. One of her overall flaps was undone and hanging loose from her shoulder. The child didn't seem aware or concerned. I thought I detected a smile when she saw me, but perhaps it was the sun that caused her face to appear brighter.

Mrs. Maiden explained to her, "Claire, this is Chancey. He'll be staying here at the Maury River Stables with us for a while, until he finds a home."

Then Mrs. Maiden instructed me, "Claire is one of my very favorite students, Chancey. I want you to be especially kind to Claire; she's having a bit of a tough time right now."

Claire reached her hand out to me. I nickered at her, hoping she would come closer. She did not come to me, but she did look up to Mrs. Maiden and say simply, "He's b-b-beautiful."

Not one to perpetuate a lie, as I would later learn, Mrs. Maiden said, "Well, he's not beautiful right now. He's a mess. You could make him beautiful, Claire."

Claire did not respond in any way, except to look at Mrs. Maiden and squint her eyes.

Three young girls, obviously just arriving for their riding lesson, strode over to us arm in arm. Claire stepped out of their way. To me they appeared nearly indistinguishable from one another, turned out just exactly as every little barn girl I had ever taught, wearing crisp white shirts, brand-new riding pants, and leather paddock boots. Each of the three wore her hair in a long ponytail. Though I suppose I shall never tire of giggling girls in jodhpurs, I rather preferred the likes of Claire already.

"Hi, Mrs. Maiden," the girls sang in unison. Though the girls looked to be Claire's age, they did not greet Claire, except for the smallest girl, who waved. Claire waved back and smiled.

"Good morning, ladies," Mrs. Maiden boomed. "Go get tacked up quickly. I'll join you in the ring shortly. Stu is up there now with the beginners."

The girls skipped off to the barn with their arms still linked. I continued watching Claire; she showed no interest in joining the trio now preparing to ride.

Claire dropped her head to the ground and quietly said to herself. "Ch-Ch-Chancey's already a gorgeous pony. He d-d-doesn't need me to make him beautiful."

Mrs. Maiden turned her attention from the girls back to Claire. "Oh, but he does, Claire. He does need you. Chancey's been through so much. So much that we could never possibly begin to know, and it's all bottled up inside of him. Look at him. His coat is matted, and his mane is knotted with burrs thicker than my fist." Mrs. Maiden tugged on my forelock and lifted my mane to show Claire its horrendous condition. Then she pointed to my cheek.

"The poor horse's face is cut so badly it's as if someone slashed him with a knife, though I suspect he somehow got tangled up in barbed wire. That's exactly why you should never fence horses in barbed wire — ever! And look at his legs, all swollen and cut, too. Claire, when was the last time you saw a horse this thin? Even with his winter coat, he's nothing but bones. Run and get a bucket of grain; he can eat while we're cleaning him up," she instructed Claire.

Claire returned in an instant. I waited but long enough for Claire to step away from the bucket before I began to consume the grain. How I had missed the taste and texture of sweet feed! I had not forgotten it, but I had beaten my palate into disciplined acceptance of whatever I could forage from the ground. I devoured the grain with such speed that it must have been shocking for Claire to watch.

"Oh, my gosh. He's so hungry, Mrs. Maiden. I'll help him," Claire told her. I stopped licking the residue from the bucket and lifted my head to the girl. She scratched my ear.

"This horse needs a friend like you, someone he can really count on. Chancey needs a girl who will love him for who he is and accept everything he has to offer—then the world will see the horse you see."

Claire stepped closer to me and tentatively reached both arms around my neck. She held me ever so lightly; I felt her eyes close against me.

"Claire," Mrs. Maiden said. "Why don't you ride with the girls today? It's been a while since you've ridden with them."

For barely a second, there was excitement in Claire's voice. "Ride Chancey?"

Mrs. Maiden shook her head. "Not yet. You know he's not ready, don't you?"

Claire nodded, her eyes welling up with tears. Mrs. Maiden squatted down to eye level with the girl. My muscles, the ones with any feeling left, ached deeply. My heart, which had fallen into a very deep sleep over the winter, began to stretch itself awake. I leaned more toward Claire.

Mrs. Maiden put her arms around Claire and pulled her little body in close. Claire wiped her eyes and nose with her hand.

"I want you to listen to me. I know you are hurting right now," Mrs. Maiden said. "Divorce is never easy. I've been there myself and even though it was the right thing, it hurt my two boys badly."

"You have ch-children?" Claire asked.

"Yes, one is grown up now. He lives in Roanoke," Mrs. Maiden explained.

"What about the uh-uh, the other one?" Claire asked.

Mrs. Maiden did not answer right away. Claire did not ask the question again but began picking the mud and rocks out of my feet. Over the years, I have observed that most little girls protest vehemently about cleaning a horse's feet when they are as unsightly as mine were on that day. Claire did the task as if it were only casual work to busy the hands. Not once did she say an unkind word. She had finished with my feet and brushed my entire right side before Mrs. Maiden answered her question.

"My younger boy died when he was thirteen."

Claire placed her hand on Mrs. Maiden's shoulder. "Oh, that's sad," she said.

"Yes, I will always be sad," Mrs. Maiden replied. Then Mrs. Maiden perked up. "You see Daisy over there?"

Claire nodded.

"Daisy was my son's first horse. Boy, were those two a pair; they were inseparable. Here's what I'm trying to tell you, Claire. There comes a day when you have to let go of the pain and let love come back to you. That might just be why Chancey came here, to bring love back to you." She kissed the girl on top of her head and turned back to the business of restoring me.

"Claire, bring me a fly mask from the tack room," Mrs. Maiden said.

"Why?" the girl asked. "The f-flies aren't, aren't out yet."

Mrs. Maiden motioned for Claire to come nearer. "Come here; I'll show you why."

Claire, eager to know why I ought to have to wear a fly mask in March, ran to Mrs. Maiden's side.

"Look at Chancey's eyes," Mrs. Maiden instructed. "What color are they?"

"B-blue," answered Claire, not yet making the connection.

"Yes, they're blue. They're blue, just exactly like yours are blue." It gave me immediate pleasure to know that the girl and I shared something already. Mrs. Maiden continued the lesson. "Now, look at the skin on Chancey's muzzle. What color is it?"

"P-pink!" Claire was enjoying this lesson very much, I could tell.

"Yes, his skin is pink. And his coat is all white, isn't it? These things tell us something about Chancey; he's an albino, or a partial albino, anyway. You'll hear some people say there is no such thing as a true albino horse. Others will say Chancey can't be albino because his eyes are blue, not pink. But none of that matters to us. His eyes are blue, his skin is pink, and that tells us that the sun is harder on him than all of the other horses we know. A fly mask will keep the sun from damaging his eyes any further."

"D-does he have to wear the f-fly mask all the time?" Claire wanted to know.

"While he's with us he will, even on cloudy days, except at night. Run into the tack room now and find him one." Mrs. Maiden dispatched Claire, again, to the tack room. Claire ran off and came straight back with a dusty fly mask, torn at the clasp. She rose to the tip of her toes to adjust the fly mask over my poll. My eyes relaxed. I felt Claire's two hands fasten the fly mask under my neck. She leaned her face into my shoulder and inhaled.

"He smells good," Claire said, while Mrs. Maiden examined me for more cuts and scrapes.

"He smells like a horse, Claire."

Mrs. Maiden didn't look up from behind me. I still felt embarrassed by the condition of my feet, all four cracked and overgrown. Only one shoe remained intact, as I had thrown the others in my effort to widen the hole in Monique's fence.

"I love how horses smell," Claire told her with such pride that I forgot my distress at Mrs. Maiden spending so much time examining every part of me. Claire breathed me in again. Unable to help myself, I inhaled Claire's hair, too. She smelled like a girl.

Mrs. Maiden laughed. "He likes you! Now, grab the currycomb and see if you can get some of this caked mud off of Chancey's other side. Don't rub his face; it's chafed from wearing his halter too tight. And be careful of his legs; they're covered in cuts. We'll tend to his wounds after we clean him up."

I doubted if my great Appaloosa ancestors would have ever wanted to be pampered in this way, but I decided that I quite liked it. Claire did as Mrs. Maiden asked of her, brushing all of me that she could reach and paying special attention to go around my wounds.

"I can't reach all of him. I'm too short," Claire said matter-of-factly, but without complaint.

"Well, then go get a mounting block so you can reach his withers." That was my first indication that Mrs. Maiden doesn't believe in the word *can't*.

The two of them spent an entire morning and most of the afternoon cleaning and bathing me. They soaked my legs in a salt bath of warm water; the moist heat of the water-and-salt combination soothed me. I believe I dozed off with two of my four legs knee-deep in buckets.

Daisy and some of the other mares checked on my progress throughout the day, but no one introduced themselves. I followed the barn protocol set by the mares and stood silently in the round pen enjoying every treatment given me by Mrs. Maiden and Claire.

After the leg soak and a good warm bath, Claire rubbed me down with a towel. The little girl was so serious and devoted to the work of caring for me that I dared not flinch or kick, though her small hands quite tickled. I did flick her with my tail, thinking perhaps she might respond, as flies often do, by at least moving from one place to another. Claire, being a little girl, not a fly, did not move and seemed to delight in the feeling of my tail snapping against her, so I continued.

★ CHAPTER FIVE ★

My True Companion

From the first day of my arrival at the Maury River Stables, Claire came to care for me every day, forgoing her own riding lessons to nurse me. She changed my bandages, gave me fresh water, and convinced Mrs. Maiden to move me into a spare room in the barn, where I would be out of the sun. Not once had Claire brought out any tack—no saddle, bridle, or girth had come anywhere near me. Most girls her age would have lost interest after a day or so, preferring to return to the company of the other girls. Claire—she committed to stay with me for as long as I needed. She sensed that I needed plenty of time to heal. I sensed that Claire needed time, too.

Since our first meeting, Claire had not spoken of her family conflict nor the sorrow that filled her. Only once, in fact, did Claire speak of her father at all.

"I'm sorry you d-didn't get to meet my d-dad today, Ch-Ch-Chancey. He had to go b-b-back to work for a meeting. You'll meet him soon; I p-promise."

I rumbled my contentment at the manner in which Claire was brushing my back.

"He d-d-d-doesn't like horses as much as Mother and I d-do. I th-think because he's a-, he's a-, he's afraid. I d-don't, I d-don't see him that much anymore."

Whenever Claire tripped in her words, it seemed to help if she breathed more deeply and slowed down not her mouth, but her mind. I was glad when she leaned onto me and sighed out a long sigh. I sighed out a long sigh, too. I rumbled again. Claire set the brush down, and we leaned and sighed until Claire was breathing evenly.

Had Claire's wound been open to the bone, as was the one she was so gently tending on my leg, I don't know that it could have been any deeper. Yet Claire's wound could not be seen. I was moved to befriend Claire for as long as she needed.

We stood together in my room through the early days of spring, watching as the redbud and dogwood, barren among the cedar and pine all winter, once again bloomed, reminding us both why we loved the blue mountains so in springtime. During our time together, while Claire gazed out of my window and into the blue mountains, I began to think of my dam.

Having lost her so early in life had impacted me severely. Not only did my heart suffer, but I lost my protector. Dam admired my lack of pigment, and it hurt her deeply to see Monique reject me. I was gelded hastily to ensure that my albinism could not further dilute the Appaloosa breed. I clung to my dam and at her death, withdrew into myself. Monique could have sold me then, but I believe we were both clinging to Dam, each in our own way.

My reflective afternoons with Claire stirred in me long-dormant memories. I remembered standing close to Dam's barrel, grazing between her feet. She would push her nose under my neck to invite me to try clover or dandelions. In this same way, she steered me from the buttercup patches in our field that grew despite Monique's effort to keep them down.

While Claire applied a healing salve to my cuts and scrapes, I wrapped my neck around her and ever so lightly touched my nose to her chest. She smiled. Then the sadness clouded her face again, and she resumed her care for me.

I repeated this action of reaching out to Claire, each time softly touching her chest with my nose. Every time, it worked. The touching of my nose to her made the smile appear, and I could feel her breath release. I moved closer to her and leaned gently against her shoulder with my neck draped around her neck. She laughed.

Claire leaned backward into me, and we stood together for such a time that I was greatly content never to move. Claire brought her hand to my cheek. "You're a good, good pony." She did not trip in her words.

Claire reached down for the currycomb; I mimicked my dam's action and pushed my nose under Claire's arm, telling her that I preferred to play. Claire laughed. She reached for the hoof pick, and again I dissuaded her, as my dam had once dissuaded me from poisonous plants. Claire laughed again. I observed that when she laughed, her face held that joy only briefly. Always the grief returned, pulling Claire back into its well.

I touched her neck with my head and the joy returned, this time in a smile. I continued with this pattern until I had proven it true that Claire's bereavement could be healed with a regular, steady application of healing touch. I resolved that during our time together, I would apply frequent doses of touch in an effort to repel the sorrow and keep her spirit elastic and soft. I would recall how my dam had nuzzled me and repeat the same with Claire by wrapping my neck around hers and blowing into her nose. Always we stood this way in my room, rain or shine.

Claire preferred, I think, to talk to me of happy things, for then she did not fall in her speech. She told me of her dream of one day becoming a teacher. I nickered my approval, for I could tell that Claire's kindness and enthusiasm would serve her well in that occupation. I wished that I had been given a bit more of both kindness and enthusiasm myself. Claire described for me how she was learning to make music with a violin. She promised to play for me one day. I listened to all she had to say.

As is the case with true companions, Claire did not speak only of herself. Claire was interested in me. She asked me about life at Monique's. She inquired about my dam and wondered how I was feeling about my new home. We continued in this way of grooming and listening, but not working, each afternoon for quite some time.

Most days, Claire's mother drove her out to the barn after school just so Claire and I could spend an hour or two with each other. Claire's mother welcomed me warmly at our first meeting. "Chancey," she asked me, "are you the pony who has stolen my little girl's heart?

"Well, I'm Claire's mother." She kissed me on the soft spot between my ear and poll. She did not give her own name, and as I had only heard her referred to as "Claire's mother" by Mrs. Maiden or "Mother" by Claire herself, I simply considered her to be "Mother," as did Claire.

The two of them quickly made up for all that I had ever longed for in my life. Mrs. Maiden accused them of spoiling me, for Claire and Mother brought me not only carrots and apples but also oatmeal cookies saved from Claire's lunch at school.

"Listen, Claire!" Mrs. Maiden once reprimanded. "You don't need to feed Chancey all the time."

Claire drew her hand down the side of my body. "But Mrs. Maiden, his ribs are st-st-still showing. Ch-Chancey needs to put some weight back on, doesn't he? I'll stop giving him t-treats when he's healthy again. Okay?" Mrs. Maiden retreated and did not again scold Claire for spoiling me. After that, my treats improved in both quantity and quality.

Claire talked Mother into buying me a most satisfying treat called stud biscuits, which aren't really biscuits at all, nor am I a stud. The little balls of molasses, barley, oats, and I believe a bit of corn, too, were pure decadence for a horse who had subsisted on grass and water for entirely too long.

Mother seemed infinitely content to watch Claire

with me. She often brought a book to read or a writing tablet to occupy her time while she waited. Mother always sat some distance away, taking up neither book nor pen, but watching us. I watched Mother, too, keeping one ear always on Claire and the other turned toward Mother. Claire noticed my curiosity and confided in me, "Mother had a bad horse accident last year. She's kind of afraid now, Chancey. Don't worry, though; she'll fall in love with you, too. You'll see."

I had only a moment to wonder if the petition I had uttered in my old field, only a few weeks before, might actually have just been answered.

Claire threw her arms around me. "Oh, Chancey, I love you! I think you have come here just for me, just like Mrs. Maiden said. You're the most beautiful pony I have ever known."

Had words been available to me, I would not have corrected her that by nearly a hand I am, indeed, considered to be a horse, not a pony. The girl's heart pressed full into mine and for just an instant I felt as beautiful as I was bred to be.

Claire's sweet hand touched the raw marks on my cheek that had been cut into my face by my halter. In that instant, I remembered how ragged I had become. I supposed I had long ago earned my reputation for being hard to catch without a halter. In my alone days at Monique's, my halter had been left on me much too tightly. Had it been loosened by just a notch, preferably two or even better by three, I should not have minded its constant presence on my face. After a while, my cheeks had begun to sting, far worse than the sting of a horsefly or bee. When I had tried to break free of the halter by rubbing my face against the cedar posts and low tree branches, I expect the rubbing also contributed to the rough shape of my face.

Again Claire touched the worst of the injuries on my cheek. "How could anyone leave such a beautiful pony all alone?" she asked. Claire kissed my wound. I felt evermore aware of my condition and ashamed of how pitiful I must have appeared to Claire. Not knowing quite what to do in this situation, I pulled my neck out of Claire's hold and turned my back to her. In this second, I realized how many times in my life I had simply turned away when I felt afraid or confused.

I wished that I could be so much more for this girl—more like Dam, even more like my younger self. How could I let Claire become attached to an old, broken gelding like me? I walked to the corner of my room. I thought surely she would know that my action was meant to separate us until I was again ready for companionship. Even the most inexperienced rider knows that a swift about-face is the clearest form of communication available to a horse. Most people would have understood my gesture to mean, "Leave me alone."

I felt obligated to warn Claire of all that she could not yet see. I had often been noticed, but never mistaken for beautiful. Though my pupils studied under me for months, sometimes years, I was never loved as a child's favorite. I had known horses and people, too many to count. Yet I had never saved a life of human nor beast. I had taught many girls and boys, but never did I carry a champion on my back.

In all my days at Monique's as a school horse, I was a reliable worker but had a reputation of being difficult, even mean. Because my physical body looked so unlike the rest of my band and so unlike my mother, and because my albinism determined me a weaker individual, I was considered even worse than merely common.

And so I turned away from Claire now. I was not expelling her from my space nor my heart, but faced with my own feelings of embarrassment, I needed to escape from *me*. I turned away from everything that came with me to the Maury River Stables and from everything it would mean for me to leave the old Chancey behind.

When I turned from Claire, she did the same to me. Claire walked slowly to the opposite side of my room and, wedging herself as far into the corner as she could, said quietly, "Ch-Ch-Chancey, I thought we were f-f-friends."

Characteristically, as I would learn over time, Claire didn't give up or walk away. My ugliness—in both manner and physical state—had not scared off Claire. On the contrary, Claire had challenged me and decided to love me for everything she could see in me.

"Ch-Ch-Chancey." She called my name again. "I'm n-not going anywhere. We're supposed to be together. You're my only real f-friend here."

I did not move. I stood there in my new room, very much wanting to call out to Claire with my heart, yet unable to do so. I felt Claire approaching on my left side; she squeezed between me and the wall, fully certain that I would not harm her. Most people know that this can be a dangerous predicament; I've seen many get pinned this way, both mistakenly and with intent. I did not pin Claire, of course. Instead, I moved off the wall to give her space. Though I was unable, at that time, to recognize how much I needed to depend on someone, Claire recognized it for me.

"Ch-Chancey," she said. "Mrs. Maiden said for me to let love come b-b-b-back; that goes for you too, p-pony." Then Claire embraced me and whispered, "Don't worry. I will n-never leave you."

Age and experience had taught me by then that "never" is a word often wielded, seldom honored, by little girls. While I was, and still am, certain that the day will come when Claire in fact will leave me, her abiding devotion to me thawed me just enough. I reached my head to her chest, pressed her lightly, and closed my eyes. Claire kissed my cheek again, in the same ugly spot that previously had driven me to retreat from my shortcomings and from her. This time I did not turn away; I held my head to her heart and sighed a long sigh. Claire did the same. I decided that perhaps Mrs. Maiden was right: perhaps it was time to let love come back to me.

✳ CHAPTER SIX ✳
The Maury River Band

My days at the Maury River Stables settled into a familiar routine, not altogether unlike the way in which I had lived at Monique's. On the surface, all seemed very much like the school horse's life to which I had become accustomed. My mornings were devoted to eating and learning about my new home. The afternoons were reserved for Claire. And my nighttime hours allowed me time to reflect on each day. Aware that I had been given an extraordinary opportunity to start over late in my life, I was determined to belong, in a way that I had not at Monique's.

At Monique's, I had been unable to overcome my dam's death. That loss grew, over time, into a resentfulness that would not loosen its grip. While Dam was alive, I had lived happily among the mares. The mares knew of Monique's disappointment at my albinism, and they colluded with Dam to shield me from her rejection. As a colt, I felt protected by all of them. Had I remained with the mares, perhaps I would have found my way after all, for the mares loved me. I did not understand how different I really was until after Dam's death, when I was taken from the mares and placed with the band of geldings.

None of the geldings at Monique's were inclined to protect me. They considered my introduction into their field a direct threat and used all available means to make it clear that my place with them was at the bottom. There I remained for my entire life.

I began my new life at the Maury River Stables on the bottom as well. I had no ambition to secure the top spot in my new home; nor did I wish to live as an outcast any longer. I resolved to find my own place as a member of this band of horses.

I observed that the Maury River Stables was a small operation, with only twenty horses, as opposed to the fifty or so at Monique's. I found the facility adequate, providing everything necessary to enjoy a good quality of life. There was one large, simply built barn, which encircled a small indoor riding ring. Six rooms lined each side of the barn; every room, though small, offered a splendid view of the blue mountains. Saddle Mountain could be seen from the window in my room, for which I was grateful. There was also an indoor wash stall, a cross-tie stall for grooming and shodding, and a tack room. Plenty of barn swallows made their home inside the barn, which Monique would never have allowed. I rather liked the presence of swallows and found their acrobatic performances mesmerizing to watch, especially on days when I was forced to remain indoors.

Outdoors, as at Monique's, all the horses were divided into fields by their gender. The social complexities of geldings and mares are too burdensome for most people to manage successfully, and thus we are more easily managed if segregated. Each field had its own hierarchy of order, and the reasoning behind segregating new horses upon their arrival was to slowly allow the others to acclimate to the idea of opening up to include a newcomer. Right away, I learned that because it was small and tight-knit, the Maury River Stables was a tough band to join, especially for an older horse.

Claire, Mother, and Mrs. Maiden had welcomed me with such enthusiasm that it seemed as if they had been expecting my arrival. Among the horses I encountered some resistance, for all newcomers must endure a period of testing before some place is made. As the mare and gelding fields shared a fence, it was easy enough for the mares to pester me, and they all did, save an old Hanoverian by the name of Gwen, who appeared nearer my age than the other mares. A striking blood bay, Gwen possessed the athletic conditioning of a Thoroughbred and the imposing stature of a draft horse. I thought she represented the warmblood breeds quite regally. Though I could tell that her position with the mares was not what it once was, Gwen still maintained a strong presence among them.

The mares did not introduce themselves, but repeatedly commented, within earshot, on my wretched condition. No doubt they knew that I could hear them, and though they never addressed me directly, I understood that their insults were intended to discourage me. "Look at him; you can see his ribs." Daisy curled her lip as if my smell repulsed her, too. "Why is Mrs. Maiden bothering with him anyway? Horses like him never win at hunter shows or horse trials, and who wants an Appaloosa without spots?"

I find that Welsh cobs, like Daisy, especially the flea-bitten ones, are particularly disdainful of my breed.

A petite Arab, whose name I learned was appropriately Princess, chimed right in with Daisy. "Daisy, you give him much too much credit. He's not a horse. He's a pony, and an ugly one at that!"

"What could Claire possibly see in him?" Daisy asked. She threw her head high in the air.

The gentle Hanoverian swiftly came to my defense. Though I suspected, quite accurately I would later discover, that Gwen had lost her high placement in the mare field to Daisy some years ago, she still carried a great deal of influence with all of the mares, including Daisy.

Gwen wasted no time scolding Daisy. "Princess, I would never expect you to understand. But Daisy, I'm surprised at you. Haven't you been paying attention to Mrs. Maiden? Chancey's been brought here for a reason. Could it be that you're a bit jealous because Claire is spending all her time with Chancey and not you? God made a horse for everyone, and mark my words, Chancey and Claire have found each other, and not by accident. Now, both of you go about your business and leave the old App alone."

Gwen's rebuke quieted Daisy and Princess, but not before Daisy got in a good air kick at Gwen's barrel, obviously missing the old mare on purpose. With a soft nicker, I offered my thanks to Gwen and hoped that her intervention in my defense would bring no injury upon her from the mares.

Princess did not let pass the offense that had been directed at her, however. She grabbed Gwen by the neck and bit the Hanoverian with an unbridled wrath;

Gwen did not squeal, as most would have. She tore herself away from Princess and tore a slice of her own neck off in the process. Daisy pushed Princess into the corner of the fence. Princess had minutes earlier been Daisy's sidekick, but she had overstepped by punishing Gwen without Daisy's authorization. Princess pleaded with the Welsh, "Please, Daisy, no."

Daisy's ears lay flat against her head. I could tell, as could Princess I'm sure, that a severe punishment was about to be handed down. Daisy snorted and kicked until Princess walked farther into the corner. Now docile, Princess once more begged Daisy's forgiveness, for she knew what was coming.

"Please, I'm sorry. I didn't mean to step out."

Daisy paid her no mind; she was making a point to all of us who were watching about just who exactly remained in charge of the mare field. The transgression was serious. Either Princess would take her punishment or challenge Daisy for the field.

Daisy lined Princess up against the fence and delivered a series of rapid-fire kicks to the Arab's belly. She did not stop when Princess began squealing. She did not stop when Princess began bleeding and would not have stopped except that Claire ran out into the mare field crying for Daisy to leave Princess alone. Daisy pinned her ears at Princess, showed all of her teeth, and chased Princess away.

I'll not deceive myself by asserting that geldings are any easier to join with than mares, for they are not. The rules have been much the same in whatever pasture I have ever been placed, though, granted, the new situations that I've found myself in have been few. Regardless, all horses know the rules well.

In the gelding field, I assumed my proper position and challenged no one for a higher spot. Mealtimes presented an excellent opportunity for me to establish that I posed no threat to the status quo. At first, I did not approach the hay ring at all, but waited for the others to finish eating, then gleaned what I could. Under normal circumstances, I would have expected to lose weight right away by forgoing hay, but as I had arrived at the Maury River Stables several hundred pounds underweight, the small amount of hay I was denied did not contribute to further weight loss. In fact, I began gaining weight straight away due to the reintroduction of grain to my daily intake. I stayed away from the hay ring for as many days as necessary to establish my deference to all in the field. I was particularly mindful of the homage due to Dante, the black Thoroughbred in charge of my field.

Many benefits are afforded to the top horse. The field is yours, so you have first choice as to where you will stand, graze, and sleep as well as who you will run with. The boss is the first to be fed, can eat as much as he wants, is the first to come into the barn, and so on. I knew I did not have the strength or desire to challenge Dante or even the short, fat Shetland pony, Napoleon, for a higher field placement. Thus I stayed back at feeding time, allowing Dante to have first rights to hay placed in the ring for all of us. After a good period of showing deference and respect in our field, I finally made a friend in Macadoo.

Despite his intimidating size, Mac is the most trusted and beloved of all the horses at the Maury River Stables. Mac is a purebred Belgian draft, a blond sorrel to be exact. Except for a missing piece of his right ear, a slight flaw to be sure, Mac is a near-perfect example of a Belgian. The Belgians are prized for their considerable height and girth. Indicative of his gentle nature, Mac, who weighed close to two thousand pounds, allowed Claire, who weighed all of seventy pounds, to effortlessly navigate him. Claire liked to call Mac her "big boy." At nearly eighteen hands high, Mac more resembled a tractor than a boy.

Mac towered over Dante and could have, if he were of such a mind, brought Dante down with but a series well-placed kicks, such as Daisy had delivered to Princess. Mac is frightfully intimidating and he sounds so as well, before you come to know him. At the canter, the ground quakes beneath his feet. I have observed his approach to cause people and horses to flee, for fear of getting trampled. Once you have been blessed to know and understand Mac's nature, the sound of his joyful hooves galloping toward you more likely impels you to greet him with equal delight. Indeed, Mac is generous in spirit and eager to be of service to all in need. So gentle and calm is Mac that he is the lead horse in Mrs. Maiden's therapeutic riding school. Mac's friendship eased my transition into the Maury River Stables.

I came to enjoy my breakfast in the field each morning alongside Mac. Mac took his grain beside me, and usually by the time we had finished our grain, fresh hay had been set out in the hay ring by either Mrs. Maiden or her barn manager, Stu. My friend Mac saw to it each day to kick out more than enough hay for me.

In fact, Mac's gesture of friendship was the only reason I was able to eat in peace. Without Mac distracting Dante in the field each morning, I might never have been allowed any hay at all. Just by puffing out his chest and pinning back his ears, Mac would signal to Dante that his throne was in jeopardy. The two would race around the field while I, unnoticed, ate hay to my fill. Once I had wandered off to the back of the field, Mac would retreat, and Dante would claim victory over yet another plot to overthrow him. Such generosity typifies the Belgian Macadoo. He eased the hazing I received from the mares and geldings.

Mrs. Maiden and Stu would bring us in each night.

In our rooms, we would not sleep, but remained awake and listening to Dante kick the walls until even he could not stand his own company. I was happy that my room was next to Mac's, though I would have preferred not to be also next to Dante. Thankfully, Dante did not kick our shared wall for very long before I deployed one of my finest strategies to deflect his obnoxious habit. Though being the lowliest member of the Maury River Band did not carry many benefits, I had by that time learned a thing or two from my many years on the bottom at Monique's farm.

At Monique's there had been a malevolent top horse—a chestnut Thoroughbred—who earned all chestnuts the right to be called trouble. He tortured me day and night. I sustained kicks all over my body; he gashed me with his shoes and bit me on the neck. At every opportunity the horse terrorized me. More than once, I found myself cornered by him, unable to do anything but wait for the impact as he landed kick after kick to my barrel, all for the offense of eating from the hay ring before he had finished.

At first, I ran from him anytime I saw him coming. I hid behind trees so he would not see me. Nothing worked; the chestnut boss was determined to put me down and keep me there. I decided to try something different. I began leaving a nice trail of grain along the top rail of the adjoining wall between our rooms every night. Soon, the chestnut stopped attacking me so violently, and he made sure the other geldings didn't hurt me. Predictably this technique worked even better with Dante, and he soon stopped kicking my wall, which made it more comfortable for me at night.

Nighttime at the Maury River Stables was the hardest for me during the remaining cold nights of spring. In the blue mountains, waking to a snow cover as winter gives up to spring is not at all uncommon. Mrs. Maiden kept the barn completely closed during the coldest nights, and though I appreciated the shelter and protection offered me there, I would have preferred to stay outside. In the barn, even my window was barred shut, obstructing my view of the stars resting above Saddle Mountain. Unlike those horses with thin coats, like the Hanoverian Gwen, I thicken right up in the winter and have no need of a blanket. An indoor room is not a necessity for the Appaloosa breed. I enjoy the night very much, and if it weren't for the pain in my haunches, I should prefer staying turned out in my field on all but the very coldest nights. Even then, I would rather my window remain open for me to see the moon, the stars, and my mountains.

CHAPTER SEVEN

A Mother's Intercession

S ince my arrival, I had hoped that the Maury River
Stables would become more than a stopover for me.
As my stay extended into the spring, I believed it would
unfold that the Maury River Stables would in fact
become my new home. Exactly how this would come to
pass, I had not imagined. I knew that Mrs. Maiden and
Monique had agreed that Mrs. Maiden would serve
as the agent of my sale to a new owner, when the time
came. I saw no sign of any effort, on Mrs. Maiden's part,
to bring prospective buyers to observe me. I assumed
that the campaign to find me a new home would begin
when I was again in good health and back under saddle.

Almost every day, Claire tended to me, and I could feel all my wounds healing up nicely. Claire reported aloud on my progress during her daily examination. "Chancey," she would confirm, "I can barely see the cuts on your front legs now. And your coat has nearly grown over the chafing on your face." She continued brushing me, as was our usual routine. Though we had not yet worked together in the ring, I felt it would not be too much longer before I was ready.

Claire was ready, too.

On the first warm day of spring, she arrived to greet me wearing brand-new jodhpurs instead of her usual torn overalls. She also brought a brand-new halter and lead rope to my room. I was quite pleased to hear her say that she had picked out these new accessories especially for me. "Purple is going to be your color, Chancey. Purple is the color of kings and queens, you know. You'll be the most beautiful pony at the Maury River Stables," she bragged.

I allowed Claire to slip the halter over my face. She buckled it loosely around my cheek and clipped on the lead rope. Claire remembered to fasten my fly mask over the halter to protect my eyes. I nickered my thanks to her, for it was only while wearing the fly mask that I felt some relief from the burning sensation in my eyes.

With my new halter and lead rope, and a fine companion guiding me, I was paraded all around the Maury

River Stables. Claire permitted me to eat grass and clover wherever I liked and did not seem to be in any hurry. I grazed alongside Claire for much of the afternoon. Everywhere around us, people and animals welcomed the sunshine, knowing from years past that the Maury River would soon be calling us for a swim, with Saddle Mountain beckoning us to its peaks.

Our pastures overflowed with birds and insects who arrived all at once from the mountain forest, busy in preparation for the day when springtime would truly settle in, bringing with it more daylight and encouragement to stay outdoors. The juncos had gone, and in their place bluebirds now hopped around, collecting horsehair from the ground, then flying off home with sturdy nesting material. As is so often the case, the first days of spring teased that they intended to stay. We all knew better but gave in just the same.

The sun had warmed us enough that everyone felt frisky. Daisy and Princess raced each other around the mare field. Gwen took advantage of their playtime to eat her fill at the mares' hay ring. Daisy wised to Gwen eventually and made sure to dash off a few air kicks as she brushed passed the blood bay. Gwen responded as do all of us living at the bottom: she backed away from the hay as Daisy requested.

Claire and I did not enter the mare field or the gelding field, but rather kept outside the fence line, thus giving the mares another opportunity to taunt me. I didn't mind, for I was with Claire. The new halter and lead rope, and undoubtedly my being accompanied, aroused the mares' curiosity but not their scorn, this time.

Led by Daisy, they all clamored to inspect me. "Come see the old App!" called Daisy. "Get a look at Chancey in his new halter!" Then, for the first time since my arrival at the Maury River Stables, Daisy turned directly to me.

"Well, you sure have changed since you've met Claire. If you're going to stick around, we might at least introduce ourselves. I'm Daisy, as you must already know; I'm the most adored and respected mare here. If you have any business with any of my mares, you come to me first. That includes Gwen. Understand?"

I marveled at the change in Daisy's demeanor toward me, no doubt brought on by my new look. I decided that I very much liked my new halter and agreed with Claire that this purple should be my official color. I also decided that having had some experience with bossy mares over the years, I would give Daisy the respect that she had earned as the top mare. I simply replied, "Yes, ma'am. It's nice to meet you." I tossed my head at Gwen, who had come nearer the fence, though she still hung well behind Daisy.

Daisy had not dismissed me yet. "One more thing,

Chancey, just so you're perfectly clear. Claire's one of my girls, so don't do anything foolish."

Before I could respond, Daisy spun around and kicked her back feet out, stirring up a bit of dust but nothing more bothersome. The mare cantered away.

Claire called out to her, "Daisy, how rude! You must have a crush on Chancey!"

I whinnied across the fence after Daisy, playing along with Claire, who bent backward in a fit of laughter. Again, I whinnied after Daisy, for I liked to see Claire laugh.

Claire's presence most definitely shifted the balance of power, and so as we walked the outside perimeter of the mare field, Gwen walked with us on her side of the fence. Though neither of us ventured to openly defy Daisy, it was pleasant to graze with the Hanoverian and exchange a breath or two. Claire teased me even more after that. "Chancey, I think purple really is your color; all the ladies are interested in you today." As Claire and I continued our walk around the paddock, we drew attention not only from horses but from barn mothers, too.

"Claire, I like your new riding pants. I almost didn't recognize you without your overalls," someone called to her.

Claire did not shrink away or fall over her words; she instead stood taller and beamed. "Well, look at Chancey. Isn't he the beautiful one?"

Everyone did notice my new accessories and the purple contrasting against my white coat. "Look at you, Chancey! What a pretty pony you are in purple!" cried a barn mother who had only weeks before pronounced me depressed. In truth, the opinion of only one of the barn mothers, Claire's, mattered at all to me, and she was not among those passing judgment.

Very early one morning, Mother came out to the barn alone. She did not bring her books, nor her writing tablet. When Mrs. Maiden accompanied Mother to my room, I deduced from their conversation that Claire was spending the day in school. The two women began discussing Mother's desire to purchase me as Claire's first horse. I dared not show my excitement for fear that the greatest wish of my heart might evaporate if acknowledged too soon.

Mother sought Mrs. Maiden's opinion on the wisdom of such a purchase. I detected from the conversation that Claire was unaware of this possibility. I fully understood that Mrs. Maiden was duty bound to help Mother consider all it would mean to bring me into her family. Thus, it did not upset me when the two women inspected me in my room without Claire present.

They stood at my head, one on each side of my neck. I could see Mother best, for she stood to my right. Mrs. Maiden kept her hand on my left cheek, never lifting it, and thus assuring me of her location at all times.

Mrs. Maiden lowered her voice and confided her concern to Mother. "I want you to look at his eyes, because what I see looks like something we'll be dealing with for a long time to come. If you do buy him, you need to know that because he's older, and because of his coloring, he comes with more health problems."

Mother didn't speak; she listened to Mrs. Maiden with her head lowered. She then placed her hand on my neck with a manner of sensitivity I had not expected from her.

"Look at this. When I move my hand across his left eye, I get almost no response. I think he's going blind in this eye," Mrs. Maiden told Mother.

Mother kept contact with me through the entire lecture given by Mrs. Maiden. For it was a lecture — one on my current and future needs should I come now under Mother's protection.

Mrs. Maiden spoke truthfully. This was the other aspect of my condition that I had tried to keep hidden, even from myself, for so long. My sight had been slowly vanishing from my left eye for some time and, to a much lesser degree, also my right. I did not know why it was so. Nor did I know what, if anything, could be done to stop further loss, or perhaps restore my eyesight.

This loss of vision impeded my work and even my very movement. Over recent years, I had learned to compensate for the low vision by going slowly or even refusing to go at all if I had no trust that the rider on my back was skilled enough to keep us both out of trouble.

It was never a lack of desire that caused me to refuse. Most of the time, with enough leg and a few light taps with a crop, I would walk or trot on if asked. Jumping was another matter. Depending on how my rider had positioned my head, I often could not see the jump at all until I came right upon it. Rather than risk injury to myself or a young, untrained girl, I refused, or, more accurately, I ducked out. I was relieved that Mrs. Maiden observed and named what was happening to me. The fear of losing my eyesight had now been my companion for many years.

She suggested to Mother, "We'll need to get a vet out here to run some tests. To me, it looks like he has some kind of growth in both eyes. You can see here in his left eye; the growth has moved well onto his cornea. I noticed it the first day that Monique brought him here. That's why he needs to wear a fly mask all the time, especially in the sun. He's so fair; the sun can really damage his skin and his eyes. I don't know what the growth is, but we need to find out. This might be something serious; if so, you'll want to know before you buy him."

Mother was not dissuaded nor did she seem greatly concerned. I didn't detect, in her manner, voice, or words, any inkling that she might reconsider. In fact, once she spoke, all anxiety I may have had about not joining with Claire vanished.

Mother touched Mrs. Maiden's shoulder. "Thank you, Isbell, for taking the time to point this out to me. When you say this might be something serious, might you mean cancer?"

I did not hear Mrs. Maiden's answer, though I felt an unspoken affirmation pass between the two women.

Mother was not deterred. "I know you're right that there are tests—X-rays and such—that I ought to order before I buy Chancey—"

"That's right," interrupted Mrs. Maiden. "There's a reason for those tests. You don't want to buy a horse that's lame or terminally ill, or in any way unsound."

Often, Mother pauses for so long in her speech pattern that others become uncomfortable and speak their own piece before she has finished speaking. Mother seems aware of her awkward cadence, and I have never observed her to rush herself or stop others from talking over her.

Mother waited for Mrs. Maiden to finish and then continued, still speaking slowly and thoughtfully. "Of course, you're right. But you know and I know that Claire and Chancey have found each other because they need each other. You're the one who brought them together! Even if Claire never gets to ride him—if all she does is come here and groom him—that's fine by me.

I mean, Isbell, Claire has all but stopped stuttering—have you noticed that? She still stutters when she's really nervous, but she's so much more confident and relaxed with Chancey. Besides, what will happen to Chancey if we don't buy him?"

"I don't know. I—"

This time, it was Mother who interrupted. "Yes, you do. You and I both know the answer to that question. Here's how I look at it: the worst case is that we buy Chancey and he turns out to have health problems that are impossible to treat and we keep him comfortable until we have to put him down. Is that the worst?"

Mother did not flinch, as I did, at her statement. I have known only one horse who was put down, for a severely broken shoulder. At the time I did not understand that compassion drove that act. I know better now. I understand that a life of extreme, constant pain and forced restriction of movement is no life for a horse. Still, I preferred not to think of being put down.

"Yes, I suppose that's the worst. You have to consider how heartbreaking that would be for Claire," said Mrs. Maiden. But Mother had already considered all that needed consideration.

"Again, Isbell, the way I see it," she repeated, "buying any horse will lead to heartbreak for Claire sooner or later. Whether she loses Chancey to cancer in six months or old age in twenty more years, it will break her heart.

Besides, you've seen Chancey with Claire; he's got a lot of life left in him. Don't you agree?" Mother leaned into me and brushed her face against my neck.

"Smell him," she invited Mrs. Maiden. "He smells so good." Mother breathed in a long inhale.

Mrs. Maiden laughed. "I'm not going to smell him, Eleanor! You're just like Claire! She always smells him. 'Sakes, he smells like a horse!"

Upon hearing Mrs. Maiden call her "Eleanor," I considered whether I ought to refer to Mother this way myself. She was not, after all, my mother and she did have a perfectly suitable name for a woman with equal measure of strength and grace. She leaned into me and kissed me in what was becoming her customary kissing spot, near my poll. She breathed me in again.

"Chancey doesn't smell like just any old horse. He smells like our horse," she said. I dismissed the notion of calling her "Eleanor." "Mother" it would be.

Horses can detect truth easily because truth is conveyed with not only words, but also with body and heart. Though admittedly, I had not a heart connection with Mother, as I'd had with Claire from the very instant of our meeting, I never doubted that Mother could, herself, see that Claire and I were our very best selves together. Though no money or paper had changed hands, without further inspection or deliberation, I joined with Mother and Claire.

⋆ CHAPTER EIGHT ⋆
A Fine First Horse

Mrs. Maiden negotiated my permanent transfer. For some amount unknown to me, the right to call me personal property passed from Monique to Mother. While the papers bound me to Mother officially, it was Claire to whom I now belonged. Neither Claire, nor I, needed a piece of paper or monetary exchange to seal our commitment.

Early one morning, Mother came out to the barn and brought me in from the field without Claire being present. For once, I welcomed the chance to spend the morning in the barn. Our pasture had so trapped the moisture rising off the Maury River that the day already felt very much like the sticky days of summer to come. Flies of every sort and size had turned out in grand numbers to celebrate the return of their kind of weather.

In order to best understand my conditions and needs, Mother had arranged for a collection of professionals to assess my health. Mother and Mrs. Maiden accompanied the experts, with Mother taking copious notes during each examination.

My day began with the dentist, who examined my teeth and then gave no more an exact accounting of my age than I could have determined myself. The dentist explained to Mother that my teeth showed greater depth than width, a triangular shape, and spacing in between. He deduced from these findings what I already knew — that my age was reliably between twenty and twenty-five years, give or take.

"I'd estimate he's about twenty-two," the dentist told Mother.

With that assessment, my official age became twenty-two. Finding no trouble with my teeth, other than their having grown a bit too long, the dentist left for his next appointment with a promise to return soon and give me a proper teeth floating.

I next stood for the veterinarian, whose exam took quite a bit longer than the dentist's. I very much liked the manner of the young doctor. He appeared to have a genuine affection for horses and took several minutes to speak to me before beginning his examination. I learned from Mrs. Maiden that his name was Russ, and his family had kept horses for his entire life. I thought to myself that it must have taken an awfully large horse to comfortably carry a man of such girth and height. I suspected that even as a boy he would have been most at home atop a broad draft horse, such as my new friend Mac.

Doctor Russ's first order of business was to measure me from ground to withers. I recall this precisely because by this time into my residence at the Maury River Stables everyone but Mrs. Maiden had grown accustomed to calling me a pony. Doctor Russ measured me twice and spoke my height out loud, for all to hear. "About fifteen hands," he determined, and made a written note on his clipboard. As the line between pony and horse is drawn at fourteen hands two inches, I was happy to hear that all could now definitely put the matter to rest.

Doctor Russ was pleased with my weight and overall health. He patted my neck. "All right, Chancey. Way to hang tough, boy." He turned to Mother. "Everything this guy's been through? Being abandoned with no supply of food or water all through the fall and winter? I think his weight is fine. He's remarkable—extraordinary, really. But that's an Appy for you, right, Chancey?" He patted me again.

I decided that I liked the intelligent Doctor Russ very much. He seemed a good measurer of horses and quite educated in the distinctive biology of the breeds. The doctor encouraged Mother and Mrs. Maiden to continue generous portions of feed, with the addition of electrolytes to encourage me to drink water.

The constant pain in my haunches and stifles was easy enough for Doctor Russ to diagnose. Without much effort at all—just by feeling me and lunging me through my gaits early in the morning—he gave my pain a name: arthritis. He did not seem concerned that this disease presented any imminent danger, but he gave Mother specific instructions as to its proper management. He told her that I was to be stretched and thoroughly warmed up before riding. Doctor Russ also explained to Mrs. Maiden that for pain treatment I would need a daily supplement added to my grain and a stronger medicine on the days when the pain seemed most severe. The matter of my eyes was determined to be somewhat more complicated, and much more serious.

Mrs. Maiden showed Doctor Russ the growths that she had noticed on my first day at the Maury River Stables. He nodded to her as if he had already intended to tackle this problem. I remained quiet and cooperative. The vision in my left eye had decreased to near blindness; I still could detect some movements, but only from changes in light and dark. I could feel the blindness reach also for my right eye, though not nearly to the same degree as had already occurred in my left.

Doctor Russ explained that he preferred to draw tissue samples to determine the nature of the growths. Mother consented for the doctor to take his samples immediately. I did not move. He proceeded to apply a numbing agent in both eyes, so that I would feel nothing when he inserted his needles. Drawing upon my Appaloosa genetics, I calmly accepted the discomfort, for I knew that no one around me wished me any harm. Doctor Russ removed a stick from his bag and then disappeared into my blindness. Though I could not see him or feel the stick, his presence so near my eye did agitate me.

Mother detected that my anxiety was growing. To her credit, she stayed by my side throughout each step of testing. Had she not been aware of my apprehension, from her own intuition, my involuntary and violent expulsion of loose stool provided evidence aplenty. Involuntary expulsion is a natural tendency for horses in a heightened state of worry.

The compassionate Doctor Russ did not linger a moment longer than necessary. He swabbed both of my eyes quickly, placed the samples in a small tube, and then spoke candidly to Mother and Mrs. Maiden.

"I hesitate to diagnose this before the lab results come back. You can see for yourself that Chancey has something growing on both eyes. Those are tumors. They may be benign, or you may be looking at a horse with cancer. I can tell you this: whether it's cancer or not, Chancey's going to need surgery. Even so, one or both of the tumors will return in time," he predicted.

Doctor Russ left the decision to Mother. "How would you like to proceed? Do you want to wait for the lab results or have me go ahead and schedule something with the eye clinic?"

Mother did not seem at all surprised, nor did I detect any increased anxiety from her. She did not stutter, nor did I hear Mother's stomach rumble, as my own had been since the doctor's arrival. She remained standing near me with her hand calmly resting on my neck and hesitated not a moment before answering.

"If the tumors need to come off, then let's do it. Go ahead and schedule the operation," she consented.

I greatly appreciated Mother's aggressive pursuit of treatment on my behalf. I felt that blowing on her was too ordinary, too common an expression of appreciation. I wanted Mother to understand that my gratitude was sincere, so I licked her. I licked her hand because it was closest to my mouth. I tasted no lingering essence of peppermint or stud biscuit even, only skin. Mother startled before collecting herself.

"Oh, Chancey," she said. Her eyes misted. "Sweet boy." She patted my neck.

Doctor Russ then explained that he would arrange for the operation to take place in Albemarle County at the hands of two eye surgeons. Until then, I did not even know that a special eye doctor existed for horses. Doctor Russ explained that Mrs. Maiden and I would need to make a trip over the blue mountains to an eye hospital for horses, where I would be expected to spend two days before coming back to the Maury River Stables. My anxious stool erupted up again, despite my best efforts to remain calm. Mother kissed my poll.

Mrs. Maiden, having known Doctor Russ and used his services exclusively at the Maury River Stables for a number of years, then asked for the doctor's frank opinion. When Mrs. Maiden inquired, he more willingly speculated a prognosis than he had with Mother earlier in my exam. He did not withhold his belief that my eyes showed cancer, explaining that the shape of the tumors and my lack of pigmentation both contributed to that opinion.

"If this is cancer, do you think surgery will take care of it?" Mrs. Maiden asked.

"Ehhh," he exhaled. "Don't ask me that." Mrs. Maiden and Mother kept silent and waited for his response. Finally he answered: "Depends on how far this thing's advanced. Might be nothing to worry about, or could be we'll need to do more than surgery to keep from losing the eyes. Let's keep the fly mask on him — that's for sure."

Mother agreed to do just that and relayed again her intent to offer me the best care within her means. Doctor Russ left plenty more instructions for Mother and Mrs. Maiden. Most important to me, other than my eyes, my arthritis, and still being somewhat under-weight, he pronounced me perfectly fit to serve as Claire's first horse.

"Chancey's got some health challenges, no doubt about that. But if we take good care of him, Chancey'll make a fine first horse," were the wise doctor's exact words. I took satisfaction that he again made a point of calling me a horse, not a pony.

The doctor and the dentist were new acquaintances of mine, and I had liked them both just fine. Now it was time to turn our attention to my badly overgrown and sore feet. I hoped that the farrier would be just as ami-able. Farriers are a transient lot, more transient even than horses. I have heard Mrs. Maiden say that there are as many as forty different farriers working around the blue mountains.

As yet, Claire and I had not begun working together under saddle and certainly we had not started a course of training, as I was recovering from Monique's unin-tentional, but now evident, neglect. One result of my abandonment in the field was that my feet were so badly overgrown that I had none of the balance required to carry out a rigorous training program with Claire. Even in the field, I had begun to use great caution to avoid stumbling.

When my old farrier, John, showed up, he was a very welcome sight, as was his corgi, Katie. She is a pleasant and encouraging assistant who stays near her owner and never frightens me or disrupts John's work. I have observed, on multiple occasions, that people and their animal friends occasionally reflect one another physically and often also in manner. This was true of Katie and John the Farrier, both reddish in complexion and friendly in countenance.

John the Farrier was deeply committed to his trade, and so comfortable was I with his easy rhythm and solid support of my body weight that it was my habit to sneak in brief naps while he attended to my feet. My bowels had relaxed considerably from Doctor Russ's visit, and I settled right down while John got to work. Mother took great interest in the farrier's craft, and as he began, she offered her assistance to hold me.

"Nah, you won't need to hold Chance. He'll try to fall asleep, so just don't let him fall down on me. He's a good boy. If you ask me, he's as good a horse there ever was. I'd trust Chancey more than any horse I know, except for my own, of course." John the Farrier, I knew for certain, rode a Thoroughbred–quarter horse cross, called an appendix, for I had galloped a field or two on the trail with that red mare.

Despite John indicating that it was unnecessary, Mother held me anyway. She cooed at me the entire time, and while I appreciated her attentiveness to my care, I was sorely lacking sleep and had hoped to get some shut-eye while the farrier worked. Being new to the gelding field, Dante was intent on testing me throughout the day and night, and consequently I was exhausted.

On this visit there was only one old shoe for John to remove, for I had seen to remove the other three on my own when constructing my path through the barbed-wire fence to the river. John clipped all four of my feet and filed them down to perfection. Katie was delirious with joy at the size and volume of my hoof clippings and, being quite the little scavenger, made off with a generous helping of them before choosing one to chew while she watched her master complete his job. John gave me only two new front shoes and told Mother that we could add shoes to my back feet later, if needed.

After he finished, John asked Mother if he could turn me out himself. I was delighted to walk a bit with Katie and John. John praised my purple accessories and let me graze the fence line.

"Chancey," John told me before opening the gate to

the gelding field, "you've found a good home here. I think you're going to be real happy."

I nickered good-bye to John and Katie and hoped that by the farrier's next visit he would see for himself evidence of my happiness. For despite the news that a cancer was likely growing inside my eyes, I knew that something even stronger was now growing inside my heart.

CHAPTER NINE

Beyond Saddle Mountain

The return to a regular feeding schedule, the added pain supplement, and, I believe, the companionship of my new friends all served greatly to restore my health. Our only remaining worry was the condition of my sight; the doctor's test confirmed the presence of cancer in both my eyes, a cancer directly related to my absence of pigment and prolonged exposure to the sun.

How many days did I stand in my field in the full sun, feeling it well on my withers and loving that feeling? Yet every day the sun and my eyes waged battle with one another. Undoubtedly, I will someday lose this battle, for no being on this earth is stronger than a star. Knowing the cause of my encroaching blindness, I thought I began to feel my cancer stretching its roots deeper into my eyes, and beyond, with every ray of sun that touched me.

Though no one had offered any hope of improved vision in my left eye, all believed that with aggressive treatment, the remaining vision in my right eye could be preserved for some time. We would need to prepare for a lifetime of surgeries to remove any future carcinomas should they return, as Doctor Russ predicted. To have the malignancies removed, I was to be transported away from the Maury River Stables, beyond the blue mountains and into another valley farther away, in Albemarle County, where cases such as mine were handled every day.

It was an act of true compassion when Mother suggested that Mac accompany me to Albemarle. Claire did not want me to be alone. Mother consented to pay the trailer fee and all lodging costs for Mac to board with me at the hospital that was to save what remained of my sight. Mac gladly agreed to travel with me. I could think of no one besides Mac who would give me greater comfort, except of course Claire herself.

Mother withdrew Claire from school on the day I left the blue mountains for my surgery. Claire did not seem afraid for me and of that I was glad. She spent the morning preparing us for our departure. Claire made a big fuss over Mac and me, grooming us both and treating us to more stud biscuits than was customary. Mrs. Maiden and Mother couldn't help but fawn over us, too. Claire readied the trailer by mucking out dung from a previous trip, filling the hay nets with plenty of fresh hay, and stringing the nets side by side in the trailer, should we feel like eating along the way. When the trailer was ready for us, Claire clipped the lead rope to my halter and walked me inside. Mother followed behind with Mac.

Claire had drawn a picture for me, too, which she had secured to the wall of the trailer. The drawing showed the peaks of Saddle Mountain grandly filling the page, with two friends standing in the saddle between the peaks. The friends — a girl and a horse — nuzzled each other face-to-face. Claire pointed out to me the shape of a heart rising between the two. Then she made Mrs. Maiden promise to keep the picture with me in my room at the hospital. Claire nuzzled me. "When you feel scared over there, just look at the picture and remember me and Saddle Mountain. We'll be here when you come home."

Mother had wet eyes; Claire did not, but stood smiling and blowing me kisses until Mrs. Maiden shut the trailer windows, leaving only a sliver of light visible to me.

Though I could only see slight glimpses of her,

I could hear Claire running beside the trailer all the way down the drive. "Bye, Chancey! Bye, Mac! I love you both! Come back soon!" Claire's words did not stumble once.

I whinnied a loud good-bye and hoped she could hear me, too. I'm sure that Claire stood at the end of the drive waving at us until we were long out of sight. I did not have enough time to say a decent farewell to Claire and Saddle Mountain. The narrow road switched over and back onto itself, and soon nothing of Saddle Mountain was visible. I had lived every day of my life standing within sight of it. Even on the days when its peaks hid under a blanket of fog or behind a blinding white snowstorm, Saddle Mountain and I stood together.

As Mrs. Maiden drove farther away from the Maury River Stables, I lost my breath and could not find it. For many miles, I strained to see something familiar out the window slot. My nervous bowels began to rumble. Mac nickered to me, "You're okay, Old App. The mountain will be here when we return, and so will your girl." I found my breath and sniffed Claire's drawing of us; it still smelled of Claire.

The surgery at Albemarle required only an overnight stay. Again my strong Appaloosa breeding aided me in recovering quickly. Of the surgery itself, I remember only that the nurses spoke very kindly to me just before I felt as if my legs had stopped working and I were going to fall down.

Mac's presence soothed me greatly, for when I first woke up from surgery, I could see nothing at all. The Belgian remained attentive, ready to explain the situation to me.

I feared I would never see again. "Mac, everything is completely dark now. Has the surgery failed?"

"No, friend. Your eyes are both heavily bandaged. I heard them say you'll have the right eye; they don't know about the left. But you will see Saddle Mountain and you will see Claire, very soon."

"Mac?" I asked. "Are you an old horse? You look very young indeed, but you seem older than I am at times. Are you old?"

"Not very," Mac replied. "The dentist says I'm eight."

"I think you are older than your teeth, Macadoo. How did that happen? What brought you to the Maury River Stables? Were you abandoned in a field, too?"

"Get some rest, Old App. We'll have plenty of time to talk when you're well."

I did rest. Mac stood watch over me until Mrs. Maiden came to drive us back to the Maury River Stables. With bandages still on both eyes, I finally returned home. Claire greeted us at the gate, just exactly as she had promised she would.

✳ CHAPTER TEN ✳
Under Saddle

U pon my return, Claire threw herself enthusiasti-
cally into leading my recovery and treatment. Her
concern for my comfort never waned; Claire remained
as attentive to me as she had been from our first meeting. She checked with Mrs. Maiden to be sure that my
medicine was administered properly. She took her role
as my friend and caretaker very seriously, and as much
as anything, I believe this is what eased my suffering.
My eyes healed quickly, and soon enough Claire and I
were ready to take our first lesson together, and indeed,
our first ride, too.

First Claire took extra time to stretch me, just as Mrs. Maiden had shown her. She leaned her small frame into me, lifted a foreleg at the cannon bone, and then ever so slowly stretched it out fully until I took the leg back from her. After completing each of my legs this way, Claire wrapped both her hands firmly around my tail, braced her legs, and pulled with all her strength. I, in turn, pulled my weight forward, until Claire released her hands.

During our first lesson, we did not jump or practice dressage tests. Instead, Claire asked to practice our flat-work bareback. "I'll feel Chancey's rhythm better if I'm riding free, Mrs. Maiden."

Mrs. Maiden obliged, "Excellent, Claire! Riding bareback will strengthen your legs and core, too."

I, too, preferred carrying Claire without a saddle, as it was easier on my back and joints.

In our first lesson, there was no guessing as to what would come next, or what was expected of the other. Claire asked for a working trot and a working trot I gave her, right away. Claire naturally rose to the trot pre-cisely in time with my outside shoulder. She touched down lightly on my back and without the slightest bounce. Together we two moved in delightful tandem. Claire needed no stirrups, no saddle, no whip, or no spurs. Claire needed only to be Claire. I will say that for the entirety of our first ride I thought only of Claire and what she might ask of me next. I found a new energy, a new appreciation, and a new joy in riding with Claire.

I kept my focus on Claire and tried to forget about the cancer in my eyes. Thanks to the skills of my Albemarle surgeons, my cancer had been halted for the time being. I maintained sight in my right eye, giving me a fair line of vision of nearly 180 degrees, as I had learned from Doctor Russ's follow-up examination. I am faithful to the belief that, had my tumors been allowed to grow unchecked, I would have quickly succumbed to complete blindness. Though I could feel that the cancer remained hidden within me, I could also feel that it had been driven away for the present. In any event, our training had to take into consideration the near total darkness in my left eye.

While neither Claire nor I were beginners, we knew we would have to work hard if we were ever to compete together. Most of my career as a school horse had been spent teaching novice riders only the very basic skills. By the time Claire and I joined, she was already an accomplished horsewoman, as she had learned to ride on Daisy. From the time she was five years old, as Mac relayed directly to me, Claire had spent as much time as possible with horses.

For the first time in my twenty-two years, I felt a sense of purpose in training with one student devoted solely and only to me. Mrs. Maiden set for us a goal of showing in the late-summer series of local hunter shows. Though Claire and I were both experienced, Mrs. Maiden insisted that we start out together in the most elementary of classes — Short Stirrup Walk-Trot. With her undeniable talent for persuasive argument, Claire secured an accord with Mrs. Maiden that if we worked on our equitation without complaint, we could also compete in a jumper class over two small fences. With several months available to train, Claire and I were confident that we would be ready by the end of August.

The focus to our training surpassed any lesson that I had given as a school horse. Claire had chosen me as her companion, and together we worked every day. With the new supplement arriving in my morning grain each day, I felt freer of pain than I had for some time. As Claire and I were not jumping too aggressively, I felt certain that I could tolerate well this degree of soreness and aches. Indeed, it would have been more painful to deny, to Claire or myself, the satisfaction of becoming a team.

True, Claire and I were only jumping small eighteen-inch fences and, at most, a course of two outside lines. But it was a joy for me to be with Claire no matter what we were doing. We progressed easily from taking the little jumps at the trot to taking them at the canter.

We quickly found that I needed to be very nearly completely retrained to jump. As a way of compensating for my poor eyesight, I had long refused or ducked out of jumps. As everyone now understood the reasoning, no one — not Mrs. Maiden, Mother, or Claire — seemed the least bit dissuaded from the effort it took to retrain me. My refusal behavior was treated as an entirely natural consequence of my visual impairment; no one accused me of a poor attitude or nasty temperament.

The burden of retraining me fell primarily to Claire, under the guidance of Mrs. Maiden, and with the encouragement of Mother, who no longer kept up a pretense of reading or writing at the barn. In fact, Mother joined us in the ring by taking lessons, using Mac as her teacher. Mac rather enjoyed this phase of Mother's. He is known to adore human females and is rather boastful of the fact that he has never, accidentally or with intent, allowed one to slip out of the saddle, even at times at his own peril. Mother and Mac got on sweetly. Though they did not train together as Claire and I did, they appeared to enjoy each other's company, and Mother grew comfortable enough with Mac to call for the canter herself every now and then.

The presence of Mac and Mother in the ring, along with Daisy and her new student, Ann, helped us prepare better for showing than if we had undertaken our training privately. As is sometimes the case with bossy mares, one must use extreme caution when approaching from behind. In Daisy's case, she is hardwired to kick out behind her at the slightest detection of another horse. This posed no problem for Claire, or me, for Claire had years of experience as Daisy's primary student. She was well informed of Daisy's invisible bubble and the consequences of violating said bubble. Daisy herself gave off plenty of warning by pinning her ears flat back as soon as any horse even approached her. Daisy's presence in the ring with us simulated the very conditions under which Claire and I would be competing, assuming I could be retrained to jump consistently and safely with Claire.

To help me undo my bad jumping habits, Mrs. Maiden constructed several exercises. First, she began placing dollar bills between Claire's calves and my barrel. Claire was then instructed to ride our entire lesson, even over jumps, without losing the bills from under her. This was necessary, explained Mrs. Maiden, because a strong leg is the best aid a rider has to communicate with her partner. Furthermore, Mrs. Maiden told us that in my case, Claire's legs needed to compensate for my poor eyes.

She said, "Claire, blind horses can compete in Grand Prix events, if they're matched with the right person. Chancey's not completely blind yet; there's no reason he can't do anything you ask him to do. You just have to consistently ask him. If you ask with your hands but not your legs, he's going to have to guess what you mean. Sometimes he's going to guess incorrectly. But if everything about you — your eyes, your legs, your hands, your heart — are telling him the same thing, then it's just as if you were talking to him, like I'm talking to you now. So we'll work on your legs first."

Claire picked up the reins and held the dollar bill tightly against my barrel. For a girl her age and size, Claire already possessed a strong leg; the dollar-bill game only added to her strength.

Mrs. Maiden also had Claire count our strides out loud on the approach of every jump. Beginning about six strides out, Claire would count us over the jump. "One, two, one, two, one, two, jump!" This was begun entirely as a finishing technique for Claire, but we all soon realized that hearing her helped me compensate for my shortcomings. In our training, I learned to keep my ears turning always toward Claire's voice, readying myself for her cues.

"Trot, Chancey, trot!" Claire invited me.

For most of my life, it had been fundamentally contrary to my philosophy to respond to voice commands

* 89 *

only, except for the command *whoa,* which I had taken quite seriously. I suppose one of the characteristics that had contributed to my reputation as an obstinate horse was that I required much more of my students than the simple voice command to walk, trot, or canter.

I firmly believe that children don't learn well on push-button ponies, or automatic horses, and so I myself had always determined not to be automatic in any way. Children deserve to learn the basics upon which a strong foundation is built, and that cannot be done through voice command alone, in my humble opinion.

But Claire was different. In working with Claire, I did not feel I was giving her lessons, but learning to move with her as if we were a single being.

"Trot, Chancey," she said again. I obliged. I picked up, and held, an easy trot while Claire performed around-the-world by turning herself around and around in the saddle while I circled the entire ring at the trot.

"And, whoa," Claire sang as she directed me toward Mrs. Maiden, who was still standing in the ring.

A barn mother, watching from the fence yelled, "He's gorgeous. He doesn't even look like the same horse; his coat is so shiny. They look beautiful together." Claire and I came to rest with Claire sitting backward in the saddle. Mrs. Maiden got back to the lesson.

"Okay, Claire, enough play. Let's practice the outside line."

We worked hard to correct my bad jumping habits in time for the summer series. Claire's strong legs became most important to our training. Mrs. Maiden worked us both hard, always pushing us each to do our best individually and to do our best as a team. She liked to pull us into the center of the ring for an explanation of the task before she set us loose to attack the jumps.

"Claire," Mrs. Maiden would say, "you've got to hold him up with both legs. He's not Daisy, remember? If you drop him, he's going to want to duck out, but don't let him. Don't get ahead of Chancey, and don't fall behind him. Use your legs to tell him when it's time to jump. It's almost like you're going to lift him up with your legs, then hold him up the whole way over the fence. He'll listen to you once he knows he can trust you. Remember, he can't see out of that left eye. You've got to see for him."

I learned, with Claire, to wait for that moment where together we would defy gravity. We would canter around half of the ring, with Claire counting my strides on the approach. I felt what was coming from the shift in Claire's weight and the tilt of her head. I felt when it was time to fly.

Claire would rise up from her seat with just enough spring. Steady with her entire leg, and with both of us looking far beyond the fence into the mountains, we would hover for an eternal instant. Once over the jump, Claire would always laugh out loud, delighting in the thrill of jumping with me. She held me straight, and cantering away from the first fence, we would soar, again, over the second fence in the line. We touched the ground, rounded the corner, and again and again we flew over the two small fences, each time with less effort and more lift. During those early days of jumping with Claire, I felt that if I had wings, they would be named Claire.

We progressed rapidly together. My desire to be a great first horse for Claire, combined with my stubborn insistence that arthritis and blindness were mere annoyances, meant that sometimes I pushed myself too far.

Once, after an outside line, Claire reached down and patted my neck, just as she usually did after a clear round. "Let's go again, Chance."

I was already tired and breathing heavily. I didn't want to go again. I wanted Claire to take off the saddle and let me graze in my field while she rested on my back. I preferred to watch the sun set while listening to Claire practice her choir songs. Yet for as much refusing as I had done in the past, I could not refuse Claire. She asked for the canter, and I stumbled.

"Claire," Mrs. Maiden warned, "Chancey's worked hard today. Why don't you walk him down to the barn? You can jump again tomorrow."

Claire's confidence was back; she wanted to jump all night.

"Please, Mrs. Maiden? We're just getting the hang of it together, and I haven't ridden like this in such a long time," Claire begged. "Just one more outside line? Then we'll stop."

Just as I had, Mrs. Maiden also had difficulty refusing Claire. She gave in. "Okay, one more line. Take your time and use your aids; Chancey's tired."

Claire asked for the canter again. This time, I threw my weight into her request, getting the correct lead despite feeling sore and exhausted. Claire counted on our approach and gave me equal support with both legs.

I was not the only one who was tired and needing to rest. I felt Claire's legs evenly on my sides, but then on the approach, she looked away and dropped her right leg. She opened the door for me to duck; I thought I was supposed to go out and so I relaxed, sure that Claire had changed her mind about the prudence of taking these last two fences. I did not expect her to come up into jump position, but she rose into her two-point, ready to jump. I tried to stop myself, but it was too late. I ducked out to the right.

Claire, who was already in jump position, fell up

onto my withers and over to my right. As soon as I felt Claire falling, I stooped and slid my neck and shoulders under her to keep her with me. That save would have made Mac proud.

Mrs. Maiden wasted no time in correcting us. "You dropped him! That wasn't Chancey's fault, Claire. What happened? What did you do wrong?" she asked.

Claire knew her mistake right away.

"I looked down at the ground."

"What else? What did you not do?"

"I didn't hold him up with my right leg," Claire confessed.

"Why not?" Mrs. Maiden always pushed her students, especially Claire, to think about their riding and find their own answers.

"I was losing my stirrup on the right, and I was trying to get it back."

Mrs. Maiden was waiting for that exact detail from Claire. Once she knew the cause of Claire's mistake, she set about fixing it.

"Okay, I know you're both tired, but let's end your lesson right. Try the outside line again. This time, no stirrups." Through our combined willpower only, Claire and I cleared the outside line.

For many lessons after that, we jumped without Claire's feet in the stirrups or hands on the reins so that Claire and I could learn to succeed without them. And so it went, with Mrs. Maiden pushing Claire and me to become a solid team. Only once in all of our training did I let Claire off of my back.

Our mistake occurred on the second in a series of two jumps. We approached from the left, and though I knew in my muscles and memory that there must be a second jump following, Mrs. Maiden had paced it differently; I panicked when I failed to hear Claire's counting.

I ducked out again—in the instant before the jump, I grew impatient, old fool that I am, and second-guessed Claire, whom I had come to love and trust more than any person. This time I was unable to scoop her up, and she fell abruptly off of me, brushing my outside foreleg on her way down. I managed to lift my back leg high over her body, and so we avoided what could have been an accident of serious consequence for Claire.

I knew right away that I had lost her and trotted immediately back to her. I dropped my head down and blew into her face. Claire laughed and blew her own breath across my cheek. "I'm okay, Chancey. Don't worry, boy."

Claire picked herself up and together we took the line again; this time Claire guided me perfectly through both jumps. After our lesson ended, Mrs. Maiden lectured us before letting us out of the ring.

"Claire, you're so good for Chancey. And he's so

good for you. You've really grown together over the last few months. I'd like for you two to show in the short stirrup division next week at Tamworth Springs."

Claire squealed and patted my neck. "We'd love to go! We'll be great together; won't we, Chancey?"

"Hold on, Claire," Mrs. Maiden continued. "If you're going to show Chancey, you're going to have to concentrate. He loves you and he listens to you. Sometimes, though, you get too distracted by other things. Chancey is a good horse; he might even be a great horse. But you've got to help him be great. He needs you to count his strides, and he needs you to concentrate."

Mrs. Maiden let her words sink in before asking, "Can you do that?"

Claire did not hesitate. "Yes! We can do it; I promise."

"You're used to Daisy, Claire. Chancey is not Daisy; he is his own horse. Daisy will jump over anything you point her at. That's why beginners ride Daisy. You and Chancey are a team now; you've got to help each other."

I don't think Claire heard a word of Mrs. Maiden's lecture to us; she walked me down to the barn, all the while making preparations for Tamworth Springs. Claire untacked me and rinsed me off with a cool bath, which I welcomed. She rubbed my entire body with a dry towel and walked me around the paddock before turning me out. We had worked so hard that Claire took extra care to stretch me out again after our lesson.

I leaned into Claire's shoulder with each leg she pulled, enjoying the full extension of my muscles. I looked at Claire, so petite, yet so strong and confident. I realized then as Claire held me, unafraid of taking my weight and holding me in balance, how delicate the matter of balance really is.

When we missed the second jump and I let Claire fall, we lost our balance in an instant. Whether I had dropped Claire or Claire had dropped me made no difference. We had recovered and resolved to go forward to our first showing together. I had never felt better; Claire's confidence was soaring. Our sights were set on Tamworth Springs.

CHAPTER ELEVEN

A Fancy Pony

Claire and I spent the eve of our Tamworth Springs debut together turning me into, in Claire's words, a "fancy pony." I am not a fancy pony. Technically, I'm not a pony at all. Claire prepared me for our little show as if it were a rated show at the horse center in Lexington, where horses from all over the country come to compete. I've been to the horse center, and I'm not the least intimated by the fancy horses and stately brick barns.

As much as I looked forward to our daily grooming before lessons, the beautification that is required to turn out well for a show is something else altogether. Show turnout is a routine that I've been through many, many times with many different riders. You don't get to be a twenty-two-year-old school horse without having your mane pulled now and again.

Claire readied me for the show with a demeanor that I had not seen since that first day of our meeting when Claire barely offered me a smile. I could not relate this girl to the same lighthearted girl that Claire had become. I asked myself, could this serious little Miss be the same one who loved to ride me backward in the saddle? Was this somber girl really Claire, who in the middle of a lesson, would often stop to remove the saddle because it felt freer to ride bareback? My Claire was nervous. She did not speak a word out loud, but the racing of her heart told me so.

Claire dragged the mounting block alongside my right shoulder and began pulling my mane to get it short and even for the show. While Claire silently wrapped thin strands of mane around the braiding comb and then yanked off the ends to make for a uniform length all the way down my neck, Mother worked on removing knots and briars from my tail, which had grown so long that it dragged the ground. Claire and Mother pulled briars and mud from my mane and tail with such steady and even rhythm, I felt almost as if I might melt in their hands. Feeling secure in the crossties, I even allowed myself to enjoy a light sleep.

Neither of them spoke a word. Mother, standing directly behind me so that I could feel her presence, knew that I would not kick. With no tentativeness about her at all, she had me detangled in a matter of minutes using both a comb and her fingers. Claire still had not spoken a word, and Mother, too, seemed content to work in silence.

I could hear all of my friends eating their dinner. The familiar smell of beloved sweet feed filled the barn. Though I knew grain and fresh hay would be waiting for me when our work was complete, I felt it more important to stand quietly while Claire and Mother finished than to dance around insisting that I have my hay and grain at once. I liked standing between them, feeling both of them attend to me together, and yet lost in their own thoughts. I liked it very much. Never, I thought, had preparing for a show been so enjoyable.

I closed my eyes and bent my head nearer Claire's heart. Despite her steady hands and quietness, her heart still beat furiously.

"Don't worry," I tried to tell her. "Don't worry, Claire. I'll take good care of you tomorrow." Claire remained too deep in her own mind to hear me.

Claire decided not to bathe me that evening before the show because I love to roll after bathing. A clean white horse will not stay clean for long, especially one who loves to roll, as I do.

There are two kinds of rolling. The frightful kind of rolling is because the pain inside you must be let out. Rolling to relieve pain is often symptomatic of a horse who is threatening to colic. But rolling in the field immediately after a bath is perhaps the most joyful kind of rolling for a horse. Extending all four legs to the sky for a good deep stretch, which then causes the earth beneath your weight to crumble into dirt particles of all sizes that massage your entire back in a most exquisite manner, is bliss itself. No other kind of rubbing or scratching can replace this rolling around with the earth

Had Claire bathed me that night, we likely would have had to repeat the exercise anyway, because I would not have even tried to resist the urge to cover myself in dirt and dung.

Show day started with a hectic pace. Claire and I were both accustomed to taking our time. We had grown used to our routine of Claire riding me bareback a bit in the field before our lesson, dawdling in my room before tacking up, and then Claire deeply stretching my legs before training. On the morning of our first show, Claire and I did not follow our usual routine. Those around us were impatient to get everything loaded, and we had much to do.

Before light—before breakfast even—Claire and Mother arrived to bathe me. A wisp of moon and one star remained lit when Claire walked into the field to catch me. She did not have to walk far in the dark as I was standing near the gate, waiting for her. After a good night of rolling in my field, Claire often jokes that I am no longer a white pony, but a red one. Not to disappoint, I was anything but white when Claire and Mother arrived on show day. I could not help but roll many times during the night.

Claire kissed my cheek and teased, "You can't be Chancey! You look like a pretty palomino. What did you do with my beautiful albino pony?"

I nickered at Claire and danced around the gate, unable to contain my excitement any longer. "Come on, boy." She pulled me out of the field. "Let's get you cleaned up; you're the reddest I've ever seen you."

Before I could even taste one morsel of my morning grain, Mother and Claire had me secured in the crossties and had begun bathing me with cold water. It made for a most uncomfortable start to my day. Claire left the bathing primarily to Mother so that she could load our tack into the trailer.

"Oh, great, Chancey rolled in poo. His whole backside is green," Mother pointed out to Claire.

Claire laughed, which annoyed Mother further.

"Claire!" Mother reprimanded. "Poo is not funny on show day. You know as well as I do that a big part of showing is how well you're turned out."

Mother turned back to me. "Let's get you white again, Chance."

She had brought with her a stack of clean towels and a special shampoo which promised to make even the dirtiest white horse glisten. Mother made no effort to help me adjust to the cold water by first starting with my legs, as Claire would have done. Cold water is more tolerable on my feet and legs; I find that if I can just have a moment to relax, I am able to endure the cold all over my body. Mother was in a hurry, however, and was disinclined to baby me.

I could hear Claire and the other girls near the trailer and could smell the hay nets being prepared for our outing. I could hear Claire, but I could not see her. In a flash of panic, I feared going to the show. I whinnied for Claire. Still wet and cold in the cross-ties, I began dancing from side to side. My nervous stomach rumbled. I wanted to stay with Claire and not let her out of my sight. My routine was off; everything seemed different to me. My bath was cold, I had not eaten yet, nor had I been stretched, and I could not see Claire. I whinnied for Claire again.

Mother tried to calm me. "You're okay, boy. Shhh, you're okay."

I did not respond to her in any detectable manner. I could not find it within in myself to touch Mother's shoulder, as I would have liked to do. I averted my face and turned away.

Finally, Mother dried me off and led me back to my room to eat. I inhaled every morsel of grain and did not pay homage to Dante by leaving grain along the wall between us. I was relieved to taste that my pain-ease supplement had not been forgotten.

Claire came and finished pulling my mane and tried to soothe the both of us. "Don't worry, boy. It's just a little b-b-barn show. There's no reason to be nervous. We've both been in bigger shows than this one, just not together. Don't worry. Everything will be f-fine."

Claire's word stumbling had returned. I sighed a deep sigh to encourage the same in Claire. She leaned against me. With Claire beside me, I breathed easier and knew that everything would indeed be fine. After all, I had many years of barn shows to my credit, though truly I had never shown with a partner for whom I felt as much affection and loyalty as I did for Claire. I touched Claire's chest with my muzzle and nickered deep to let her know that I would do my best, too.

She was not thinking of me anymore; Claire was watching Mother talk, rather animatedly, to a man I did not recognize. "That's my dad! My dad's here! I better go over there before he and Mother start f-fighting," she said. Leaving me in my room, Claire ran to her father's side and hugged him with nearly as much squeeze as she usually reserved for me.

"Dad, come meet Chancey." Claire pulled her father by his hand toward my room.

He shuffled his feet, reluctantly following behind Claire. Though of course my loyalty resided with Mother, who had saved the vision in my right eye and given me a stable home with Claire, it did surprise me that my ears, quite on their own, instinctively pinned themselves back at Claire's father. I caught myself before Claire noticed, however, and stretched my neck out toward him in an offering of friendship. He stood a step or two beyond what was necessary to make a connection.

"Come on, Dad," urged Claire. "Let him smell you. That's how horses say hello."

Mother interrupted the two of them. "Claire, your father's afraid of horses. Maybe if you bring Chancey closer to him?"

Her father stiffened. "No, I'm fine. I can see the horse just fine."

Claire resumed brushing me, chattering with her father about the classes we would compete in later and how hard the two of us had been practicing. Her father began to relax, and I was glad to have met him, for despite my allegiance to Mother, my highest faithfulness was to Claire, and the child was beaming in her father's presence.

Mother stood watching them with her arms folded across her heart. She allowed the two of them only another moment before she interrupted. "Claire, come on. Let's get Chancey loaded into the trailer."

"Okay, I'll be right there. I want to show Dad around the barn first," Claire said.

I could see that Mother badly wanted to pull Claire away from her father, but she did not. Mother nodded to Claire and walked back over to me. She hooked my lead rope to my halter and led me to the trailer. I could feel in Mother, the way she so tightly gripped the lead and yanked on my halter, that the morning was difficult for her for reasons unrelated to Claire or me. I stopped, intent that I should have a moment with Mother before loading.

Mother tugged on the lead; I refused to go. She pulled harder on the rope, forgetting momentarily that I weighed more than a thousand pounds. Mother loosened her hold on the rope and turned to face me. I blinked my eyes at her and threw my head up for her to come nearer. She stepped back to my cheek and rested her face against mine.

"It's just not fair that he waltzes in here like a big hero. He doesn't even want Claire to ride. He thinks it's too dangerous. I get tired of fighting with him about it;

anyone can see how happy Claire is out here." Mother's eyes filled up to the lids with water, which then spilled over onto my neck.

I pressed my cheek into Mother's until finally she began to breathe in an equal and deep rhythm.

"You're a good horse, Chancey. You know, you've saved Claire's life in these past few months. She has taken the divorce so hard. Without you, I don't know that there would have been any joy at all in this little girl's life right now. You've seen her through the hardest thing she's ever had to face," Mother told me. "Thank you, Chancey." She patted my neck softly in one of my favorite spots.

Claire came running up to us, and she was a sight to behold, as her freshly pressed show clothes were already disheveled and soiled from the morning's work. Still, Claire was as radiant a girl as I have ever seen. Mother observed this as well. "Claire, you're beautiful! You and Chancey are going to have a fine time today."

Mother put her arms around Claire and pulled her in so close that I could barely hear her whisper, "Have fun today, my sweet girl."

As the sun had not yet fully risen, I concluded that with Claire nearby, perhaps the sun did not need to wake so early today.

CHAPTER TWELVE

She Fell Up, Then Down

I believed Claire and I were ready for Tamworth Springs. Everyone believed we were ready. We had worked hard throughout the spring and summer, building first our friendship and then our skills. With each other's help, Claire and I had conquered our respective troubles. We were now a team, and Tamworth Springs was to be our debut. All of us certainly expected that Claire and I would compete without incident. Mrs. Maiden had even predicted that we would come back to Maury River Stables with a champion ribbon, although we were only at Tamworth Springs to get our legs under us.

Hunter shows have never been my favorite. I detest the stressful conditions under which one must compete. The number of times that I've been cut off, kicked, or rear-ended because of rude or novice horse-and-rider teams is not worth counting. But then I am not much of a counter anyway. Coaches and spectators alike move in and out of the show ring with great inconsideration and little awareness. There are those who thrive at hunter shows; I am not among them.

Daisy would rather spend a day at a hunter show than most anywhere else. Of course, because of her sacred bubble, Daisy has always been permitted to show with a red ribbon tied around her tail. Tamworth Springs was no different. The ribbon warned that all who dared to enter the space around Daisy's Welsh rear end would receive a swift, hard kick. I, without a red ribbon to excuse me, was expected to behave amid some quite poorly mannered teams.

If truth be told, hunter shows cause my stomach to clinch up almost instantly with a magnificent force. I am competitive, but prefer my competitors to meet me in an open field. Instead of measuring my worth in diagonals, leads, and head positioning, I prefer that we traverse a course designed to test not only our speed and endurance, but our command of varied and challenging terrain. An event where we are measured by our wisdom, sure-footedness, and resolve to go forward to the end, and without injury is my ideal.

That was not the measure of our challenge at Tamworth Springs. Claire and I were to compete in a most basic set of classes: Short Stirrup Walk-Trot, Short Stirrup Over Eighteen-Inch Fences, and Short Stirrup Pleasure. We expected to place well in all three classes. In some secret place in my heart, I hoped we might win.

We succeeded in placing third in Walk-Trot, a fine enough showing for our first class, though surely not as well as we could have done. There were several factors working against our success. As I've already identified, the crowded conditions in the ring presented difficulty. We did not have ample space to relax and find our spot. We just couldn't get settled. Mrs. Maiden felt the judge erred in not dividing the large class into two separate classes, as it would have improved conditions in the show ring for everyone.

Our third place in the Walk-Trot class was likely caused, in part, by a few strides at the trot where Claire rose to the wrong diagonal, though feeling the error herself, she self-corrected right away. Mrs. Maiden also pointed out that Claire's dirty riding clothes had probably cost us points; she requested that next time, Claire keep her show clothes cleaner. Further contributing was what Mrs. Maiden speculated to be the judge's bias against my albinism. Convinced that we should have placed higher, Mrs. Maiden most emphatically complained to us that this judge was known to despise what Mrs. Maiden gently described as "pink skin" in horses.

Daisy competed in the same class with her young rider, Ann, who, though the same age as Claire, was an inexperienced rider, having only started lessons at the Maury River Stables after my own arrival there. As impudent a mare as Daisy is, she is the pony of choice for graceful, but green, riders such as Ann. With a strand of Daisy's tail braided and tied with the red warning ribbon, and Ann Hayden turned out in two pigtails with red ribbons of her own to match, they presented a classically sweet image, even to my old, jaded, half-blind eyes. Daisy knows her job, and she excels under these same conditions that cause extreme digestive turmoil for me. Daisy and Ann placed fourth in Walk-Trot, a fine showing for their first time out.

Claire seemed pleased with our placement, and she happily tucked our third-place ribbon into the headstall of my bridle. Mother had emphasized to Claire, and to me, that our only charge was to have fun, and not to worry about winning. I noted, however, that Mother was beside herself that we had placed at all, so I couldn't help but believe that despite her protestations about having fun, she took pleasure in our achievement.

In our second class, over the little fences, we failed. I confess that although the entire scene remains vividly

indexed in my memory and always will, it is still difficult for me to relive exactly what happened. But for my
own conscience, I will try to reconstruct the event as
best I can.

Before we entered the ring, it was evident that
Claire's anxiety from the day before had only increased.
"I f-feel sick. M-M-other, I c-can't," Claire said.

Mother rubbed Claire's back but before she could
speak, Claire's father interrupted. "Claire, you're stuttering. You're just nervous, sweetheart. Stay focused.
Don't psych yourself out."

With the bit in my mouth and Claire perched too
high in the show saddle, which sparkled more than
either Claire or I, I had no means to assist Claire in finding her breath as I had done in our early days, when
Claire would often tumble in her words, or stutter, as
her father called it. I tried to sigh a long sigh, but with
so much dust in the ring, the result sounded more like a
cough.

Mrs. Maiden motioned for us to walk on toward the
gate. Claire patted my neck. "Mother?" Claire asked.
"Just have fun, right?"

Mother told Claire and me as we entered the ring,
"Right, have fun and be safe!" She patted Claire's leg
and then my neck.

"Number one-eighty-five, Claire Dunlap, riding
Take-A-Chance," the announcer called out as we

entered the ring. I've never been addressed by any name other than Chancey. Even my registered documentation, as far as I am aware, reads Chancey. Claire had wanted me to have an official show name; Mother had come up with Take-A-Chance. I felt as proud at that moment, hearing my new show name called along with Claire's, as I ever have in my life.

I know that we took the first jump fine. Six strides out, I saw the jump clearly and straight ahead of us. I heard Claire counting, "One, two, one, two, one, two." I had come rely on her counting to compensate for the darkness in my left eye. Claire's voice command — "Jump!" — accompanied by an even squeeze of her legs and the raising of her hands to be nearer my ears, aided me in flying over the jump, as we had practiced in our training. We attacked the fence with purpose and unison. I listened for Claire's breathing, but could not find it.

Still, our first small fence was textbook. I felt it to be so, and as we passed by, I heard Mrs. Maiden call out to us, "Perfect!"

We completed the first jump and, cantering away, rounded the ring toward the left. I did not relax a bit, for Claire had not. I listened closely for her second wave of counting. I saw Claire's father out of my right eye; I'm certain that Claire saw him, too, for I felt the slightest tilt of her head in his direction. She was so proud that he had come to see her. Claire sat higher in the saddle, making little contact with me.

Perhaps, had the two jumps been placed in a simple line with two strides in between, the day would have ended pleasantly. On the second approach, Claire did not count, and I did not feel her legs firm on me as I had at our first jump. I could not find Claire's aids—neither her legs nor voice instructed me. Nor could my right eye find the second jump, and so I wavered. Not until late in our approach did I see the jump at all.

When the fence did appear, dead-on in front of me, I panicked, unsure what Claire meant for me to do next. She failed to move into jump position. I did not refuse the jump straight on by stopping, for having gathered a nice speed, I knew that an abrupt halt, even if Claire was intending our retreat, would likely throw her over my head. Not feeling Claire's right leg resisting my duck, I did not aim to take the fence—though in looking back, I know I could have managed to barrel through it, had I kept my wits. I swerved out to the right without breaking stride and without Claire. She was so light.

To my right and just behind me, I saw Claire fall, first up and then down. I could do nothing. I heard her helmet crack against the ground. In unison, the spectators gasped for air. I whipped quickly around, but in the slowest measure of time could only watch Claire bounce off of her head and come to a rest near the jump rail.

I galloped back to Claire, slowing to a walk only when I came directly upon her. Reaching her before anyone else, I bowed my head and blew across her face. Her eyes remained closed, and nothing of Claire moved. I blew again, this time closer to her face, and waited to catch the smell of her breath back to me. I could find no breath, no smell of Claire, only a great weight in my chest. I found no voice of my own to call for help. Everyone around us moved about slowly, too slowly. In those first few moments of Claire's unconsciousness, I had no one to help me revive Claire.

Some horses beg and spend their entire lives begging. Whatever they do get is never enough and they beg for more, constantly. I have probably not asked for enough in my life. At Tamworth Springs I asked for Claire. In fact, I begged for Claire. I didn't ponder it. I fell to my knees to be nearer to Claire and simultaneously to beg my Creator, and Claire's, to awaken her quickly with either my breath or His. I lay beside Claire.

As I set my head near Claire's, again I heard the crowd suck in their own collective breath. I could not speak to Claire but with my heart, and with it I showed her everything we had yet to do. There was still Saddle Mountain to be explored. I had yet to take Claire across the Maury River. She had promised to play her violin for me. We had planned to one day gallop through the snow.

I gave my breath to Claire. I begged Claire to wake up and forgive me for dropping her. My prayers for her restoration were interrupted by a change of pace; everyone who had been so slow to reach us now descended upon us. My stomach tightened. I remained on the ground next to Claire.

"Get that horse away from my daughter," Claire's father demanded. I looked to Mother for protection, for she was now kneeling beside us. Mother took no notice of me or the command that I be removed from the show ring.

Instead, Mother began yelling for help. I stood up and with my voice strong now, joined with Mother and whinnied long and shrill to better relay our urgent need for assistance. Still, Claire did not move, nor did she answer the questions that Mrs. Maiden had begun asking to ascertain whether Claire was damaged by the impact of the fall.

Daisy, carrying Ann, stood at the entrance to the show ring, watching our attempts. Daisy tossed her head toward me, but that was of small comfort.

Claire's father spoke sharply under his breath to Mother. "For God's sake, Eleanor, I told you this would happen. What were you thinking? The horse is dangerous; he's half blind."

My chest tightened; a weakness grew there and

spread within me. I felt the brick in my stomach churn. I dropped my head down toward Claire. I wanted to roll.

Mother stayed crouched beside Claire, holding her hand. She did not look up.

Still, Claire's father persisted. "Eleanor? Did you hear me? That's it; it's over. The horse needs to be sold. He's hurt Claire. Do you understand? We're getting rid of him."

Mother said nothing. She held Claire's hand and kissed her forehead again and again.

Claire's father said to no one in particular, "Will someone get this horse out of here? He's hurt my daughter. He needs to be taken away."

Mother did not look up and did not speak. I stood by Mother, for she needed me and so did Claire. I stepped in closer, for I belonged with them.

Claire remained motionless; again I blew a long breath out, across her nose and mouth. My girl opened her eyes, but I gather was not altogether restored.

More people joined us, and the biased judge grabbed my reins to lead me out of the ring. I refused to go and sank all of my one thousand pounds as far into the earth as I could. The judge, with warmth that I did not expect, turned to face me and patted my shoulder. "Come on, fella. The rescue squad will take good care of her."

I whinnied at Claire. She did not respond. I whinnied at Mother. Mother looked up at me with her sad eyes. She smiled at me and finally opened her mouth to speak.

"Please, Eleanor, this horse has got to go!" shouted Claire's father.

He snatched my reins from the judge and began pulling on me. He yanked hard on my mouth, but for Mother and Claire I absorbed the pain because I would not leave them. Mother jumped up and took the reins from his hand. Without shouting, she faced him squarely and told him, "Chancey is our horse. You don't get to decide. He's not your horse."

Mother handed the reins back to the judge. Then she kissed my poll and whispered in my ear, her voice cracking, "You're going home now, Chancey. I'm going with Claire. You belong with us; don't ever forget that, boy."

The judge again tried to comfort me. "That's a boy; come with me. Claire will be just fine." Her voice conveyed no pigment bias toward me whatsoever. I yielded to the judge's pull and watched the rescue squad take Claire and Mother away.

CHAPTER THIRTEEN

Waiting Out the Storm

I ached to leave Tamworth Springs at the instant that Claire left, but was required to stay on, as we had all traveled there together for the purpose of allowing Claire and Ann to compete. Mrs. Maiden took my reins from the judge and thanked her for holding me. I could think of nothing but Claire. I did everything to slow my breathing, yet it remained fast and shallow.

The judge resumed her post. After a moment, the announcer started the class again. "Short Stirrup Over Eighteen-Inch Fences. Number one-eighty-six, Ann Hayden, riding Shasta Daisy."

We waited for Daisy and Ann to enter the ring. Ann wouldn't budge, but motioned for Mrs. Maiden. The child was understandably shaken up. She did not try to choke back her tears. "I want to get off now. I don't want to jump," she cried.

Mrs. Maiden spoke gently to her. "Are you sure? Take a deep breath. Trust Daisy; you'll be fine. Can you do that?"

Ann opened her mouth and breathed. She looked at the show ring and patted Daisy's neck. Daisy stood still and quiet; she did not dance or shift her weight at all. She waited for Ann to decide. Mrs. Maiden encouraged the girl to breathe in deep.

Finally, Ann said, "Okay. I'm okay." She picked up the reins and clucked for Daisy to walk on.

Daisy did her job. She was, I believe, born for the purpose of taking little girls over little fences. Ann did not count, for on Daisy little girls need only to sit deep, look graceful, and trust. The pair took the two little jumps superbly, placing first in the class.

Though I stood beside Mrs. Maiden watching the event, I could only see the image in my mind of Claire sprawled on the ground and Mother kissing her face to wake her up. There was much noise around me, yet nothing could deafen to me the sound of Claire's father saying, "The horse is dangerous. This horse needs to be sold."

The words of Claire's father and the image of Claire, whom I had hurt, began to tangle themselves together until the pain of the morning had woven itself into severe knots deep inside my gut. Reflexively, I began biting and kicking at my sides in an effort to disperse the knots and free myself from the memories of the morning. I needed to get home.

After the end of the jumper class, I began to dance around with enough fuss that Mrs. Maiden knew to take me back to the trailer. I could not watch the Pleasure class. I wanted to roll, not for the joy of rolling, but to break up what had become the constant cramping in my belly. Right there at Tamworth Springs, I badly wanted to roll and never get up. I did not give in. I waited at the trailer for my teammates' return.

Though it may have appeared that I waited quietly, on the inside I twisted with pain and regret. Every second that passed was more horrific than the one that preceded it, for it brought no relief from the tangles, no relief from the guilt, and no relief from the certain knowledge that my future with Claire was in jeopardy.

When it came time to depart Tamworth Springs, I loaded easily into the trailer as is mostly my habit anyway. Daisy, Ann, Mrs. Maiden, and I drove back to our barn without Claire. In the trailer, Daisy tried to comfort me. "Don't worry. Claire's a tough little girl. I've known her a long time. She'll hold no grudge against you."

I appreciated Daisy's sympathy, and it softened me toward her greatly, as I confess, I still held sourness in my heart concerning the flea-bitten Welsh.

Though I would have preferred that Macadoo, my friend and fieldmate, the Belgian who had traveled with me to Albemarle and who had helped me find my place among the geldings, be the one to see me in this state of vulnerability, I found myself in such desperate need of assurance that I willingly risked reaching out to Daisy.

"Daisy? What if the girl's father is right? He said I am dangerous. He said I need to be sold." I rumbled softly, feeling some relief at letting another know what had occurred in the show ring. I hoped I was not foolish to seek some affirmation from the mare.

Daisy moved closer to me. She offered no comforting exchange of breaths. Nor did we touch noses.

"You know you'll never be a jumper of the caliber that I am. That's a fact you have to face. The sooner you do face it, the better for you and for Claire. Claire should do her jumping with me. I've said that from the beginning."

Her words stung like a hard rain striking into my eyes. I moved away from Daisy as far as the cramped trailer would allow. Had there been room to entirely turn away from Daisy, I would have shut the conversation down completely. I had, indeed, been an impulsive fool to reach out. Daisy had won; I had no energy to argue. Daisy and Claire's father were right.

Then Daisy spoke again. "Chancey, I've got to face the facts, too. Claire's father can't see the truth right now. I couldn't see it at first either. Gwen was right; Claire is your girl and you are her horse. You can't give up on her now. If you think you will be sold because of what happened today, I think you are underestimating Claire and her mother. If you are willing to give up so easily, then you are not the horse everyone's been trying to convince me that you are. And if they do sell you, then so be it. We will all go away one day."

Daisy leaned over the railing between us. "I know this, Chancey. In my lifetime, I have belonged with someone, and now he's gone. But it was worth it."

I rumbled to myself. I belonged with Claire; I could not deny that I belonged with Claire. I nipped at my belly, for the tangles would not relinquish their grip on me.

"Whatever happens, do not colic now," Daisy urged me.

I knew she was right. For no matter what the future held, every moment with Claire had been worth it. Though I wanted to acknowledge Daisy's kindness to me, I found myself unable to respond. My heart ached; the brick in my belly had increased in size. I could not reciprocate.

Daisy recognized my condition and did not require that I respond in kind. She leaned across the gate between us and blew on me. "Do not colic. Do you hear me? That little girl will need you when she recovers. Do not colic!" I knew that Daisy was correct: Claire needed me.

I do not pretend to have a medical understanding of how colic endangers horses. Nor am I well versed in its causes. I am well aware that colic is life-threatening. I know firsthand that it can arrive without warning, and that, even with ample warning, there are times when colic cannot be stopped. I can tell when it is imminent. Having colicked once in my life, I know what it is to face the possibility of such a painful death.

I was just a colt when my dam sustained a fatal injury; she had been defending *me*. A new mare had been introduced to our field and had challenged my presence there. Dam suffered greatly from a break in her shoulder. She could not have recovered. I know this now. Though I have lately heard of a horse that recovered from such a break, after surgery, it was not even a consideration those many years ago. I was a colt and I could not save Dam. Nothing could have saved Dam. My dam was resting in the field, stoically accepting her pain, waiting until they could come to take her away, as she knew they would. I stood vigil, protecting her as she had done for me so many times.

Dam knew that Monique would soon come to put an end to her suffering, and my dam was accepting—I think, grateful. The other mares visited Dam. One by one, each of them closed their eyes and whispered a final blessing across Dam's face. Even as the last mountain breeze she would feel waltzed around us, I begged Dam not to leave me. I was just a colt.

My dam did not turn back once Monique arrived to take her from the field.

"Come on, Starry; let's go now." Monique spoke tenderly to Dam. I whinnied and paced the fence line, urging Dam to turn around. I stood at the gate calling for her to look at me once more, for I knew if she did, she would come back to me. Though in grave pain, Dam walked on with Monique as if she were only going to be shod and then return.

I cried out for Dam morning and night, all the while fasting from food and water, so badly did I wish her with me. I was presently seized with a pain tangled deeply in my bowels. The knot clenched its grip on me forcefully and repeatedly, until I too lay down, ready to accept the consequence. I was just a colt.

I yearned for my dam; I lay down in the spot where she had lain. The grass was still matted from her weight, and something of her smell lingered there, too. I closed my eyes and wished for Saddle Mountain to bend over me and swaddle me so tightly that I would disappear into it forever. But mountains do not bend.

I writhed in the wet grass until finally I heard, "Get up." The mares had come to me, but they did not whisper their last blessings.

"Get up, Chancey. Get up and walk," they ordered me.

By turns, the mares pushed me up to my feet and, in pairs, boxed me between them. The mares tended to me by forcing me to stand up and move about until the tangled knots passed through me. I soon drank and ate again. But I was not the same. I was just a colt when my dam left and I colicked. I had not expected to ever love or depend on another as I had my dam. But I had not yet met Claire.

Returning from Tamworth Springs, I fought against colic for the second time in my life. I badly needed relief from what had ahold of me, just as badly as I had needed relief as a colt. I told myself that I would roll just once, just once for a second of peace. I dropped to my forearms. No sooner had I given my mind over to this urge than did the sky open up with such a forceful rain and wind that I instinctively rose to seek shelter in the run-in. Finding it crowded with the other geldings, I moved on, for upon seeing me, Dante pinned back his ears and would not allow me to enter the shelter.

There was one spot in my field, from which if I stood just so with my head held rather up, I could see the entire line of Saddle Mountain. Being that the spot is high on a hill in the far corner of my field, it took some effort to reach during the storm. It was there that I gave up. For the second time in my life, I then gave in to colic. Its grip was too tight; I could do nothing but roll and seek relief. Either the tangles would pass and I would live through the pain, or the tangles would win and I would die alone in the storm. I dropped to the ground and opened my belly to the sky. This time, there were no mares to tend to me. There was only the wind and the rain. Just as before, Saddle Mountain waited for the colic to run its course in me.

My mind began to create nonsense out of the wind. "Get up," I heard. Certain that my mind had now joined my eyes in a state of decline, and this voice was mere evidence of a new impairment, I whinnied to drown out the voice.

"Get up! Get up!" I heard the demand again, only in a much louder and firmer tone than either the mares of my youth or than I supposed my own confused mind might urge.

Softer now, more like a whisper in my ear, it was the Belgian, Macadoo, who called to me. "Get up and walk, friend." He pushed me up with his big head, and together we paced the hill in the pouring rain. Stu tried calling us in from the storm with grain buckets; Mac refused to leave my side, saying only, "I have been where you are, afraid and unsure of tomorrow. We will walk through the night together."

Through the storm we walked; I fought off the urge to fall to the ground and roll. We could not see Saddle Mountain through the sheets of rain. The wind threw branches and sticks to our feet, but I did not drop. The rain quickly filled the dry ruts in the field, and new rivers rushed down all around us. At times, the field turned so thick with mud that we sank down to our fetlocks. Still, we kept moving. Mac would not let the colic win.

When the danger of colic had passed, Mac and I stood together under the row of cedars at the fence line, waiting for the morning. I felt thirsty; I grazed on the wet grass and it caused no cramping or pain. Mac detected that some anxiety still lingered.

"What is it, friend? Why are you afraid?" he asked.

"I am not afraid. I am not afraid of hunger or cold or being beaten. I am not afraid anything. I am an Appaloosa; have you forgotten?"

Mac nuzzled me as a mother would do. "Chancey, it's me." He asked the question again, "Why are you afraid?"

I considered resisting Mac, but thought the better of it, for the Belgian had saved my life. As surely as the mares had saved me when I colicked at Dam's death,

Mac had saved me when I colicked at the thought of losing Claire,

I decided to speak the truth. "I am old, Macadoo. I am old and have been called dangerous for all to hear by Claire's father. He has even publicly called for my sale. I am afraid of myself. I am afraid to go back to that barn. I am afraid of Lynchville. I fear going blind; I fear I will forget the blue mountains."

Mac tossed his head back and forth. "My friend, you are carrying a great burden. Why don't you set it down now? There's no need to clutch it any longer. Have you not noticed? You live among friends now. You are loved."

I dropped my head to the ground, for the weight of these worries did, indeed, feel heavy. We grazed in silence under the stars. The force of the storm had moved farther south. From our hilltop we could appreciate its beauty as we watched it circle around the valley.

"Did you mean to hurt Claire?" Mac asked me.

"I am bound to Claire forever," I answered. "I would never hurt Claire."

"Do you enjoy jumping? Is that your purpose in life?"

I had never considered such a question. I ate some more grass; I was hungry. I knew not to eat too much until I could drink water and pass a normal stool.

I answered, "I love Claire, and Claire loves to jump. I'm not a jumper; it hurts me to jump. I love the open field. I can see better there, and my other senses can more easily help out. I love to teach. When a student is open, like Claire, I do love to teach. I love these blue mountains more than anything, besides Claire. Claire wants to be a teacher, you know."

Mac tossed his head, then touched my neck. "Well, there you are, Old App. You must stop jumping right away. Do not spend another moment jumping, for every moment jumping takes you further away from your purpose of teaching and showing students the joys of riding in these mountains."

I will admit that the burdens that had locked my stomach so tightly and forced me to the ground now vanished. I passed a very satisfying round of gas. Mac grazed beside me as if all had been happily resolved.

"Mac, what if the father is right? What if they sell me?" Mac looked up at me with a mouthful of grass. Our field was so wet from the storm that a foam of grassy residue had formed around his entire muzzle.

"Chancey, I have gone to auction twice in my life, yet I stand here before you a horse fulfilled. Both times, I endured and witnessed beatings by ignorant men. The first time, I was a yearling and had no one to protect me. Hundreds of others were lost to kill buyers in an instant. Despite their fine breeding, many finer than I, they were sold at a price measured per pound. Do you know what that means?"

I did not respond for I knew well the answer. I walked away from Mac to the other side of the hill, following the track of the storm below us. Mac followed me.

"They were eaten, Chancey. When the value of a horse is measured in his weight, Chancey, by the pound, it means he will be eaten. I was sold to a gentleman farmer, a gruff old man with a kind heart and a bad leg, for one thousand dollars flat. I survived. I am blessed and haunted by it daily. I had only a vision, placed on my heart by my mother, of a greater purpose for my life. Had I fought them at auction, I would not be here. Had I given myself over to them completely at auction, I would not be here. Acceptance is not the same as giving up. You seem to be giving up."

"But I am old. At auction, I would surely be sold for meat." I quivered at having finally named that which frightened me the most. Mac lost his patience with me. He reared up slightly.

"You must lead Claire and her mother to a new vision, Chancey. What is it that you want? Jumping is but one way to be a girl's horse. Has the father the final say in this matter? At the show, what did Claire's mother say about all of this?"

I thought back to Tamworth Springs. Mother was so quiet and lost in Claire's injury that I had lost her in my own recollection of the day. Claire's unconsciousness and her father's condemnation of me as a dangerous horse had overshadowed Mother, who in her grief, I now recalled, had spoken to me as the judge led me out. I tried to remember.

"Yes," I finally told Mac. "Mother did speak to me. She told me something very important. She whispered to me, 'You belong with us; don't ever forget that.'" Mac whinnied at me. "And I seem to have forgotten right away."

"Take heart, Chancey. Your work here is not completed. Only now are you ready to begin."

I stood with Mac in the gelding field that night and did not sleep at all. Claire did not come the next day, or the next, or the next, for her recovery took some time. While I waited, I forced myself to return to Mother's words—"you belong with us"—each and every time I became anxious.

Though neither Claire nor I realized it, the calamitous jump at the Tamworth Springs show would be our last jump together for some time. While our love for each other would grow deeper and stronger, this aspect of our working—training together as a hunter team—had come to an end.

CHAPTER FOURTEEN

Ode to Joy

A week or more had passed, yet Claire still had not returned to the barn, nor had I any word of her condition. One afternoon, Mrs. Maiden came to me. She related to me that Claire had suffered a concussion, and though Claire was expected to make a full recovery, she would not be fully well for several more weeks. Mrs. Maiden's voice cracked when she spoke, and thus I could tell that she had been worried, too.

Though still under her doctor's care, Claire successfully prevailed upon Mother to bring her to the Maury River Stables just to see me. Claire insisted that the doctor's order of no riding did not mean no visiting. Tenderhearted Mother not only allowed Claire this occasion, but she believed that a visit would hasten Claire's recovery. This was reported directly to me by Mrs. Maiden, who not only informed me of Claire's impending visit, but showed me a great kindness by taking the time to groom me in preparation.

I appreciated this kindness very much, not only because it helped me to feel my very best for Claire, but also because it was the first time that Mrs. Maiden had expressed a true fondness for me. Make no mistake: the care that I had received, and receive to this day, was expression enough of Mrs. Maiden's deep love of all horses. But our grooming time, as we both waited for Claire and Mother, was Mrs. Maiden's first real display of personal affection for me, Chancey.

Mrs. Maiden set my brush box beside my front feet; it will come as no surprise to those familiar with the habits of girls that the brush box Claire had chosen for me was also purple. Starting on my left side, Mrs. Maiden began to brush my coat, talking to me the entire time. I enjoyed the sound of her voice, not just for what she told me, but for the fact that even though I could not see her, I could feel her at my left side and so never felt surprised at any action that she took. Mrs. Maiden is a kind woman, but she does not always feel as relaxed as she did on this morning. Understandably, with her great responsibilities of providing safety and protection to children and horses, as well as a few barn mothers like Mother who ride, she is often too preoccupied to relax.

With the same warmth that she uses only for the very youngest of her pupils, Mrs. Maiden said to me, "Claire's on her way, handsome boy. I know you've missed her. Claire's mother thinks a short visit will help her feel better."

Mrs. Maiden used a soft brush to clean my face; I closed my eyes and let the dirt fall from them to the floor. She lowered her voice and, touching my cheek, spoke again. "You know, sometimes little girls are hurt more inside than outside after a fall like Claire's. I bet her mother's right: a visit with you is probably just what she needs."

Mrs. Maiden fluffed my forelock and tucked our third-place Walk-Trot ribbon into my halter. Standing there in my room with the late afternoon sun streaming in the window and resting on my crest, I gave thanks for Claire's health and the many days we would have together.

Claire appeared at the door to my room just as Mrs. Maiden finished up. "You're gorgeous, Chancey! Did you get dressed up just for me?" Claire asked me.

Before I could manage any kind of an answer, Mrs. Maiden blurted, "Claire! You sure didn't get dressed up for Chancey. You're in your pajamas!"

Claire seemed not to hear Mrs. Maiden, for she did not answer her but threw her arms around me. "Oh, Chancey. I missed you so much. I don't even remember what happened the entire day. Mother said we got third place in the Walk-Trot class."

Noticing the ribbon, Claire observed, "The yellow ribbon looks pretty on you." She took the ribbon in her hands and confided in me, "I don't remember anything about the show. I only know I fell because Mother says so. I'm sure it was all my fault. Don't worry, boy, we'll be riding again soon. Mother and the doctor won't let me jump for a while. But we'll be together soon, I promise."

Daisy was right; Claire harbored no blame or resentment about the accident. Had my Creator given me tears to cry, I would have shed them all at that moment, so relieved was I that Claire did not intend to give up on us. Mother, I was also relieved to observe, seemed to share happiness at our reunion.

I listened closely to Claire's voice, as she told me how we would win our next show. She continued planning and dreaming of how high we would be jumping by the end of the year. I listened, but did not allow myself to dream with her. Claire rested her head on my shoulder and told me, "Chancey, you are everything I've ever wanted in a pony. Thank you for trying so hard, and for always being here for me."

Mother interrupted Claire's dreamy plans. "Claire, when you do return to jumping, we can't ask Chancey to jump with you again." Claire stopped breathing.

"Wh-what? But he's my pony. I don't want to ride anybody else, just Chancey." I moved closer to Claire, for I felt this same wave of sickness myself.

"I know, sweetheart. We have to honor Chancey and recognize his strengths and talents. It hurts him to jump. He tries so hard because he loves you so much, but it's not easy for him. To ask Chancey to jump higher and higher because you want to jump higher and higher is very unfair and very unkind. And one day, it could be very dangerous for both of you."

"Oh." Claire leaned into me. She rested her head on my shoulder and smelled me. "Oh." Claire nuzzled her face in my coat.

She began to cry. "D-D-D-D-Dad said we're selling him. I'll run, run, run away if we sell Ch-Chancey."

Claire clung to me and cried, hiding herself in my neck. "Please, Mother. Let me keep him. We don't have to j-jump. I love him so much. We can trail ride. I can practice my dressage. I can take him on a hunter pace. Please, he can do so many things."

Mother wiped Claire's face. "Claire, we will never sell Chancey. He is our family."

Claire laughed out loud and began crying again. I pressed my head close to my girl's heart and at the same time, flicked Mother with my tail.

Mrs. Maiden laughed, too. "Chancey is an amazing horse, Claire. He's just not a jumper, that's all. But he has so many other talents. When you're all better, you and I will find the perfect job for Chancey. In the meantime, let me take care of him and let your mother take care of you. Is that a deal?"

Claire hugged Mrs. Maiden, then Mother. "Deal." She nodded.

"Claire," Mrs. Maiden said, "let's turn Chancey out for the night. Would you like to lead him?"

Claire nodded furiously. "Could I?"

Then, as if it had almost slipped her mind, Claire asked permission to do something quite different. "Mrs. Maiden, I brought my violin to play Chancey a song. I've been practicing. Will that be okay?"

"What a nice idea, Claire—horses love music. In fact, why don't you go on and take him out to the gelding field and play there so Chancey and all of his friends can enjoy it?" Mrs. Maiden smiled.

Claire led me out to the field, with Mother following behind us. I noticed then that Mother held in her hands a black bag of sorts. As the three of us approached the gate, Dante, Napoleon, and Mac crowded the fence to greet Claire. Daisy, Princess, and Gwen all cantered along our adjoining fence line to greet her. I was not the only one who had missed Claire.

Dressed in her pajamas, Claire looked very much smaller than I had remembered. As is often the case after a storm, the entrance to our field was a mud pit, made worse by Dante's incessant pacing back and forth, guarding the gate, presumably against some unseen enemy. Claire and Mother seemed oblivious to the condition of the field and to their own ill-suited attire.

I stuck close to Claire as she unbuckled my halter. Mother opened the black bag and handed Claire what I presumed was the violin. I remembered how Claire had told me of her music when we first met. I nickered for Claire to show me the instrument.

Sensing my curiosity, Claire held the violin out to my right eye for inspection, for Claire was well aware not only of my blindness in the left but also of the narrow blind spot directly in front of my nose. Then she lifted the violin to her chin and with a stick of sorts began drawing out a low, sweet sound. I moved in closer to Claire's playing arm. She paused and encouraged me to thoroughly examine the stick.

"Chancey, this is called a bow," she instructed me.

With the ability to draw such rich notes from a hollow, wooden box, I should not have been surprised to find, as I was, that the stick, or bow as Claire called it, was strung end to end with strands of horse tail. I blew onto it.

"You're such a smart pony, Chancey. Of course, you're right. The bow is made from horsehair. So you see how horses and people make music together?" I nickered at Claire, encouraging her to continue playing.

My girl closed her eyes and brought the violin to her chin once more. I found that the notes appealed not only to me but, as Mrs. Maiden had predicted, to all of the geldings. All of us encircled Claire and Mother, getting as close as possible so that we could hear and see the fine gift Claire brought us.

I noticed that almost directly behind me, even the mares had lined the fence separating our two fields. They had stopped gossiping and gathered around to listen. I turned my head slightly toward the mares, to encourage them to come even closer, yet remain quiet. I am always amazed, and grateful, at the connection Claire and I have and credit the depth of this connection entirely to Claire's open heart and keen skills at observation. She saw, or felt, me indicate direction to the mares and ever accommodating and while continuing to play, Claire walked closer to the mares' fence so they, too, could share in the sweetness.

The geldings and I moved with Claire, as she now played to nearly twenty horses. We remained quiet, hoping that our stillness might consent Claire to play on. She played for us, without interruption, through many songs, occasionally asking Mother's advice as to which tune should be played next. Finally, Mother indicated to Claire that the time had come to leave.

Claire is as gifted in the art of managing Mother as she is in riding or playing music. She pleaded, "One more song, okay? What should I play?"

Mother indulged her without any sign of irritation or impatience. "Okay, one more song, Claire. Play 'Ode to Joy'; you've been working hard on it."

Again, Claire closed her eyes and poised her elbow in the air while she took in a deep breath. The cedar and river birch, all of us in the field, reached out to the sun, now falling behind the blue mountains. As Claire's bow pulled across the strings, the sun made one last rally, splashing our field with its easy afternoon light. I leaned in closer to Claire, grateful that she had not been irreparably harmed by the accident, and grateful that she was standing here with me. The storm had indeed passed; I wished for this song never to end.

When Claire finished playing, all of us remained standing near her, wishing, I think, for one more song. She handed the violin to Mother, then walked back to me, her pajama pants covered in mud. She stroked my neck; I felt content to be near her.

"Chancey, I have to go now. I love you, pony. I'll be

back soon, when I'm all better." Claire kissed me on my cheek, as little girls are fond of doing to horses.

Then she ran to catch up with Mother. Mother protectively slipped her arm around Claire's waist; Claire pressed her head into Mother's arms and leaned full into them. Mother nuzzled Claire's face, then opened the gate. I watched them walk all the way to the barn. Claire turned back several times to wave and blow me kisses. I nickered good-bye as she and Mother disappeared into the barn. Then, from the barn, Claire turned back once more and shouted to me, "I love you, Chancey! Sweet dreams!"

I was glad that we were still on evening turnout. Once the weather turned cold for good, we would again spend evenings in our rooms. The early autumn stars came down so close to the field, I felt sure that, from my spot on the hill, if I stretched up just a bit more, I would find myself among them, and perhaps I might find Dam there, too.

I stood all night watching for just one fire star and fell asleep waiting. No stars raced through the sky. Instead, the stars gathered close around me and held me in my sleep. When I awoke, in the morning, I understood. Dam had long ago told me that the stars said something special was planned for me. Finally, I understood.

In the morning, the gelding field looked very much the same as it had every day before, green and open with steps of granite boulders rising to the blue mountains. Napoleon was hiding under the cedar trees at the fence line; I could see his fat legs sticking out from under the branches and his long, blond tail sweeping the grass. Dante paced the gate, waiting for more hay to come. Mac grazed beside me, passing over the chickweed in search of any remaining clover. The mares were fighting over the morning's hay.

The world had not changed overnight, but I had. I had felt outcast among people and horses for much of my life. Even so, I had devoted twenty years to teaching. I had developed a strong habit of showing up and carrying on even though I hurt, even though I could no longer see well. Claire had shown me the most important lesson of all—that love grows when you give it away. Now, at last, I was ready to accept my calling. An extraordinary new beginning lay only a few months ahead for Claire and me, and it began with a gunshot.

CHAPTER FIFTEEN

A Bombproof Pony

Guns don't frighten me, though I am aware of their capacity to harm animals and people. While I have no firsthand knowledge of a horse being mistaken for a deer, there are certain seasons when the threat does exist. It is uncommon for hunters to shoot near horses or cattle, so if we remain in our fields, we remain safe. The deer, of course, know this undisputed rule and thus often does, and occasionally bucks, will seek refuge among us. I can't say that I blame them at all. I might well be terrified myself if every second of daylight brought the threat of armed pursuit with intent to kill me.

Here at the Maury River Stables, Mrs. Maiden runs a special type of riding school, which she calls therapeutic. This school is indeed therapeutic for all involved in its operation, though I believe that the term *therapeutic* refers to the needs of the students enrolled. Mrs. Maiden chose me for the program not long after a rather disturbing incident in the gelding field one morning during the deer-hunting season. No one was hurt, and the day turned out quite well for me and opened the door to a future with a purpose so rewarding that I could not have imagined it for myself.

Before I describe my display of courage that drew Mrs. Maiden's attention, I must explain that I had encountered hunters and their weapons on two prior occasions. Both occasions, no doubt, drilled into me the response that Mrs. Maiden had found so admirable.

I first witnessed the power of guns at Monique's barn during the deer-hunting season some years ago. Monique was born with a good deal of fight in her; if she were a mare, she would undoubtedly be the boss. I admired this quality and sometimes felt that she recognized a bit of herself in me, which, despite a somewhat difficult two decades together, contributed to our long union. I remember one morning a deer herd, having been driven out of the forest by hunters, arrived at the mare field seeking asylum. Half as many men as deer soon followed and took it upon themselves to set up on

Monique's land in order to run the deer out of the field, in spite of clear trespass notices along the tree line.

Not surprisingly, Monique directly confronted the party of hunters, who had arrived with no shortage of guns or egos. It was an easy enough confrontation to predict, knowing Monique's strong distaste for hunters on the eastern side of her property. It should be noted that for many years, Monique granted exclusive rights to an older gentleman and his grandson to hunt the western side of her property with no restrictions save one—to give up the chase, even if in hot pursuit, if it meant coming into any of the fields with horses standing. I relay that to establish that, in fact, Monique held no prejudice against hunters, but did hold a strong prejudice about hunting her land without permission, especially too near her mares.

As Monique approached the hunting party, with commensurate gun and ego in tow, she neither flinched nor hesitated. She walked with sure stride, her gun pointed toward the ground, to the truck where the hunters had gathered. I was able to observe the incident, as the entire scene unfolded where the mare and gelding fences converged. Monique asked the hunters to leave, explaining that not only were they trespassing, but they were frightening her mares. The hunters laughed. I shook my head at their underestimation of Monique.

Monique did not laugh, but demanded that they

vacate her property immediately. There was no stutter in her voice; no syllable remained in her throat. One of the hunters adamantly claimed his right to engage because of hot pursuit. At that, I distanced myself from the dispute to create a safety buffer between us. The other geldings and mares followed suit.

Monique pointed her gun to the sky and fired it, startling the mares, the deer, and the hunters, who promptly left. No one was harmed, and our fields soon returned to normal. Thanks to Monique and her gun, we did not have such trouble again.

I have witnessed Mrs. Maiden make good use of her gun as well, again in defense of mares. It is here that I must stop and share my opinion that if Mrs. Maiden, or Monique for that matter, had considered placing a stallion, or even a strong gelding, with the mares, there might be no need for such protection, as that is the role of a strong male. I digress.

Though coyotes are not native to Rockbridge County, or the blue mountains, they have immigrated here and seem intent on settling. Horse farms, such as the Maury River Stables, haven't as much to fear from these rascally canines as do our neighboring cattle and sheep farms. Coyotes will, on occasion, however, intrude upon our mares, just for sport, I believe. This doesn't happen often, and again the placement of a strong male could deter this kind of taunting. Often, once the mares have banded together and threatened death by stomping, the coyotes will leave of their own accord.

Only once have I seen a coyote fail to respond to well-directed kicks and bites from our mares. That coyote, foaming at the mouth, met his death quickly, though I doubt painlessly, by the hand of Mrs. Maiden. She was alerted to the security breach in the mare field by my desperate calling to her. Upon seeing the coyote tormenting the mares, Mrs. Maiden retrieved her shotgun and, without a trace of fear, marched into the mare field, yelling at the coyote to distract him.

Though not all coyotes are call-shy, not even the most curious, if sound of mind, would have mistaken Mrs. Maiden's vocalizations for anything other than a threat. In the case of our rabid coyote, Mrs. Maiden's yelling had the effect of causing the coyote turn to away from the mares and set his course upon her.

Daisy and the mares cowered in the far corner of their field; Mrs. Maiden stood in the middle of the field, yelling and cursing the coyote. The words that shot out of Mrs. Maiden's mouth are the same words forbidden around the barn. I have seen Mrs. Maiden discharge from her employ more than one foulmouthed, defiant stable hand for such conduct as she displayed toward the coyote. Mrs. Maiden fired off every one of those words, and, indeed, her projectile of cursing seemed to draw the coyote closer to her, which was, of course, Mrs. Maiden's intent all along.

When the beast reached a proximity of about six paces—though you must understand that I am as poor a measurer of distance as I am a keeper of time—Mrs. Maiden simply aimed her gun, cursed at him one last time, and shot him between the eyes. The coyote may have yelped; I can't be certain of it. I am certain that a follow-up shot was unnecessary.

So, you see that I had twice witnessed the power of guns, and their usefulness, in times of danger to horses and people. I had not expected that the firing of gunshots would have led to a new and rewarding career for me. At my age, not much startles me, gunfire included, and that is what led to my recruitment into a new position at the Maury River Stables.

On the day of which I speak, three deer were grazing in the gelding field with us, enjoying quiet refuge from the forest full of hunters. The deer—two does and a young buck with perhaps half a dozen points on his antlers—behaved as if siblings. I had waited patiently for two seasons to lay eyes on the buck; his presence in the blue mountains was well known, for he was an albino, like me.

One should never really be surprised at the exquisite beings that are born of the blue mountains. The does who accompanied the buck seemed oblivious to his unusual coloring and unaware how his presence made them all stand out. Stu, who is a devoted hunter, had himself spoken reverently of the albino buck, whom he had seen and had opportunity to kill but, fearful that taking a pure-white deer might render him cursed, could not bring himself to fire upon. I wrongly assumed that all hunters believed, as Stu, that when our Creator grants us the privilege of sharing our space with a fine and rare creature, such as the white buck, the appropriate response is reverence. I believed the albino buck to be safe within our fence line.

I heard, then saw, on my right, four hunters crouched at the back fence, guns drawn. When I saw them so near our field, I believed they would refrain from opening fire, as the trajectory would have endangered the geldings. They readied their weapons. I lifted my head and turned my right eye more toward them to be sure that I had seen accurately. I confirmed their position and subtly, with only a slight movement of my head, relayed the location of the hunters to the three deer, out of courtesy.

My warning immediately sent the two does racing toward the safety of Saddle Mountain. The white buck remained with us. I moved between the hunters and the buck, though I failed to fully conceal him from the hunters' line of sight. He was too precious for me not to intervene; I expected the hunters to walk away.

What happened next shocked me; I have never known men to shoot so near horses. These men seemed oblivious to us geldings and irreverently unconcerned with the albino. Shooting rather recklessly into our field, they opened fire on him. This close-range firing caused great alarm among the geldings; all but Mac and I stampeded to the southern side of the fence. Fearing for their lives, ten geldings tore down the fence and galloped toward the Maury River, away from the hunting party. The buck took cover within the stampede and all escaped, unharmed.

Only Mac and I remained in our field. We called for Mrs. Maiden, who came quickly with Stu. Mrs. Maiden and Stu pieced together the chain of events quite accurately and with great speed. Wasting not a second, Mac escorted Mrs. Maiden and Stu to the fence, where they rightly observed that it been torn apart in a surge of fear by all of the missing geldings. While those three inspected the fence, I walked to the spot where the firing had begun, seeking any evidence that might be helpful to their investigation. On the ground, I spied an item similar to the residue that was left on the ground after Mrs. Maiden killed the coyote; I believed it to be a shell.

Certain that my discovery was germane to the investigation, I trotted over, nudging Mrs. Maiden to follow me back to the spot. As I suspected, the shell provided confirmation to Mrs. Maiden and Stu of the incident. They rightly reconstructed the event, though they mistakenly deduced that there must have been one deer in the field, having no way of knowing that, in fact, three deer had that day been saved. Feeling that this detail was not critical for the recovery of our fieldmates, neither Mac nor I wasted any energy on the great effort it would have taken, such as presenting the two with multiple sets of tracks, to correct the notion of a solitary deer. It must be said that Mac and I both ably directed them to every clue available, short of opening our mouths and speaking.

Before Mrs. Maiden set about the chore of bringing the ten escapees home, she turned to Mac and me and, with very apparent gratitude, gave us each a nice pat, saying, "Thank you both, my brave boys. You weren't afraid, were you?"

She turned toward the barn to retrieve lead ropes and grain to bring the geldings home. Then she turned back to me and said, "Chancey! I've got an idea! Would you like a new job? I need a good, sound horse—a bombproof horse—to help Mac, Gwen, and me teach in the therapeutic school. Ask your buddy Mac what he thinks. I'll ask Claire's mother."

This seemed a revelation as to how a new vision of belonging with Claire would come to pass. Claire and I had met just when each of us needed the other. Claire needed a companion to help her sort out her feelings and find her confidence at a difficult time in her family life. She needed a friend who would believe in her and give her the courage to be great and true to herself. And I had needed exactly the same. What we had already accomplished together was more precious than one hundred blue ribbons; I did not want to see that foundation erode over time because any future ribbons weren't the right color.

I faced the truth of the matter. Whether she knew it or not, Claire needed something that I could not give her. Claire needed to be a champion; she needed to win. Though I would have given up the last of my remaining eyesight for it, I was not the horse who could take Claire to the level that she was ready to achieve.

I suppose that I should have felt regret about this truth, but I did not. Had Claire grown tired of me or rejected me for another, stronger gelding, yes, that would have cut to my heart. But Claire would have gone right on training with me three times a week, taking me to little hunter shows, and cantering me through the mountains, without complaint. She would have kept cheering me on with every fourth- or fifth-place ribbon we brought home. In Claire's eyes, we were a team. Had either of us placed competition at the center of our friendship, I believe we would not have lasted together as long or as true as we have. From the beginning, there was something more in it for both of us. I hoped that Claire and Mother would agree with Mrs. Maiden and allow me to try this new endeavor.

CHAPTER SIXTEEN

My Training Begins

I felt it a great honor to have been recruited to serve alongside Mac. Although less than half my age, Mac agreed to act as mentor to me as I prepared to enter service in the therapeutic school.

Mac had worked in therapeutic service since he was purchased at auction by Mrs. Maiden for that very purpose. To Mac this was not a menial position; it was his life's work. He spoke lovingly of his students and cautioned that should I accept the opportunity offered to me, I could no longer save the best of myself only for Claire. If I were to become a therapeutic school horse, I must withhold nothing and give myself to every student as if each one were, in fact, Claire. "There must be no favorites, my friend. To succeed in this work, each must become your favorite," he advised me.

According to Mac, each of my students would need something different from me. While one student might desire to gain muscle tone in her back, which had been ravaged by a disease of the muscles, another might wish to increase concentration in order to find a moment of peace from acute misfires in his brain. Still another student might work on improving his gross motor skills, which had been slow to develop. Mac impressed upon me that I must be ready to love each of my new students as deeply as I had come to love Claire. I vowed to welcome each student just exactly as I had been welcomed and nurtured.

When I arrived at the Maury River Stables, I too was in desperate need of restoration. Mrs. Maiden devised a plan specific to my needs. We worked to manage the pain from my arthritis. We salvaged what we could of my eyesight and used a variety of techniques to help me find new ways to see. Most of all, I finally found purpose and joy in my life. It was no accident that Claire was assigned to oversee my nourishment back to health. Mrs. Maiden gave me Claire because Claire was the person I needed in order to become whole.

It would be the same in return with my new students. Mrs. Maiden, together with each of my students, or their families, would create a plan for healing and strengthening. Through barn skills and riding, we would work in the therapeutic program to nourish body and soul, just as Claire had nourished me. I gathered that for therapeutic riders, horsemanship was a means to restoration. Whether to body or soul, my job would be to help restore each of them. I was eager to get started.

Mac assured me that proper training would equip me with the skills that I needed. He warned that therapeutic service, while rewarding, was also challenging. The training program on which I was about to embark posed the first challenge for me to overcome.

Mrs. Maiden had recruited me into my new position fully aware of my age and my conditions. It was Mrs. Maiden who had first observed the tumors in my eyes. Of course, Mrs. Maiden had also witnessed my refusal to jump with Claire because of my increasing blindness. These facts did not diminish Mrs. Maiden's faith in me, but I believe these were cause enough to put me through an intensive training with Stu.

Stu's charge was to increase my capacity to remain brave and calm under any and all circumstances. Courage has never been lacking in my spirit, thanks to my exceptional breeding. My dam was not only the most striking Appaloosa I have ever known; she was also the bravest, most serene being that I have yet to encounter. Dam was my first teacher in matters of courage.

I am not frightened to hear the wind tearing through our forest, even when there are few leaves to soften its howl. I am not afraid of other horses, be they moody mares or scowling, hot Thoroughbreds. I don't spook or dash away at the sight of a red umbrella, as do some others. A chair that was upright yesterday does not shatter my confidence if it is upside down when I encounter it today. Nor do I bolt when an engine backfires. I dare say neither friend nor foe can detect fear in me, ever. This courage was the trait admired so by Mrs. Maiden on the day the hunters fired upon our field.

Tolerance was to be my lesson. I quickly deduced, from listening to Stu and Mrs. Maiden plan my course of study, that increased tolerance was to be the primary aim of my training. By eavesdropping, I learned that Mrs. Maiden doubted not at all my bravery or my ability. She wanted to increase my tolerance to be able to accept the often unpredictable, erratic actions of some therapeutic students. I further overheard that I would not be immediately placed into service as a teacher. I would spend the rest of the fall and all of the winter learning to welcome intolerable and unexpected stimuli. Stu was to be my teacher, Mac and Gwen my mentors.

In addition to being the barn manager and a trainer at Maury River Stables, I am of the opinion that Stu was Mrs. Maiden's special companion. On a number of occasions, how many I cannot accurately state, I witnessed with my own eye a physical closeness between the two, the likes of which I have yet to see between other people. Their intimacy rivaled that of Claire and Mother, but at the same time was very different indeed. Having observed Stu's capacity for tenderness, I placed my complete trust in him and, in fact, welcomed him as my teacher. I felt certain that Stu would allow no harm to come to me, if for no other reason than his profound devotion to Mrs. Maiden.

Like me, Stu also battled arthritis. The disease had rendered his hands so twisted that the act of buckling the girth around me was very nearly impossible for him to complete without assistance. Yet he never winced or cried out. I saw how he rubbed his hands when the task was done. In this way, too, Stu trained me, through his example, to better tolerate that which aimed to distract me.

I was not surprised to find that Gwen, the old Hanoverian, along with Mac, was a star in the therapeutic school. There was no gentler mare in all of Rockbridge County. More than once, hearing Claire singing in the mare field, I had trotted over and found Claire sitting in the grass with Gwen's big, warmblood head resting in her lap. Claire held no fear of Gwen, who at seventeen hands high is a great deal larger than I am. I never disturbed the two of them at such moments, nor did I allow them to detect me as I watched from behind the cedar clump in the gelding field. Gwen's gentle spirit was well suited for teaching, particularly in the therapeutic school.

Before we started our training, Stu tied my lead rope to the door of my room so that I was facing the indoor riding ring. He proceeded to bring Gwen into the middle. She wore no bridle or halter and could have bolted from him at the moment of her choosing; she did not bolt. She appeared bored. Her breath warmed the air and formed a cloud around her face as she blew toward Stu with her standard greeting of exchanging breath.

With no warning or verbal cue, Stu reached back to his belt loop, then threw open an umbrella directly into the old mare's face. She blinked at him once, but made no sound or movement. She did not spook. She stood square in the same bored way as she had started out.

"See that, Chancey, my friend? That's you when we're done," Stu told me. Then he reached in his pocket for a treat, which Gwen gladly received. Ultimately, I was to achieve this same level of tolerance.

My formal training consisted of repeated conditioning to every unusual, unexpected sight, sound, or feeling that Stu could imagine. Stu started our work together by crumpling paper bags near my ears and face. He popped balloons next to my ears. Had Mac not opened my heart to the higher purpose of this most irritating training period, I may well have been put off and refused to accept these distractions. Stu dragged ropes and twine across my withers and barrel. He waved the rope around my face and rear. I did not react.

With no evidence that I understood his words, Stu explained to me that each lesson was necessary to simulate sensations that I might encounter with my new students. Stu's goal was to condition me to expect anything. When I had passed each test, Stu always made his satisfaction known to me with the same three words: "That's right, Chance." I came to expect that hearing the phrase signaled that we were ready to move on to the next challenge.

Throughout the winter, we trained everywhere. Our lessons were held in my room, the indoor ring, the out-door ring, the cross-country field, and, if Stu desired maximum distraction on any given morning, in the mare field. I may be gelded, but the mares still distract me like no other living beings. All over the grounds of Maury River Stables we worked for two sessions daily, in the morning after breakfast and again at midday.

Claire came most every day after school. Gradually, we all but stopped our own equitation training in exchange for taking quiet afternoon trails together. The winter ground was hard and crunched beneath my feet; I did my best to keep Claire warm, though I did not mind the cold as much as she did. Some days we had no need to talk at all and would only walk through the many miles of hills or alongside the river. Other days, Claire gave me detailed reconnaissance from Stu and Mrs. Maiden about my progress as a therapeutic horse.

"I'm so proud of you, Chancey. Everyone is proud of you, especially Mother. She gets all choked up whenever Stu tells her about how well you're doing."

In time for my evening meal, Claire would walk me back to my room. "I love you, pony," she'd say. Often Claire would return more than once with an extra carrot or apple to place in my grain box.

Mealtimes and after dark were the only hours I spent in my room while I was training. I can't say that I missed my room during my training as a therapeutic school horse, for I did not. I desired to pass as many hours as possible outdoors while I could still see. I knew that blindness would one day close the mountains to my eyes for good, for cancer knows not compassion. I knew there would be enough time for standing in my room, one day.

In order to build camaraderie, Mrs. Maiden had relocated Dante to the other side of the barn and now cradled me between my two mentors, Gwen and Mac.

To further cultivate an *esprit de corps* among us, she had sectioned off a new field in order that we could establish an unbreakable bond that would carry over to our work with the students. As Gwen was the oldest and most experienced in the therapeutic school, she easily and without fight became the lead horse in our paddock. There were occasions when, because of the shared fence line, Princess still assaulted Gwen. At those times, Mac or I were only too happy to race to Gwen's aid and slam our back hooves into the fence with such force and reverberation that Princess would not only scamper away, but squeal, too, as if she herself were the injured party.

At night in our bordering rooms, we three would whisper until early into the morning. Gwen and Mac made me repeat to them each exercise and aspect of my training progress; they then explained to me its purpose and described what I might expect the next day. I had easily passed the first phase of my training; still, Mac said even more was necessary before I could begin my work with students. Gwen rightly foretold that Stu would introduce me to more unpredictable stimuli than simple bags or colorful balloons. Thus, I was not at all alarmed when Stu showed up for my lesson with a pack of beagles.

CHAPTER SEVENTEEN

Canis Familiaris

Though I had exhibited great courage, enough to be recruited by Mrs. Maiden, it would be another month or more before Mrs. Maiden actually allowed me to teach in the therapeutic school. This next phase of my training would test me to the limits and ultimately desensitize me to loud noises and erratic movements. All of my senses would be reconditioned for extreme tolerance. I would have to learn that I could not bolt or squat, rear or buck, in retaliation of any stimuli. I would learn to accept, as had Mac and Gwen, that neither fight nor flight could ever be an acceptable response for a horse in therapeutic service.

Stu arrived at my room with all of his hunting beagles at his side. He hoped that using his dogs in my training would speed my progress. During the deer-shooting season, I had seen the dogs out on several occasions. As was customary, Stu began our lesson by greeting me in my room and offering me a peppermint from his pocket. A young beagle, whom I had not seen before, showed great interest in the candy and snatched it out of Stu's hand before I could take it myself. Stu lowered his voice. "Tommy!" he scolded. "Tommmmmy, that's not nice."

The puppy dropped his head apologetically, leaving the candy on the ground. I quickly scarfed it up for myself. I sniffed Stu's jacket, certain that I detected at least one more candy piece. Stu reached in his pocket and then handed it to me.

"Chancey, meet the new pup. His name is Tommy. His Latin name is *Canis familiaris*. He's going to help us today. If you like him, I'll bring him with us every day." I lowered my head to see the young dog, whose only interest was how much horse dung he could eat. Tommy took no notice of me whatsoever.

"Tommy, meet Chancey," Stu continued. "His Latin name is *Equus caballus*. Chancey's studying to be a therapeutic school horse," Stu told the dog. He patted me on the neck and added, "You didn't realize that I know Latin, did you, Chance? It's always good to learn something new. Keeps you alive."

I blew on Stu, for even though I had no interest in Latin or beagles, Stu had won a secure place in my heart precisely because he credited me for having such interests. Tommy remained obsessed with the ground.

In the cross-country field, Stu and his unrelenting hunting dogs set to work on me. It must be noted that I was never in any danger or under a threat of physical harm from the beagles. The dogs did not bite or nip at me, and I returned the favor by neither biting nor nipping at them. They did annoy. The beagles jumped and yelped. They crawled under me and used my rear and chest to prop themselves on two legs. Stu seemed to find their behavior endearing. I did not.

To keep myself focused, I played a concentration game with myself during these arduous sessions. I set about documenting and remembering my home so that even long after I had completely lost my sight I would still remember the Maury River Stables. I tried to completely tune out the dogs by imprinting the details of my surroundings onto my heart. I stood in our field, with hunting dogs bounding all around me. I could just see the tops of the sycamore trees lining the left bank of the river. While the dogs set about distracting me, I turned my mind toward the Maury River, and Saddle Mountain just beyond.

I recalled how when I first arrived at the Maury

River Stables, I visited the Maury River often and cantered alongside it searching for some clue as to where the river had been or what it was rushing to find. After a rowdy storm, the Maury might flow muddy and fast, pulling downstream an entire chestnut tree, or some such debris, which it had ripped from the banks upstream.

While the beagles lunged at me and pestered one another, I listened for the river. I confess that a part of me desired to break from Stu's dogs and gallop toward the sloping river birch that in the dead of winter marked the Maury definitively with its bright white bark. I knew the beagles would stay right on my heels if I attempted such a break.

Only once during this daily practice did the beagles successfully break my concentration. We had enjoyed an unusually high occurrence of rain; I knew the river ran high and fast, for I had no trouble at all hearing it rush by us, beyond the gelding field. I judged the electric fence to be approximately three feet high. As a young horse, I had successfully cleared more than three feet, but only a handful of times, if that, since coming to the Maury River Stables. Both the cancer and the arthritis had by then contributed to the demise of my jumping career, but logic had no such hold on me that morning.

Tommy began jumping at my left side, and I could not ascertain his intent. Though he stood no higher than the top of my cannon bone, his vertical range reached much nearer to my cheek than I had expected. I felt Tommy there, bouncing up well past my forearm, but could not see him. I could hear the pup; it would have been impossible not to hear him. I could smell him, too, for this young beagle had no bladder control whatsoever and in his excitement, he covered my feet in the contents of his bladder more than once. Though it had been almost a year since my first tumor was removed in Albemarle, and I had by then grown accustomed to complete blindness in my left eye, I panicked that I could not see but only feel Tommy there at my side. I tried to ground myself with my remaining good eye.

Tommy then launched himself above my head. I cast about for the sound of the river. I was sure I could clear the electric fence. I flicked my tail at Tommy and began to dance. I pinned my ears back, a fair notice of warning. The young beagle continued, aware, no doubt, that he had gotten a reaction from me and from Stu as well. I lifted my front left foot and poised it there, giving Tommy one last opportunity to leave me alone. "Chance, you can do this," Stu urged. But it was too late; I kicked the little beagle away from me, not hurting him badly, mind you. Without question, if my intent had been to injure the pup, I would have done so with such might that little fellow would not have been able to run crying to his mother, as he did.

I knew my error straightaway and regretted it. I did not bolt to the river. I stood square in front of Stu, who just laughed. "Whoo, Chancey, he got to you. Tommy got to you."

Stu sent the dogs to the front of the field, where they obediently waited for him. He moved to my left out of my vision, and patted me on the neck. "It's your left side, I know. You've done a fine job compensating until now. Don't worry, Chance, don't worry." Stu did not sound disappointed but rather satisfied with what he had discovered about me. I hoped that my outburst toward Tommy had not eroded Stu's confidence in me.

I was comforted to walk with Claire that afternoon and relieved that she already knew about the incident with Tommy. Claire did not tack me up but walked me bareback up an old logging trail around the base of Saddle Mountain. Few leaves remained on the mountain and those that did swirled around behind us for the entire five-mile trail. We stayed inside the mountain, for neither Claire nor I dared to take on the frigid, unrelenting mountain air at the unprotected peak. On our return to the barn, Claire finally told me.

"I heard about that annoying puppy this morning. I don't blame you for kicking him. Don't worry; he's not hurt. Stu's not mad, either. He said every therapeutic horse he's ever trained has cracked with the beagles . . . except Gwen."

Claire patted my neck. "You're doing a good job, pony. Stu says you're one of the best."

Claire, Gwen, and Mac, between them, kept me motivated during my training. Without them, I would have easily become discouraged.

* CHAPTER EIGHTEEN *

Equus Asinus

Mac predicted that my training would soon extend beyond the Maury River Stables onto adjacent properties. As ever, Mac was correct. Our lessons were no longer stationary, which Mac assured me was indicative of great progress in my training. Stu intended to introduce me to companions immensely more annoying than Tommy and the other beagles. In Rockbridge County, many people keep horses, and as they all ride and love the countryside, a strong tradition of courtesy use exists for the purposes of pleasure riding nearly every day of the year, except for those days when hunters are allowed in the woods.

For our first morning ride, Stu tacked me up quickly with only a bareback pad and a lead rope tied into reins. I am always overjoyed to ride without the bit in my mouth. I don't mind the bit so much in the hands of a rider as knowledgeable and kind as Stu or Claire. Claire and I often ride without a bit or saddle and I can say, with certainty, we both enjoy that very much. In the case of Stu, unlike some of my younger and more diminutive riders, his instructions to me through his legs and seat are straightforward and easy enough to follow that the additional aid of the bit is unnecessary. Stu is not a big man, by comparison to John the Farrier or Doctor Russ; Stu's weight, because it is well balanced and evenly distributed, actually gave me much confidence and security as we rode.

Stu led me away from Maury River Stables with great purpose. My nemesis from the cross-country field, Tommy, accompanied us. To my surprise, the puppy behaved more respectfully to me after I had kicked him. He stopped relieving himself on my feet, an outcome that was well worth the mild kick I had previously delivered. Having learned his lesson, Tommy ran beside me, always on the left and well away from my feet. His panting and yelping kept me aware of his position and served to mark the left edge of the trail. I found that by keeping an ear turned toward Tommy, I was able to use him as a guide on the trail. The willing pup kept alongside me; his presence kept me from stumbling into ditches or holes. I began to warm to his personality and could see why Stu was so fond of him.

We rode away from the Maury River. Our destination was Mrs. Pickett's farm, some distance from our barn, past a neighboring cattle pasture, through an overplanted pine farm, and across the paved street.

As we approached Mrs. Pickett's farm, we moved straight along the fence line at a nice working trot. Before I could see my distraction, I heard him. His coarse voice grated my ears so badly that Tommy's yelping would have soothed me. I wanted to bolt, not from fear, but to get some relief. The honking was not altogether unlike a horse, but not nearly as refined. It was not quite a neigh and definitely not a whinny. I wasn't frightened, just annoyed.

Stu kept me trotting, again keeping the fence on my right, which I greatly appreciated. The beast, upon seeing me, acted quite as if we were long-lost brothers. He magnified his horrendous noise tenfold, alternately begging me to break him out of the fence and pleading with me to jump over the fence to live with him. He professed to be a lonely soul, certain that I had been sent by our Creator in answer to his prayers.

I did not laugh when I saw him, for I know well the

feeling of being laughed at and would not wish that feeling on any fellow being. He stood on four disproportionately short legs with a barrel almost as wide as mine. He very nearly appeared to be a horse, but a most uncommonly exaggerated one. Besides his torturous voice, his astoundingly elongated ears were his most defining characteristic; they towered above his head straight up at attention. As I moved closer to him, I observed that his nose was nearly twice as long as my own. Indeed, I had to suppress my deep urge to laugh, for he was comical in every way.

As Stu had orchestrated this gathering, he introduced us formally.

"Chancey, my friend, meet Joey. This is Mrs. Pickett's new donkey, also known as *Equus asinus*. Y'all are kinda cousins, I guess, since you're both *Equus*."

Joey seized upon the mention of a familial connection. He turned his ears rapidly to and fro, then rolled his eyes down to Tommy. He squeezed his oversize nose under the fence and said to the puppy, "Yes! Yes! We're cousins, you and I. Yes, we are."

Offended as I was at Stu's ludicrous suggestion of a genetic resemblance between Joey and myself, I was even more offended that Joey would feel elation at being related to a beagle, when an Appaloosa stood right in front of his eyes. I did not flatten my ears, though I most certainly wanted to do so.

Tommy furiously wagged his tail in circles at the donkey, eager to be adopted. Taking no notice of me, Joey invited Tommy into the family. "Hello there, little wagger. Hey, I have a tail, too. Look at my tail; look at mine!" Joey flicked his tail around for Tommy to see. Tommy barked and yelped to encourage his new cousin, *Equus asinus.*

I could take no more of their foolishness; I pinned my ears, showed the whites of my eyes, and whinnied sharply into the donkey's ear. Joey looked up from sniffing Tommy.

"Are you my cousin, too?" Joey asked me.

I then set the matter straight. *"I'm* Chancey, not him. He's not our cousin. He's *Canis.* We're *Equus."* Joey practically threw himself over the fence toward me.

"Oh, cousin! Oh, Cousin Chancey! I've been waiting for you to come. Please, don't ever leave again," pleaded Joey.

I had learned by then that the longer I held my curiosity on any new object in our lesson, the longer Stu would require me to spend on that lesson. Eager to be far away from my new cousin Joey, I feigned boredom by dropping my head to graze and passing gas. This technique proved itself as Stu picked up my head and with a squeeze of legs we set off again.

Joey begged us not to leave him. I promised we would return in the morning. Even as we cantered out of sight, Joey still called to me, "Come back! Hey, come back! There's nothing down that way but a mean, spiteful llama. Come back, cousin! Come back!"

Before we could move into a gallop, an ugly, shaggy animal with a neck longer than any I've ever seen, and even longer eyelashes, came running up beside us. I guessed this was the llama of Joey's warning. He did not appear to be mean, or spiteful, as Joey had suggested, just odd. I was most curious. As the fence line was still at my right, I was able to observe this striking animal more closely. Stu never changed his directions to me, so, lacking any perceptible shift in leg or hand, I continued to canter the fence line, with the long-necked animal and Tommy cantering along beside me. I felt the llama sizing me up with his eyes and nose. Had Stu given me room, I would liked to have shown that llama the impressive speed that Appaloosas are capable of reaching. Though the llama spoke not a word, the air between us smelled of tension.

I hadn't the chance to become too agitated, for Stu pulled me to halt. The llama halted as well. I was pleased when, at the end of the fence, Stu gave me my head to investigate. I am ashamed to say that after the long canter, I was shorter of breath than the llama, Stu, or Tommy.

Stu introduced us. "That's a llama, Chancey. I don't

know his name. I don't know his Latin name either. He belongs to Mrs. Pickett, too. We'll give him another race tomorrow."

I nodded to the llama. We stood face-to-face, yet the llama would not exchange breaths with me. I studied him carefully for some clue as to his rancid demeanor toward me.

This bushy fellow had no fine tail like mine, and really had practically no tail at all. Nor did he have any sort of mane. It struck me as especially odd that his ears stuck straight out to the sides horizontally, not elegantly tall, like mine. He was covered in a short, furry coat that made me so itchy my tail involuntarily flicked in a rhythm reserved only for the most persistent flies. Though he stood almost to my height, most of the llama's height was in his neck. I deduced that he weighed considerably less than I. In response to my greeting, the llama batted his long lashes, then proceeded to spit in my face. Then he turned his full attention to Tommy. I decided that Joey was the more tolerable creature of the two.

In the barn that evening, as I recounted the day's lesson to Gwen and Mac, I could see they were impressed with my advancement. Mac nodded toward the mares across from us. "See Princess?" Mac threw his head in her direction. "She came unglued at the llama on a trail ride last week. She nearly threw her rider and wouldn't go a step farther. The entire riding party had to turn around and come home."

Gwen leaned close to me and whispered through the bars separating our two rooms. "You won't believe this, but Dante is scared of the donkey."

I laughed. "He's frightened of our cousin Joey?"

"Shhh, he might hear you," warned Gwen. Then she continued, "It's Joey's voice that frightens Dante. He rears and bucks over there by Mrs. Pickett's. He won't go anywhere near Joey."

I cut a glance at Dante, our boss, who was too busy kicking his room door to bother with listening to us. Gwen nudged me with her nose. "And don't look at him either. Here, look at me."

I was encouraged by our conversation that evening that my formal training was coming to an end, and soon I would begin to work with students in the therapeutic school. I confessed that I was nervous. My training had gone well, but had it really prepared me for the dynamic, real-life world of being a school horse again—and in such a highly specialized school?

My mentors assured me that I would never be alone; I would work with my students in partnership with many people and other horses. Mac or Gwen would always be in the ring with me. Not only would one of my two good friends be there, but Mrs. Maiden or Stu would handle me directly for the duration of each lesson, and for added comfort and protection of the students, specially trained volunteers called sidewalkers would join me as well.

Macadoo explained that sidewalkers were required to complete a training program just as the horses were. While Stu handled the training of horse partners, Mrs. Maiden coordinated the training of sidewalkers. Each therapeutic student would be assigned two sidewalkers per lesson. The sidewalkers would attend to my students' equipment, teach them about grooming, and monitor things such as correct seat position and foot placement. Some students might require sidewalkers to hold them in the saddle and walk along the left and right side of me. Other students might need nothing more than praise and motivation. If I happened to spook—a highly unlikely scenario because therapeutic horses are dependable and unspookable—the sidewalkers would remove the rider, if necessary. If my student needed help steering, the sidewalkers would help steer. The sidewalkers would be there for whatever was needed during the lesson.

This was the first I had been told that I would work so closely with sidewalkers. My stomach rumbled. I wondered how well my sidewalkers would manage with my blind side, or if they would even welcome getting to know an old horse such as myself. My nervous stomach erupted into a very loose stool. I ignored my symptoms of anxiety; I did not share my concerns with Mac or Gwen, for I was determined to prove to myself and Mrs. Maiden that I was worthy of the therapeutic school. More than anything else, however, I wanted Claire to be proud of me. I wanted Claire, and Mother, too, to see that though I could not give Claire the championships she deserved, I was still a good, sound horse.

"Old App," Mac said one night after my last training session with Stu, "we've saved some very special news until now. We've all been saving a surprise for you. I didn't want to tell you until you had made it this far in your training program." Mac moved from his window to the wall between our rooms. Gwen came closer, too.

It was difficult to speak privately in the barn, for we had to speak in whispers. We had much freer conversations when we were turned out in the field; we all looked forward to the springtime, when we would be outdoors more. I put my ear to the bars between us to hear Mac's news.

"Your sidewalkers will be Claire and Mother." I wasn't sure I understood what Mac meant. Did he mean that I would not have to work with strangers? My family would be joining me in service to the therapeutic school? I leaned as close in to Mac as I could.

"What? Would you say it again, Mac?"

Gwen repeated Mac's news. "It's true, Chancey. Claire and her mother have been training with Mrs. Maiden while you've been training with Stu. I heard Claire say you weren't getting away from her so easily. They're going to volunteer with the therapeutic program, too. You three will be a new team. How do you like that?"

I nickered softly to Mac, then exchanged breaths with Gwen. Mac walked over to his window; I walked to mine and pushed it open with my nose. At that time, I was blessed that the vision in my right eye still allowed me a clear and fine view of the moon hanging full between Saddle Mountain's pommel and cantle, throwing off rays nearly equal to early morning sun. Mac and I did not speak; we stood in our stalls, both looking up at Saddle Mountain. I had worried about the sidewalkers for nothing.

By spring, Claire, Mother, and I were prepared to teach in the therapeutic riding school, together.

By the first day of spring, Claire, Mother, and I were working in the Maury River Stables Therapeutic Riding School. Three times weekly after Claire's school day had ended she, Mother, and I taught a lesson as a team. Though Claire was at that time only eleven, she had completed the required training and was considered a junior volunteer able to serve alongside Mother.

Our charges in the therapeutic school ranged in age from the very young, of perhaps five years of age, to much older, closer to the age of Mother. I found satisfaction and purpose in this work and felt that my entire life had prepared me to teach in this way.

My therapeutic students always greeted me with affection and treated me with the greatest respect. They often brought me drawings and paintings for my room; some gave me cookies and treats. Others, I was told, included me in their bedtime prayers, and it was for this that I was most thankful. To be so loved at such an advanced age as mine was a great motivator. Their devotion humbled me.

I returned their love fully and generously. Whether I was hot or cold, whether I was in pain or enjoying a respite free from pain, I welcomed every therapeutic student, every time.

Why some students attended the therapeutic school and others did not was not always immediately evident to me. True, for many of my therapeutic students, a physical impediment blocked their technical mastery, but that was truly the case with all my students, whether in the therapeutic school or not. Take Mother, for example: a deformity in her back impeded her technical mastery, and an unexamined fear in her mind kept her from pushing herself further. Yet Mother was not enrolled in therapeutic school as a student but as a sidewalker volunteer with Claire.

I gathered from Gwen and Mac that the therapeutic riding school served people of all ages who were in some manner wounded. Perhaps they had no use of their legs, which was easy enough to discern since in those situations, a chair with wheels carried them up a special ramp built to the height of a horse's back so that all transfers were made laterally. This removed the danger that could be caused by lifting a student up and over onto my back. Other students brought wounds that were more difficult to detect because there was no outward evidence.

I quickly observed that the most noticeable difference in most of my therapeutic students was that they possessed an uncommon openness and willingness in their hearts. I will take heart and loving-kindness over technical ability any day of the week—for a rider with an open heart allows the fullest possible joining up, whether galloping over the Maury River, slowly walking a figure eight, or merely standing in my room watching the blue mountains.

Before I started this work, Mac told me we could not play favorites in this job. I suspected Mac spoke from having learned from experience that such strong attachments eventually cause a degree of brokenness in the heart. I, however, am not ashamed to disclose that there were a couple of students to whom I was particularly partial.

One student, a girl named Kenzie, I learned after three lessons together, could not see out of either eye. At first, I had thought perhaps Mrs. Maiden had mistakenly placed Kenzie in the wrong program. She moved with such confidence and grace in the saddle and on the ground and with a heart as open and kind as any girl, save my Claire. I adored Kenzie; she was like a blast of spring, arrived in the dead of winter. Her blindness did not prevent her from placing her full trust in me or Claire and Mother, her sidewalkers.

Claire and Mother kept us moving as a team by acting as Kenzie's eyes and, of course, compensating for my own left eye. They guided us around the ring and over poles, or around a spiral of cones set up for bending practice. Truthfully, Kenzie had little need of sidewalkers in a traditional sense. Claire and Mother gave Kenzie no physical support. Nor did they make actual contact with Kenzie or me. They jogged or walked alongside me and used their voices more than anything— Claire instructing us and Mother encouraging us.

"A little more leg, Kenzie. Now close your hands around the reins, but don't pull back on them. Sit down and relax," Claire would say.

After trotting circles in our corners without breaking, Mother would applaud us both. "Beautiful, Kenzie! Beautiful, Chancey! Now enjoy this straightaway— you're doing great!"

Mrs. Maiden always kept the therapeutic horses on a lead line, for precautionary measures. After only a few lessons, Kenzie became such a proficient rider that Mrs. Maiden hardly worked at all. I listened for Kenzie's directions, and Mrs. Maiden kept the lead line slack. I certainly would have indulged Kenzie a bit more than my other students if she had squeezed her hands too tightly around the reins. Yet she held the reins with a light touch as if they were robin eggs in her palms. If, because of her blindness, Kenzie had fallen on my neck a bit more than my sighted students, I would gladly have tolerated her weight. But she kept her center of gravity fully aligned with mine.

Kenzie rode with an open heart. Like me, she used her ears, her nose, and every nerve in her body to work for her eyes. My role with Kenzie was simply to respond to her touch, her voice, and her feelings. When Kenzie brushed my body, I made a quiet, low sound of contentment so she could feel that I enjoyed her manner of grooming me. If Kenzie wrapped her arms around me for affection, I wrapped my neck around her in kind, so that she could feel my affection, too. In the saddle, I paid close attention to the directions of Claire and Mother as they instructed Kenzie which aids to deliver, so that at the slightest detection of effort on her part, I obliged. Kenzie showed me that eyes are but one way to see the world. She comforted me a great deal, and every time I spent an hour or two with Kenzie, my fear of losing my own sight lessened.

Zack, a boy student of mine, bore no evidence of

physical wounds at all, but even as he picked up the body brush to groom me, I sensed that his wound hid deep within his mind and so prevented him from enjoying or experiencing much of anything for more than the briefest measure of time. With Zack, my task was to reach deep enough into that wound and give it a soft enough interruption that it did not send Zack's sparks flying. With Zack, I strove to relax him enough that his concentration would increase over time.

Zack's nature was such that he took in too much information, too quickly, and then became paralyzed by a jungle of stimuli. When Zack started with me, he would regularly melt down, as Mrs. Maiden described it. I know that to a stranger looking at our progress, or perhaps trying to chart Zack's progression as a rider, it may have appeared that we were slow to advance. But I am proud to say that we made extraordinary progress together. Eventually, Zack could hold his mind quiet and groom my entire right side before he disengaged again and had to be redirected to the task by Mrs. Maiden. Frequently, Zack would stand near me and take in only the feel of my mane or the touch of my nose to his neck for some time before he became distracted again. It was several months before Zack made it out of my room and into the ring. To understand our accomplishment, you would need to feel what it is like to be Zack.

When we did begin our work under saddle, Claire and Mother had a much different role as Zack's side-walkers than they did as Kenzie's. At our first lesson, Zack was frightened to be in the saddle; he screamed and thrashed around. He was unable, however, to calm his mind enough to get down or get help getting down.

"I want down! I want down! I want down!" Zack screamed.

I stood square; I did not dance. Tommy, who had been trying to stir up trouble in the mare field, heard the commotion and ran over to the edge of the lesson ring. I blinked my eyes at Tommy and pinned my ears back, warning him to stay out of the ring. I knew Zack didn't like dogs.

"Down! Down! I want down!" Zack began kicking his legs and pulling wildly on my reins in an effort to free himself from the saddle. There were too many places of connection: two stirrups, two hands on the reins, and several feet between him and the ground. Zack didn't know where to begin. Claire interrupted the boy's thought process.

Claire clapped her hands. "Zack!" Zack turned to Claire.

"Do you like ice cream? Chocolate ice cream?" Claire asked him.

He forgot that he wanted down. Mother lifted the boy out of the saddle and placed him on the ground beside her. I turned my head back to see if he was all right and touched my nose to his shoulder.

"Hi, Chancey." Zack waved at me. "I was way up there." He pointed to my back.

Claire held her hand out.

"Zack, come with me. We're going back down to the barn to teach you emergency dismount on a barrel. That way you'll know what to do if you ever freak out on Chancey or any other horse."

"Okay, Claire. What about the ice cream? Do we get ice cream after I learn emergency dismount?"

Zack never forgot emergency dismount and, in fact, he used it at every lesson. He said it made him feel like a superhero. Claire, Mother, and I learned to be on guard at any point in our lesson to hear Zack shout out, "Ready y'all? Emergency dismount!" I would halt immediately. Then Zack would fling himself out of the saddle, just as Claire had taught him to do that day in the barn. Mother was always there to spot him and give him an able assist to the ground. Mrs. Maiden learned to keep chocolate ice-cream bars in the freezer, for Zack always asked for ice cream after emergency dismount.

Once, after a lesson, I heard Zack's father say that the boy had brought home a B in one of his classes at school, which meant nothing to me in and of itself. But I saw Zack beam at his father's pride. I heard the child tell Mrs. Maiden, "Now, when I get overloaded, I think

of brushing Chancey. Then it's easier to calm down."
Zack has taught me that no achievement is to be over-
looked or undervalued.

Yes, Kenzie and Zack gave me many hours of satisfaction and joy. I eagerly anticipated our meetings each
week and was not surprised to find that I grew as much
as either child. I loved Kenzie and Zack very, very
much. Still, neither was my favorite. Two years would
pass before I would meet that student.

CHAPTER TWENTY

A Child Like Me

Trevor Strickler could see with his eyes perfectly well, excepting the long bangs that hung in his face, not unlike the unkempt forelock sported by Napoleon the Shetland pony. Trevor also was capable of a deeper, longer concentration than most adults whom I have taught.

Trevor was like me, only Trevor was not old, and his cancer did not take his eyesight first. His whole body was filled with cancer. A bit younger than my Claire, Trevor was, in his own words, "too old to be treated like a baby and forced to take riding lessons." My job with Trevor was to find joy. That was my sole task, to help my friend feel joy.

I could feel my own cancer, behind my eyes, growing deep within me, waiting, I believe, for my work to be done. I know that Mother and Doctor Russ had kept my cancer at bay for as long as possible. Over the past few years, I had submitted to eye surgery as a matter of routine, to remove the cancer not only from my left, but also my right eye. Doctor Russ confirmed that I was slowly losing vision in my right eye, but with surgery, he was able to slow down its pace. Doctor Russ regularly pointed out to Mother that I was, after all, an old horse.

When I first met Trevor, he wanted nothing at all to do with me or any horse. Though enrolled in the therapeutic school and assigned me as his horse, as he did not participate in lessons, there was no need for sidewalkers. In fact, Trevor refused to acknowledge me in any way. He would not pick up a brush or a currycomb. Mrs. Maiden, Trevor, and Trevor's mother would stand in my room for an hour, once a week, waiting for Trevor to show an interest. Trevor would stand with his back to us all, kicking the wood shavings against the wall of my room.

I ignored him because that is what he desired: to be left alone. Having turned my back on many, it's a gesture that I understand fully. When an about-face like Trevor's is deployed with such conviction, it is prudent to honor the request to be left alone. I did not judge the boy in his anger, nor did I take it as a personal affront.

I didn't feel the urge to defend myself against his out-bursts, for they were directed at the wall, not me. Besides, Claire was plenty equipped to defend my dignity.

Though Claire had advanced in her jumping and dressage well beyond my abilities, she refused to give up her riding time with me. Claire's attachment to me, and mine to her, allowed us each to feel secure in pursuing our separate paths confident in the knowledge that we were eternally bound. I loved our work together in the therapeutic school and our riding time in the mountains.

Claire and I had kept an easy routine of taking to the trails in the afternoons. We often strolled down to the Maury River in order to cool down from the hot after-noons. After wearing ourselves out in the water, Claire would sit on my back drying off while I grazed the lush banks of the river.

"See Saddle Mountain up there, Chancey?" Claire would ask. "One day, I'll take you up there again. We'll canter all the way to the top, then look out at everyone we know. They won't see us or know where we are. It will be just the two of us, looking out at the whole world, together."

I did not doubt Claire that one day we would find ourselves on the highest peak of Saddle Mountain. I looked forward to that day and hoped it would, indeed, come to pass. I had by then grown accustomed to Claire riding many different horses and this did not concern me or detract from my love for her, or hers for me. Claire and I had saved each other, and I knew, truly, that our love for each other grew even deeper as our training together came to an end.

I was happy that my therapeutic service did not supplant my time with Claire. Once a week, my trail time with Claire followed immediately after my lesson with Trevor, which could not be accurately described as a lesson, but more precisely standing-around-in-my-room time with Trevor. One afternoon, Claire arrived at the barn early, at the request of Mrs. Maiden. She had asked Claire to come out early to pick up registration forms for the Ridgemore Hunter Pace, a cross-country race of sorts that I very much hoped would be the event where Claire and I would finally win our first blue ribbon together, and my first blue ribbon ever.

Claire and I had not entered a competition together since Tamworth Springs. With Daisy, Claire had won every hunter show on the circuit. The pair brought home champion ribbons regularly, and Claire always came straight to my room afterward to tell me stories of the day. I did not miss the stress of hunter shows, and was glad that Daisy was the one to take my place. Daisy and I had come to appreciate each other; the mare excelled in hunter shows. Still, I longed to compete just once more with Claire and thought the hunter pace a perfect setting to do so.

Mrs. Maiden had convinced Claire that I would excel at a hunter pace. Though the course would include optional jumps, each jump would offer a go-around. Together, Claire and I would ride as a team over seven or eight miles of open pasture, up into the blue mountains, crossing over the Maury River several times. We would join with another horse and rider to form a team of four—two people, two horses—in a challenge to ride not the fastest, but the closest to the time the judges had determined to be optimum—a time that would not be announced until after the event had ended. The hunter pace was designed to test endurance, speed, agility, wit, and sportsmanship—all characteristics bred into me and highly developed among all Appaloosa horses.

Neither Claire nor I had dared utter aloud our hope that we might win the hunter pace, but we needn't, for it was there in both our hearts. Though the event was still several months away, Mrs. Maiden preferred her students to register early for purposes of scheduling trailerloads and finding substitute trainers to teach in her absence.

Claire picked up the form and, as was her routine, brought her tack to my room in preparation for the trail. There we all stood, Trevor, with his back turned; his mother, absently brushing my neck in the same spot over and over; Mrs. Maiden; and Claire.

Mrs. Maiden introduced Claire to Trevor and his

mother. "Trevor," she said, gesturing to the boy as if he were really listening, "this is Chancey's owner, Claire."

Then she told Claire, "Trevor rides Chancey every Friday right before you do."

Claire did not know, as did I, that it was perhaps not a lie, but at the very least an extreme exaggeration to state that Trevor had ever ridden me, for he had refused to even interact with me.

Mrs. Maiden seemed rushed. "Claire, I am kind of in a bind today with the farrier coming to shoe and the vet coming to give shots. Could you help Trevor tack up, please?"

Trevor's mother opened her mouth to protest, but Claire answered too quickly, "Sure!"

Mrs. Strickler placed a protective arm around Trevor's shoulder; he did not turn around. She smoothed the back of her son's shirt. She pushed his long bangs out of his eyes.

Mrs. Maiden took Trevor's mother by the elbow and escorted her out of my room, saying over her shoulder, "Thanks, Claire. I knew I could count on you."

Claire moved toward Trevor as if it were perfectly expected that he would be tucked into the corner of my room.

"Come on. I'll help you." Claire did not know that Trevor had made a practice of angrily kicking my wall for several weeks in a row. I could have told her that he had no intention of tacking me up.

Trevor lashed out at Claire. "I don't need your help! And I don't want to ride your stupid horse."

If Mrs. Maiden heard the outburst, and I believe she did, she did not turn back, but busied herself in the tack room preparing for John the Farrier and Doctor Russ.

Claire did not require adult intervention. She responded to Trevor with equal venom in her voice. "Why do you even come out here? Why don't you just go back to wherever you came from? Go play baseball or something. Geez."

Claire turned her back to Trevor and began grooming me—a little more forcefully than usual, I might add.

Directed at any other student, I would have appreciated Claire's zealous defense on my behalf. But Trevor was different; slowly, we were working toward an understanding of each other. Undoubtedly, Mrs. Maiden and the boy's mother could detect no change in his demeanor, as he did stand in the corner every week for one solid hour. I could tell he was softening to me; he was opening just enough. He kicked out less and less each time. He had begun to sneak glances at me. He was behaving much like a horse. He needed to be left alone for long enough that his curiosity would overcome his anger or fear. We were making progress; I worried that Claire's harsh words might close Trevor to me for good, before I had come to know him at all.

The boy, at least, was interested enough to fight with Claire. He had held so much inside for so long, I suppose, that I should not have been surprised that Claire had opened up a rather clogged pipeline of emotions.

Trevor said nothing after Claire's outburst. He kicked the wall hard. Then he kicked it again. Down the line, the other horses danced around and gave half-hearted whinnies of displeasure. Across the way, Dante began kicking his own wall.

Claire brushed me roughly then turned to face Trevor. "And Chancey's not stupid! You're stupid!" She turned her back on Trevor.

All of the other horses turned to watch my room. Mrs. Maiden did not emerge from the tack room, nor did Mrs. Strickler. Stu, who had been mucking stalls, parked the wheelbarrow outside of Gwen's room, next to mine. He listened and watched but did not intervene.

Trevor did not hold back. He screamed at Claire, "My mom makes me come to this stupid place! I hate it here, and I hate your horse!"

Claire spun around to face him, but Trevor didn't let up. Trevor's lips sprayed saliva on my muzzle as he spoke. "It's an old, stupid, smelly horse. I wish it were dead!"

For the first time, Trevor stood right next to me. I could not see him, but felt and smelled that he was at my left cheek. He smelled precisely of an oatmeal cookie. In fact, I was certain a cookie, or part of a cookie, remained in his shirt pocket. Claire moved closer to my face and closer to Trevor. I had no trouble hearing either of them.

"Shut up! Shut up and leave Chancey alone, or you're going to wish you were dead!"

I nickered at Claire, trying to calm her down. I feared she had gone too far, but it was too late. The boy had egged her on purposefully, it seemed. In fact, I sensed that he needed someone, like Claire, to give him room and reason to say what came next, for he said it without anger, without any emotion, really.

"I am going to be dead. I have cancer and I am going to be dead. Don't say you're sorry, either. Don't say anything."

Claire did not speak, at first. She picked up a curry-comb and began circling it on the dirtiest part of my body, starting at my neck. Trevor remained in the room with us, and he did not turn back to the wall. He stood facing Claire, waiting for something. Finally, Claire spoke to him.

"Don't just stand there; pick up a brush. If you're going to come every week, you might as well have fun."

Trevor didn't budge.

Claire kept talking to him anyway. "When I first met Chancey, my parents were getting a divorce. I hardly remember anything about that time it hurt so bad every day. Everybody at school and at home started treating me differently, like they felt sorry for me or something. Even though I felt like a different person, I wanted to be the same person, and I wanted everybody to treat me like the same person. Does that make sense?"

Claire did not wait for Trevor to respond; Trevor remained silent. Claire had rarely spoken of her parents' divorce, though I knew her heart ached because of it. Claire continued talking to the stone wall of Trevor.

"What I do remember is that Chancey was always there for me. If I needed to talk, or be goofy and ride him backward, or just stand in his stall and smell him, it didn't matter. I was always his Claire, the same Claire every day."

She turned to look at Trevor, still silent. Claire kept talking to the air. "I know a divorce is not the same as cancer. For me, though, it's the hardest thing ever in my life. I miss my dad a lot when I'm with Mother. When I'm with Dad, I want to be with her. I know it's not the same, but it still hurts."

Trevor's posture softened. He put a hand on my cheek. Claire rested her head against me, perhaps remembering the day we met.

"Mrs. Maiden told me one time, 'Claire, you need to let your pain out and let love come back.' All I'm saying, Trevor, is the same thing. Chancey is good at letting love in. He will love you as deep as an atom is small, if you let him."

Claire put her arms around me and held me close. Then she turned and looked at Trevor. "Besides, Chancey has cancer, too. Y'all have something in common." Then Claire ignored him.

She had learned, from fraternizing with horses for so much of her childhood, that if you ignore us, our curiosity will almost always demand that you not. Neither Claire nor I were surprised when Trevor picked up the body brush and began brushing my neck alongside Claire.

"Slow down," corrected Claire. "Here, brush him like this, softer, in long strokes. See how he closes his eyes? That means he likes it." I closed my eyes again to demonstrate for Trevor.

Finally, Trevor spoke. "Does it really have cancer?"

Claire put the currycomb in the brush box and turned to Trevor.

"His name is Chancey. Here, I'll show you."

Claire moved around to my right side and pulled the lid of my eye down toward her hand. I stood still so that Trevor could see my cancer.

"See that kind of white-pink blob right there? That's

cancer. He has it in his left eye, too, but you can't see it because we had the tumor taken off that eye last month. But the cancer's still growing. He'll need another operation at some point. He's probably had six operations since I got him three years ago."

Claire released my eyelid and kissed me on the nose.

"Can it see?" Trevor asked about me.

Claire patiently repeated, "His name is Chancey." She waited for Trevor to repeat the question satisfactorily.

"Yeah, whatever. Can it see?"

"No, not 'yeah, whatever.' Chancey is his name; don't call him 'it.' To answer your question, *he* can't see on his left side, but *he* seems to see all right on his right. We did have to take a tumor off of his right eye last year, and this one will probably come off soon."

I had not let on to Claire that my right eye's vision had begun its deterioration. Mac and Gwen knew, and they covered for me quite well by always staying nearby and giving me guidance whenever I got into trouble in the field, mostly at night.

"Can you teach me to ride him?" Trevor asked. "Can you teach me to ride Chancey?" He repeated the question again with my name, to show Claire his sincerity.

"Sure! I'm an awesome rider and Chancey's an awesome horse. I'll teach you to ride, no problem. You'll be winning ribbons before you know it," Claire boasted.

The smells of sugar, oatmeal, and raisins right under my nose had caused me too much agony already. I nudged Trevor's shirt pocket very gently, certain that the remnants of an oatmeal cookie with raisins waited inside and hopeful that it waited for me.

Claire cocked her head. "What, Chancey?" she asked me, tickling my chin. Then Claire laughed. "Trevor, did you bring Chancey a treat?"

Trevor reached inside his pocket and pulled out half a cookie. "Oh, yeah. I don't like oatmeal cookies. So, I, uh, well . . ."

"You did! You brought Chancey a treat! You were going to make friends with Chancey on your own, weren't you?"

Trevor pushed his bangs around and stood looking at me. He made no move for the pocket that contained the cookie. I nibbled at his shirt. He laughed and reached inside.

"No, not like that," Claire ordered him. "Hold your hand out flat."

"You're so bossy," Trevor told her. "Are you always this bossy?"

He did as Claire told him, held his hand flat, and fed me the oatmeal cookie. I rested my head on his shoulder. He exhaled and began to breathe evenly.

The boy grew quiet. "Claire, I might not be able to get good enough to win a ribbon. That takes time."

Claire understood, as I did. Trevor meant he didn't have the time it would take to become an accomplished rider. Claire, being Claire, had no problem making big promises.

"Trevor, it won't take long at all. We'll have to pick the right event and you'll have to practice, but sure, no problem."

"Really? Like you think we could be champions?"

"Definitely, you two could be champions. But you have to promise two things. One, that you won't call Chancey stupid ever again, and two, that you'll try to have fun." Claire stuck her hand out to Trevor. Trevor accepted the deal and we set to work that afternoon.

CHAPTER TWENTY-ONE

Under Claire's Instruction

Over the summer Claire began working closely with Mrs. Maiden to teach Trevor to ride, forgoing her own time with me to focus on instructing Trevor. Despite his illness, Trevor was still a strong boy. Like Claire, he asked to learn everything right away. While Claire was content to just be near horses, whether mucking our rooms or feeding hay, Trevor was impatient to learn to ride and to win a blue ribbon. Having never won a blue ribbon, I had just about given up that goal for myself.

Claire never let Trevor cut corners. Whenever Claire would make Trevor go back to the barn to stretch me before riding, he would get frustrated. Trevor's impatience would show.

"Claire! We only have one hour; can't I just ride?"

"Okay, if you just want to argue with me for the fun of arguing, we can argue the whole hour. Or you can start stretching him right now and be done with it," Claire would insist.

She always won, and soon enough, Trevor did not forget to stretch me. Though I understood the boy's urgent need to learn quickly, I very much appreciated Claire's insisting that he care for me properly.

The first time he was in the saddle, Trevor kicked me hard in both ribs and shouted, "Yah, boy, yah!"

I did not move. I blinked my eyes twice to show Claire that I understood Trevor's request but would not respond.

"'Yah, boy'?" Claire laughed so hard her face turned dark. "Where'd you learn 'yah, boy'?" She tried to catch her breath.

Trevor giggled and squirmed around. "I've just always wanted to say it, that's all."

Trevor was motivated and fast to pick up the technical aspects of where to place hands and legs. For the first few weeks, Claire worked with him from the ground, teaching him to find his seat, making sure he placed his legs just behind the girth. He quickly grasped the idea of rising to the trot in time with my outside foreleg. He had more difficulty learning to ride with an open heart, but Claire was insistent that he must learn this, as well as how to post on the correct diagonal.

"Trevor, you're straight as a board. Relax. And don't forget to breathe. You're holding your breath," she scolded him. He did not immediately experience the contradiction of riding with a posture both straight and relaxed.

"You said, 'Sit up straight and tall.' I am sitting up straight and tall," he complained.

"Try this, Trevor. Sing your favorite song while you're riding. That will help you relax, and plus, you can't hold your breath while you sing."

"I don't have a favorite song," he protested.

"Seriously? You don't have a favorite song?" Claire was incredulous. "Do you know any songs?"

"My mom always sings a stupid one to me." He resisted Claire's suggestion.

Claire did not cut Trevor any slack, ever. "Everything can't be stupid all the time, Trevor. Okay, sing your mom's stupid song, even if you hate it. Sing it while you ride. Go ahead, sing."

Trevor asked for the trot and held his breath.

"Sing!" Claire screamed at him. She threw her arms in the air.

"All right, Claire. You can't get me to relax by yelling at me."

Claire laughed at Trevor because she knew he was right. "If you would just do what I say, I wouldn't have to yell."

That made Trevor laugh, and he began to sing his mother's song. "'Tis the gift to be simple; 'tis the gift to be free.'"

Right away, I felt Trevor relax. He loosened his hands, which had been tightly gripped on the reins; his back softened. Trevor began to breathe.

He sang on. "'Tis the gift to come down where you ought to be. And when we find ourselves in the place just right, 'twill be in the valley of love and delight.'"

People are often astonished at the nearly imperceptible movements and shifts that are felt by horses of their riders. I can feel where my students' eyes are looking. The slightest fidget of a seat feels like a tremor to me. I felt Trevor smile. We remained at a posting trot many times around the ring. Claire called out our instructions: "Now, add circles in your corners, but keep singing and keep posting."

Trevor's shoulders opened up, and he sunk deeper. What had been a tentative effort turned into a full serenade. "'When true simplicity is gained, to bow and to bend we shan't be ashamed. To turn, turn will be our delight, 'til by turning, turning we come 'round right.'"

"Now you've got it, Trevor. That's perfect," Claire praised him. She called for him to halt, which he did smoothly and gracefully. I squared my legs, so that Claire would compliment Trevor again.

"Look at you, Trev," Claire said. "Who taught you to halt Chancey square like that? I think you're ready to go on the trail. Hop down for a sec."

Trevor lowered himself to the ground tentatively and patted me on the neck. "Good boy, Chancey. You're making me look good to Claire."

One afternoon toward the end of August, after Trevor had been riding but three weeks, Claire unbuckled my saddle and hung it over the fence. She cupped her hands tightly together and gave Trevor a leg up.

Without a saddle, his rhythm improved and Trevor was able to mold his body to mine more easily. As Trevor felt the warmth of my own body, he relaxed the tension in his legs and core. He held my mane tightly with both hands, while Claire led us away from the ring and down to the river for Trevor's first trail ride. Though Trevor did exactly as Claire asked him to do, I could sense his uneasiness; Claire could, too.

"Relax, Trevor," Claire encouraged him. "Close your eyes and grab mane. Let Chancey carry you all the way down to the river. Don't be scared, okay?"

"Chancey," whispered Trevor. He held my mane in his hands and leaned forward to my neck. "I've got you, Chancey. I'm not going to let go, either."

We walked through a field of brand-new saplings of

every hardwood of the mountains, all fighting for their share of sunlight. I looked up and could tell by the bend in the canopy which direction the river flowed. Even if I could not have seen it, I would have known by the cool, damp change in the air how to get to the Maury River. I found that if I listened beyond the wind and the song-birds, I could hear the Maury River long before I could see it. Claire heard it, too. We halted.

"Listen," she told Trevor. "What do you hear?"

Trevor stretched out on my back; he took his time answering her. "I hear a woodpecker drilling that dead tree right there."

"What else?" Claire wanted him to name the river.

"I hear those annoying geese honking at each other," he answered.

"Hmmm. I hear them, too. What else?" she asked again.

This time Trevor heard the river. "Water. It sounds like cars driving by, but softer. That's the river."

Trevor sat up and again grabbed a handful of my mane, this time with only one hand. He shifted around excitedly.

"Look," Trevor shouted, "a belted kingfisher! My favorite bird! I like that spiky hairdo."

I turned my head far to the left to give my face full exposure to the right bank of the river. The kingfisher sat perched on a sycamore limb, searching for trout, a sure sign that the river was running clear.

Claire tied the loose end of the lead rope to my halter. "Scoot back," she bossed Trevor. "I'm hopping up there with you. I like being up high when I come up to the river."

Trevor slid back all the way to my tail to give Claire enough room. She grabbed my mane and hoisted herself up. Trevor moved forward and held Claire's waist.

"Will you sing that song for us the rest of the way?" Claire pleaded with Trevor.

"Claire, stop making me sing. I just want to sit here on Chancey."

"But your song is the most beautiful song I've ever heard and besides, Chancey likes it."

Trevor laughed at Claire, and began his song anyway. Just as the undergrowth of saplings gave way to tall, thick grass, the Maury River appeared. Claire let me stop and graze while Trevor finished his song. The wind from the river kept most of the flies away from me. The shade from the birch, leaning out far beyond the bank, protected my eyes from the sun.

"Have you ever been swimming with a horse?" Claire asked Trevor.

"You're such a show-off, Claire. You know I've

never been swimming with a horse. You've been with me every time I've ever been on a horse," Trevor teased.

"Okay, I was just asking," Claire said, pretending to be hurt. She thought for a moment, then rephrased her question to him. "Trev, what I meant was, do you want to go swimming with Chancey and me, right now?"

"Sure," Trevor answered. "If you think it's safe."

"Geez, Trevor. Stop being such a fraidycat. Hold on."

Both children slipped off their socks and shoes. Claire squeezed her legs and gave me a little kick. Claire clucked to encourage me, but it was an entirely unnecessary aid. I, too, wanted to swim. I walked slowly into the water, allowing plenty of time for my legs, and the children's, to adjust. Claire and Trevor both sucked in their breath the moment the river slapped their legs. I waded slowly out to my neck; Claire stood on my back and dove into the river. Trevor did not need coaxing from Claire to do the same.

The river was slow and seemed ready to fall asleep as we three splashed the afternoon away. We stayed in the water together until the breeze blowing off it became too cold for Claire. She started to shiver, and not liking to be cold, tied my lead rope back into reins. I carried the two of them back to the barn. For what was left of the summer, this became our habit. Trevor would arrive for his lesson with Claire, and we would end our time together with a trail ride to the Maury River.

Once summer turned to fall, Trevor was ready for a greater challenge—taking me on the trail without Claire at the head. Claire would accompany us on Mac; her goal was to simulate the conditions of the hunter pace that would occur at the Ridgemore Hunt in Rockbridge County at the end of November. Though I had hoped I would be paired with Claire for the Ridgemore Hunt, I considered it an honor and a privilege to carry Trevor.

CHAPTER TWENTY-TWO

The Ridgemore Hunt

At the start of the Ridgemore Hunter Pace, Mrs. Maiden tied our team pinny, number sixteen, around Claire's waist. Trevor and Claire looked very much the team, both turned out in what appeared to me to be matching jodhpurs, and both sporting brand-new Maury River Stables team jerseys, given to them by Mrs. Maiden. I swelled with pride; I could imagine no better teammates than Claire, Trevor, and Mac.

Practically the entire barn family, it seemed, had turned out to cheer us on. Mother, Stu, and Mrs. Strickler were all there to help out. Even my canine friend Tommy had joined us. As I had come to expect, Mother reached to my neck and gave me a pat; she did the same with Mac and Claire. "Be safe; have fun!" she said. Mrs. Strickler seemed nervous. She smoothed Trevor's shirt, brushed his bangs out of his eyes, and fidgeted with my bridle until Trevor made her stop it.

Our team was barely out of the start box when we came upon trouble with some young horses. Some of them refused to cross the brook at the start of the course. Horses and riders were backed up twenty deep; the situation was tense not only because of the green horses but also the green riders. Trevor wisely asked me to move around the trouble. I thought it quite brave of him, really, and was proud of the way he tried to over-come his own fear, which of course I felt because he stopped breathing.

Trevor held his breath, tightened his legs, and instructed, "Walk on, Chancey," with such resolve, that even if I had not already been intending to move away from the catastrophic backup at the start, I would have walked on anyway at the urgency and intent of his request. He glanced back at Claire and Mac and urged them to come with us. We both felt Claire move out, and so proceeded up the hill, leaving the green horses and their people to fret over a bit of cold mountain water running across the course.

The moment we reached the top, Trevor and I both realized that in our haste to break away from the others, we had allowed Claire and Mac to get cut off by a loud, domineering woman trying to organize the field of novices. I called down to Mac, "Come on! Don't waste any more time. You've placed Claire in harm's way. Walk on!"

Mac called quickly back to me, "The girl on the bay's the problem. She's having trouble."

I could see for myself that the situation at the brook had deteriorated. I was glad to be at the top of the hill, looking down, though I desperately wanted Claire and Mac beside us. The girl and her young bay causing the trouble were so worked up that panic was spreading like a wildfire through all of the horses. Green horses, especially green fancy horses, are rather unpredictable. Green girls, especially fancy girls, are rarely prepared to lead such horses, as was the case at the brook.

Mac and Claire, I could see, remained calm. I could hear Claire pleading with the hunt mistress to let them cross. Mac called to me regularly, letting me know the status of their progress up the hill. All of the horses below were dancing wildly, except for Mac, who stood, observing and, I could see, thinking of how to get around the situation, which was becoming more dangerous by the minute.

When the bay not only refused to walk on, but reared

up on her hind legs, the girl dismounted—a wiser decision than I had credited the young lady with the capacity of making. I hoped the young rider might lead her green mare across the stream and get back in the saddle once the mare understood that the water would not harm her. I was sure the incident would now be resolved.

My judgment was premature. Once on the ground, the girl took hold of her stirrup iron with a grip of such force that I had only seen prior in our John the Farrier at home when removing old shoes. She struck her horse, no doubt thinking that this beating might persuade the mare to eagerly cross the brook and win the race. The mare cowered, and from the top of the hill I could see her fear growing, for her ears were now pinned flat back, and from way atop the hill, the white of the mare's eyes was unmistakably visible even to me.

When the iron struck the mare the second time, I vehemently objected to the brutality. I neighed shrilly as if my doing so would sway the girl to stop. When the girl struck the mare a third and then a fourth time, I lost my composure and reared up, both in anger and in alarm, issuing a call to end the cruelty and also, again, urging Mac to get Claire safely up the hill. The green girl had just injected the mare with a lifetime fear of water. The mare would now associate crossing water with pain and a beating.

Yet again, the girl hit her horse with the stirrup iron,

only more forcefully did she strike. I reared once more. It was at the top of my second rear that Trevor, so patient until then, made his own fear known to me. He leaned his weight full into my withers, forcing all four of my hooves to the ground. It was the right thing for him to do, for it pushed me back to earth. Trevor was scared, and without Claire, forced to make all decisions by himself.

Trevor pleaded quietly in my ear, "Please, Chancey. Remember, I'm not Claire. I'm afraid now, so I'm getting off of you until you stop it. You're behaving too recklessly!" With that assertion, Trevor jumped out of the saddle and began leading me around, turning me away from the harsh scene below.

I felt ashamed, if truth be told, that I had frightened Trevor. And I felt relieved that he had turned me away from the beating so that I did not have to watch any longer. Trevor talked to me as he led me around the hill, telling me that Claire and Mac would join us shortly. He commented on the clear day and warm late-autumn air. It did feel almost like summer. My coat was already thick in preparation for winter to come. The air felt good while we were standing still at the top of the hill, though I knew that by the end of the race, Trevor and I both would be lathered and breathing fast. Trevor was already breathing too fast, but at least he was breathing. He started singing to slow down his breathing and gather back his courage. Claire had taught him well.

Trevor and I were relieved when Claire and Mac reached us. Trevor wasted no time—again I thought him quite brave—in jumping onto my back by using his own strength and determination. I rumbled at Mac and looked Claire over; both seemed well and ready to go.

Claire's strategy, as explained to us prior to the event, was first and foremost to get out of the start quickly and stay well away from the other teams. She aimed to keep our riding conditions as much like a trail ride as possible to minimize distractions for Trevor. Originally, she had planned to keep us trotting for much of the course, except at the hills, which we would canter up. Because of the early mishap, Claire now said we would need a much faster ride than any of us had planned.

She changed our strategy and relayed to Trevor and me, "If we're going to have a shot at this, Trevor, you've got to canter a lot more than you ever have done. Don't be scared; just trust Chancey and let him go. Chancey will stay with Mac and me. You stay with Chancey. Can you do that?"

I could feel Trevor's hands, already wet with perspiration, shaking on the reins. "I think so." I nickered at him to tell him I would not let him down, or off.

"Okay." Claire looked at Trevor directly. "Are you ready then?"

Trevor stalled. "No. I don't think I can do it, Claire. Forget it. This was a stupid idea."

Claire and Mac looked as though we had all the time in the world and this was just another day of trail riding in the mountains. Claire tried to convey her surety to Trevor. She backed Mac up until they stood right next to us.

"Shhh. Don't say that, Trev. We're a team, all four of us. Who cares if we win or not? We're going to finish together, and you can do it."

Trevor nodded.

Claire smiled at him and asked, "If you feel off at the canter, what are you going to do?"

"Uh, grab mane?" He sounded so unsure.

"Yes! Grab mane. Chancey won't let you down. Now, let's go—we have a hunter pace to win!" Claire and Mac cantered away. Trevor moved his right leg behind my girth; he did not have to ask for the canter, for I was determined to stay with Claire and Mac. Halfway across the field, Claire turned back and shouted, "Are you okay?"

Trevor could not speak, for he was not breathing. He did manage to nod. I did not break our canter until Claire and Mac slowed to a trot. Claire waited for us to pull alongside her. She was such a good leader, letting us know of every twist and turn and challenge in the course and how we could best take it as a team.

"We're going over the Maury next, but it's shallow and narrow. Breathe, Trevor, and chill. Chancey loves water; just stay with us. I want to get us out of this big group and by ourselves again."

Trevor again nodded. His head darted around, looking left, then right, at every other team near us. As his head turned, so did his shoulders, his hands, and his hips. It was difficult for me to keep from dancing around, for with each nervous movement the boy made, the bit in my mouth followed likewise. I could tell that being close to so many other horses had unnerved him. I knew, however, that his excitability was not to be mistaken for intentional communication with me. I followed Claire's instruction on the course. Once Trevor refocused, though his hands gripped the reins tightly, he posted expertly in good time with me.

When the course entered the forest for the first time, I felt sure that we must be nearing the halfway point. Up until then, the entire route had been up and down through open fields, much like our trails at home. As we entered the forest, we realized that the terrain had been deceitfully comfortable. None of us had anticipated a steep and slippery cliff down so far into a ravine that the bottom could not be seen.

Our competitors, evidently, had not anticipated this obstacle either. The forest floor was muddy from several days prior of rain. Only a few strides into the woods, the forest floor dropped off so steeply that I could not see below to the point where it would level off again. A gray pony in front of us lost her footing in the mud and fell to her knees before stabilizing and bolting through the trees, off course. When the pony bolted, she caused a cedar branch, rife with berries, to snap back into Claire's face. Claire did not lose her seat or her courage.

Claire may well have been afraid, but she did not choose fear as her advisor. She called back to Trevor, "Chancey's an App; he's made for this stuff. Do what I do: breathe and lean back. Lean way back. We're going down one step at a time."

Trevor breathed in deeply. He gave me my head and leaned back, keeping his center of gravity weighted exactly with mine. Had he been too far forward, no doubt, I would have slid easily. There was a point in our descent where both Claire and Trevor were stretched out flat on their backs, loosely holding on to Mac and me, allowing us to do the work. Neither child panicked once. I was proud of them both, especially Trevor.

Some horses behind us whinnied and bolted back up the cliff. I heard a rider thud to the ground. Trevor began to sing; he was breathing. Mac and I did not speak, but head to tail, we got down the cliff together. My Appaloosa feet served my team well. There was no hint of slipping or sliding, only an easy, steady walk in the forest. Trevor did his job of staying relaxed; I did my job of keeping Trevor safe.

When we reached the bottom, Claire turned back to us. "Awesome! Y'all are awesome!"

For the first time on the course, I felt Trevor relax. "We did it, Claire!" He patted me on the shoulder. "Chancey, we did it!"

Claire brought us back into the open field. "Don't get too fired up just yet. As soon as we're totally out of the forest, we've got to canter up that hill. Then we'll need to stop at the checkpoint and get our halfway chip. It doesn't count as a finish unless we turn in the chip at the end. Come on, let's go!" Claire and Mac cantered away, and I stayed right with them.

Finding the spot in the saddle that is secure and balanced is not easy. Claire is the only one I've known to find that spot right away, without effort and without fail. It's a spot where I feel the legs of my rider secure against me, almost holding us both up, moving us both forward together and in good time. If my rider can find the spot and hold it, we can achieve a unison that is not dependent on my eyesight. We can move together, galloping up hills, through forests, and over streams as if we are welded. Claire knows this spot on me, and I suspect on Mac and every other horse she has ever joined.

Trevor was a different story. He was, at times, consumed so greatly with his own fear that he failed to realize even the most obvious mistakes, such as placing the bridle on me upside down, in a convoluted mess. Often he sat high, perched up in the saddle, with all his weight gathered atop of me in a compact triangle on the saddle. Carrying Trevor sometimes felt as I imagined it would feel to carry two or three hay bales all stacked up on the saddle, and I was constantly shifting my own weight to keep the unstable tower from toppling over.

The hunter pace was the occasion that presented a perfect teaching moment to show Trevor how it felt to ride together, moving as a team. On one of the final hills, we cantered at first, and as I moved into a gallop, Trevor's imbalance caused him to grab my mane to keep from falling. Thankfully, he did not lean his weight onto my neck, nor did he pull back on the reins. He grabbed a handful of my mane to steady himself, and, as I had by now several times witnessed his courage, I was not surprised that though feeling unbalanced, he did not ask me to stop.

What I did next was risky to be sure, but I felt for the first time that Trevor was feeling confident. He was breathing. I could not see it, but I believe he was smiling. On this day, Trevor was riding with heart.

What I did, actually, was to lob him into the perfect spot. If I could have used words, I might have told him to sit deeply, close his knees around me, and drop his pelvis into me. I did not have words available to me, and, truthfully, Trevor had heard these words from Mrs. Maiden and Claire many times in his own lessons. He needed to feel what the words meant. I wagered that if I got Trevor into the spot on my own, he would feel it and know it was right. It happened just like that.

Midway up the hill at a gallop, I pushed Trevor into the right place. He stuck to me; he let go of my mane.

Trevor hollered through the wind to me, "Woohoo! We're flying, Chancey!"

He stayed in the right place throughout the remainder of the course, only once losing his left stirrup and even then not losing the spot. When I felt the loose stirrup slapping my barrel, I slowed enough for Trevor to pick it back up. As he did, he yelled to me, "Good boy, Chancey. Go on — I've got it!"

Trevor was one of two boys his age that I had observed on the field that day. The other boy and his paint pony each carried a girth that far exceeded that of anyone on our team, save Mac. As we neared the checkpoint, the chunky pony and her boy cut us off, inserting themselves directly behind Claire and Mac. Claire and Mac stretched out beyond us, not realizing that Trevor and I had been left behind. The pony and her boy challenged us to race them up the hill at a gallop.

Trevor, with his newly found confidence, leaned into

me and whispered, "Yah, boy! Yah!" I understood his command, and this time I welcomed it. Though already at a gallop, and nearing the end of my capacity, I reached down into my reserves to give Trevor the extra bit of speed that a command such as "Yah, boy" deserved. *This,* I thought, *is the greatest contest of my life.*

We galloped away from our challengers and caught Claire and Mac, who were waiting for us at the checkpoint. Claire encouraged Trevor to take the chip, so that he could officially represent our team at the finish.

"Are you sure?" Trevor asked Claire.

Claire nodded. "Come on, we're almost there!"

Trevor yelled over to Claire, "That kid was trying to race me! Did you see him?"

"The boy on the fat pony?" Claire gobbled up the challenge. She collected Mac's reins and dug her heels into his side. "Ever race a paint before, Trev? Easy peasy. There's no way he'll catch us."

Trevor pressed his heels into me with conviction. He clucked at me and yelled into the wind, "Yah, boy!"

The rest of the course was open, flat field, with only a few small hills left. Claire and Trevor galloped to the end, and both children hollered wildly when we spotted the Maury River Stables delegation standing near the finish, waiting for us. Mrs. Strickler and Mother were jumping up and down, clapping their hands together and holding on to each other like old friends. Mrs.

Maiden threw her head back and laughed. Stu pumped his fist in the air to show his support. Tommy tore away from his leash and ran up to me, sniffing each of my legs for a replay of the course we had run. I whinnied my gratitude to them all. Mac echoed my sentiment then and together, we four crossed the finish line of the Ridgemore Hunt unharmed and grateful for a victorious ride through the blue mountains, for, ribbon or no ribbon, all of us had ridden the hunter pace course exactly as it was meant to be ridden: with confidence, patience, strategy, and endurance.

Our fine team was exhausted after the Ridgemore Hunt. For the entirety of the race, Claire and Mac led the way through seven miles of beautiful gallop hills. All four of us needed refreshment. Claire hitched Mac and me to the trailer; Trevor tied fresh hay nets nearby. Trevor and Claire ran off together, still giddy from our race. Tommy curled up in the shade underneath me and took a nap. I felt quite content that day. Claire and Trevor, I knew, would soon return.

I was proud of Trevor and his many displays of courage throughout the difficult course. He had trusted me, and I had trusted him. I knew the boy was tired and was glad that Claire had taken him off to find food and water. I finished off the last of the hay in my net and remembered to thank Mac for taking such good care of Claire. He rumbled, but did not stop eating.

"We were a good team this morning, Macadoo. We should do this more often," I said, ignoring my quivering haunches. I tried to catch my breath. Mac was tied to the right of me, and though he was on my good side, I could hardly make him out. I attributed my clouded vision to the perspiration still running into my eye, as it had from our first canter up a hill. Mac must have sensed my difficulty, for he did not reciprocate the congratulatory praise. He inquired, with concern in his voice, "How are you, Old App?"

I had no opportunity to reply or form a response, for the children came sprinting back, bursting with some news.

Trevor and Claire each clutched a blue ribbon in one hand. The boy threw his arms around me. "Chancey! We won! We won the hunter pace!" Claire was laughing; she came to me first.

"I knew you could do it, pony. You're the best friend in the world. I knew you could do it! You made Trevor a champion!"

Then she whispered in my ear, "Next time, I'll ride you myself, like we planned."

She kissed me, then congratulated Mac and tucked her ribbon into his halter.

Trevor, likewise, tucked his blue ribbon into my halter and, more to show off his win than anything else, I'm sure, he untied me and we walked to the watering place. Seeing no one else around but some mares from the course, Trevor shared his grand news with them. "We won! Chancey, Claire, Mac, and I won! I've never won anything; I won today!" I rumbled low and affirmed my own elation. That day to one boy, I became a champion.

CHAPTER TWENTY-THREE

Yah, Boy!

After the hunter pace, throughout the fall and into the winter, Trevor continued to come to the barn for his weekly riding lessons, but he did not ride. He resumed his earlier habit of standing in my room; this time I stood beside him. Trevor leaned his head out of the window, as is also my habit. I recognized that he was trying to catch the wind and nickered softly to him, letting him know he was welcome to remain as long as he liked, for Trevor was a champion; he had won us a blue ribbon. Claire often stayed in my room with him, and she never pressed him to ride.

"Look how blue the sky is, Chancey, and not a cloud to be seen. Snow will be here soon; can you smell it?" Trevor asked me.

I looked at Trevor, turned out in fresh riding clothes that smelled of plastic, not hay or dirt. I understood then that our riding together as a team had come to an end.

I was content to stand with him, noting every change in the sky and clouds for many days in a row. He loved to describe for me every hawk and pileated wood-pecker he spotted. He explained to me that which I already knew—how the river birch, clustered just below the gelding field, told us in which direction we would find the Maury River.

Trevor also told me much that I did not know; I was happy to listen to all he had to say, and so was Claire. During these times, Claire spoke not a word, but would sit atop me or lean against me and listen to Trevor teach us about the natural world around us.

"Chancey, did you know that in some other moun-tains, far away in Utah, there lives a stand of forty-seven thousand aspen trees that are really all the same organ-ism? That's the largest living organism on Earth. Can you believe it? I've been there myself, and it's amazing to think that all of those trees grow from the same exact root system: all one tree. If you cut one down, it wouldn't die; another would grow in its place."

Trevor closed his eyes. I closed mine, too, in order to imagine such an aspen grove. He leaned into me and grew quiet. Then he whispered, "I wish I could see Utah again."

We never competed together again, but the three of us often walked down to the river together. Whatever the weather, we three enjoyed the trail to our private spot. Trevor usually sat on my back, while Claire was content to lead us both, as long as Trevor would promise to sing. Even though it was too cold for swimming, the two friends would hop across the rocks, Trevor always on the lookout for the belted kingfisher.

My eyes were failing me more than I had revealed to anyone. Even Claire did not realize the loss that I had endured. So strong was my trust in those around me — Claire, Mother, Stu, Mrs. Maiden, Tommy, Mac, Gwen, and even Daisy — that it was easy to hide the truth of the darkness that had taken over my right eye.

Before anyone else noticed, it was Mac who witnessed me walking into fences and gates. He never let on, but he did keep closer to me at those times of the day when we were either being turned out or brought into our rooms. When Mac was near, I could smell sunflowers on him. Like me, Mac received special supplements to his grain twice daily. Mine was to ease my pain; Mac's was to keep his coat shiny since he was showing nearly every weekend. Had I not been able to smell my friend, I would have felt the ground tremble whenever he came galloping up to me.

"This way, Old App. Come this way." He would guide me through the gate or toward fresh hay. We never discussed my worsening condition, but Mac surely knew first.

I found it fairly simple to continue my routine with almost no interruption. In my therapeutic work, the sidewalkers flanked me on both sides, guiding me around the ring and through simple courses. While Claire and Mother were still my sidewalkers, Mrs. Strickler had also become certified and occasionally replaced Claire in the ring. None of my therapeutic students were trotting or cantering, and I had long ago retired from jumping. In fact, the last jump I had attempted was at Tamworth Springs. No one had realized yet how rapidly my eyesight had declined, though none would have been surprised to learn of it, for we all had expected this day would come.

While Mac may have been the first to detect the true state of my eyes, Claire was the first to speak of it. Claire's discovery came on a day of sorrowful circumstances for us both. It was the afternoon that we received the news Trevor's cancer had returned full force.

One late winter afternoon, as we eagerly awaited the day when springtime finally returned to the blue mountains, Claire was in my room grooming me. She did not intend to ride, only to pamper me a bit. We had no show to prepare for; Claire was pulling my mane because she knew I would enjoy it. In fact, I had nearly dozed off when Trevor's mother appeared at my door, without Trevor.

"Hi, Mrs. Strickler," Claire said. "Where's Trevor today?"

Mrs. Strickler walked into my room and patted me on the neck. She did not answer Claire's question; instead she asked, "Claire, how are you?"

I felt Claire step back from Mrs. Strickler. I turned my head to Claire's voice. "Wh-what's that in your hand? Why do you have Trevor's blue ribbon?" Claire stopped breathing.

"Claire." Mrs. Strickler moved closer to me and steadied herself on my neck.

She started again. "Claire, Trevor wants Chancey to have this ribbon. I promised him I would bring it over today." Mrs. Strickler tucked the ribbon into my halter. She patted my neck again, then smoothed her hand over the ribbon. I recalled how she had smoothed Trevor's shirt in much the same way on the day we won.

Claire's hand breezed by my face; she snatched the ribbon out of my halter. "No! This is Trevor's ribbon; he won it. I have a blue ribbon from the Ridgemore Hunt at home, and T-Trevor, Trevor has one."

I felt Claire's hand shake beneath my mouth, as I stood between the two. "H-here, this is Trevor's." Again, she tried to make Mrs. Strickler take the ribbon back to her son. Mrs. Strickler was silent. I could feel the two of them looking at each other.

Mrs. Strickler sighed and softly placed the ribbon back in my halter. She touched the ribbon again, and ran her hand slowly from my neck to my withers. Then she addressed me, not Claire.

"Chancey, Trevor is going home soon. He wants you to have this ribbon. He hopes that you will remember how the two of you beat the boy on the fat pony. He especially asked me to give you a message."

Mrs. Strickler put her mouth to my ear and whispered, "Yah, boy, yah."

Then she turned back to Claire and took my girl's hands. Her voice barely made it out of her throat. "Thank you, Claire, for treating Trevor like Trevor. He asked me to give you this. . . ." Mrs. Strickler leaned across me and kissed Claire's face. Then she left my room.

I heard Claire turn away from the door and walk to the window in my room. I moved toward the sound of her breath and waited for her to call me nearer. I did not wait for long.

"Chancey?" Claire called. "Pony, we're not going to see Trevor again."

I took two steps and bumped into Claire. I blew a long breath out. Claire blew back into my nose.

"Come on, Chance. Let's go for a ride."

She did not tack me up with a bridle or saddle or even a bareback pad. Claire clipped a lead rope to my halter and escorted me out of the barn. She walked at an urgent pace past the mare field. Daisy and Princess cantered up alongside us, eager to know where we were going. I whinnied my uncertain reply. We passed my paddock, where Gwen and Mac were already turned out; they called out the same as the others.

Claire stopped at the gelding field; Dante threatened to block our entrance. Claire popped Dante's rear hard enough to make him whinny and canter away. I waited for Claire to guide me through the gate. She clucked at me to hurry up, but I could not see my way through. As she had done so many times in our friendship, Claire tied my lead rope into reins, grabbed hold of my mane, and pulled herself onto my back. When she was a little girl, she would wiggle and writhe to make it up without help. Now she pushed herself up with ease. She squeezed my barrel and called into my ear, "Yah, boy! Yah!" We cantered away.

For the length of the gelding field, Claire never allowed me to break stride. Her calves stayed firmly planted, and she leaned forward, asking for a gallop.

"Yah, boy!" she called again. The other geldings whinnied at us to stop. From our field, Mac called out to me, "The fence, Chancey! She's running you into the electric fence!"

I thought surely Claire could see the fence, for I could not. She began counting, "One, two, one, two." Claire intended to jump the electric fence. I readied myself, knowing there was nowhere for me to duck. I listened for my cue. My muscles remembered what it felt like to jump, and they began to twitch. "One, two, one, two, one, two, *jump!*"

Claire held me tight, rose into jump position, and lifted me up over the electric fence. She gave me my head, and though I could not see it, I felt that we had easily cleared the height. The geldings galloped right up to it and called out to us. We did not turn back. Claire galloped me through the river where we had swum so often with Trevor. She held her legs firm and stayed right with my center of gravity, encouraging me to scurry up the river's right bank. Claire was taking me to Saddle Mountain.

We cantered up the old logging trail, never stopping until we had almost reached the peak. Claire jumped down and untied the lead rope, allowing me to graze what grass and sarsaparilla I could find. I kept near Claire, and when I could no longer hear her breath, I rumbled out to her. "Up here, Chancey. I'm sitting up here." I walked on until the terrain became rockier and I smelled Claire directly at my feet. I dropped my head down to her, and she wrapped her hands around my neck.

Claire was shivering cold. I tossed my head up and down to indicate that we should head back; Claire did not budge. She sat, freezing on a boulder, and, I can only presume, looking down at the Maury River Stables below us. I positioned myself to guard Claire from the wind. I felt the shadow of storm clouds gather around us. The air had grown damp and thick; I could taste that we were standing in a cloud. Claire's teeth knocked against themselves violently. She would not leave.

I pushed my nose under Claire's arm; she rebuffed me. "Stop, Chancey." I pushed against her again.

"Stop it, I said. Stop."

Now Claire was turning away from me. I wondered what would have happened that day many years ago, when I first turned my back on Claire, if she had left my room as I had asked. She might never have come back. I might never have lived this life at the Maury River Stables. I tried to recall what she had told me that day. "Let love come back," Claire had said. "Let love come back to you."

I rested my head on Claire and gently nodded into

her shoulder. She paid no mind to me or the winter air. Appaloosa horses grow fine, thick coats; I was happy to share mine with Claire. I moved closer in to her so that I could protect my girl from the harsh wind blowing across Saddle Mountain. So deep were we in winter that the trees atop the mountain could not deter the winds from ripping into us. Claire had never liked the cold.

In the shelter of my withers, Claire grieved for Trevor. I grieved with her, though it would be false for me to claim that I did not also rejoice, for Mrs. Strickler had told me herself Trevor was going home.

Finally, Claire stopped shivering. She held me to her face and warmed her bare hands against my coat. "I love you, Chancey. Let's go back."

Claire dried her eyes on my neck, stood up, and tucked her body close into me, seeking warmth. Again, she pushed up onto my back. I waited for some direction from her, for I could not see. The mountain was pulling at me to go down, but I could not determine how steep the grade. Earlier in our friendship, I would have done all the work and carried Claire back to the barn without any need of direction whatsoever. Claire had steered me up Saddle Mountain; Claire would have to steer me down.

"Come on, boy, go on," Claire urged. Yet she did not pick up the makeshift reins. I did not move. I waited for guidance from Claire. She grew impatient with me, which I understood, for she had yet to realize that I needed her to be my eyes now.

"What's wrong, Chancey? Can't you see I'm ready to go?" I did not answer, and I did not move.

"Oh, no. Oh, no." Claire jumped off me, not on my left side as is customary, but on my right. She stood next to my face, I could feel her there.

"Oh, no." I felt her arm jerking back and forth.

"Can't you see my hand?" Claire cried. "Can't you see my hand?" I rumbled softly into Claire's ear. There on top of Saddle Mountain, Claire discovered that I was now blind. She did not panic. Claire grabbed my mane and jumped up again.

I felt her legs even and firm on my barrel and her steady application of evenness from both hands. She pushed gently with her seat.

"Walk on, pony. Walk on."

I stepped out, tracking straight until Claire invited me to turn right. Claire was riding as she always did and I trusted her, as I always had. She led me down the mountain, encouraging me every step. "I've got you, boy — don't worry." I was not worried; I was with Claire.

As I stepped into the Maury River on our return home, a light snow began falling on us. I heard no birdsong, nor did Claire sing for us—only the sound of my hooves splashing in the river interrupted the silence.

The mares and geldings all stood lined up along the fence watching for our return home. Stu was there, too, to disable the electric fence and allow us to walk over it. As Claire and I walked through the gelding field, each of my former fieldmates offered a word of welcome to me. Gwen and Mac rumbled affectionately, glad to have Claire and me safely back before the snow picked up. We made our way to the barn. There at the end of the line, in the mare field, stood Daisy, who announced for all to hear, "There goes a great horse."

CHAPTER TWENTY-FOUR

Fulfillment

Have, then, Dam's prayers for me been answered? When I pass through every memory, as far back as I am able, I arrive at only one answer to this question. My life itself has been a long, prayerful response to my Dam and the fire star. In thinking back to the first echo of my heart, I do not find Monique and her disappointment in me. Nor do I even find Dam and her protection. I find the blue mountains.

I was born here and am grateful that, though I was nearly forced once to leave, I shall remain here forever. Though I will never travel through all of them, I have traveled the mountains enough, along the Maury River and beyond, to know that what can be seen from my room is only their beginning. I am sure the blue mountains go on and on. It comforts me to know that whether I can see them or not, I will always be surrounded by the mountains and the river.

These mountains have watched me grow blind. Yet in the time it has taken me to become an old and failing horse, the mountains have aged but a second. I cannot see, and I am not afraid. Standing here now, in my field with Gwen and Mac, some greater vision has replaced my eyesight.

Here, at the Maury River Stables, is where I will remain for as many more days as I am granted. More than once, I have heard Mother instruct Mrs. Maiden that I am to always occupy the corner room because of its ample space. I have no anxiety about my future and the care that I shall receive, nor do I need to search for food or water, as once I did. I fear nothing and am certain that of the many horses whose end will come in Lynchville, or some similar place, I shall never be among them.

Though I am now entirely blind, I do not lack a meaningful purpose, for I am surrounded by friends. I cannot see them, but I know when they are near. I continue my work with the therapeutic school; my students continue to pray for me every night, and I for them. My former student Kenzie comes often, too; she is helping me learn to be blind. Even Zack has been known to stop by for a visit.

Claire and Mother still agree that though Claire's talent has surpassed my own, we are family and will remain bound forever. Now that Claire is away, studying at a university at the edge of the blue mountains, Mother comes most often to hold me for the farrier or pull my mane. These days, sleep comes easiest to me when my mane is being pulled. I can smell when it's Mother coming up behind me. She always carries a stud biscuit in her pocket. Mother's skin smells cleaner than the sweat and grain that Mrs. Maiden wears on her skin. Even if I could not recognize Mother from the smell of her skin, I would know her by the way she sneaks around my face and reaches above my cheek to kiss me.

She speaks quietly to me. "Oh, I love this soft silky spot. That's my spot." She presses her lips deep into my head the same as she has always done.

Claire continues to visit me as her school schedule allows. When she comes home, she takes such an interest in grooming me herself that I confess there are times when I indulge in rolling deep into a briar patch without fear of being admonished. Claire still seems especially content to pull the briars out of my forelock, as she has done for so many years now. She is unfazed by my blindness. Where once she came to me, a small child with a big spirit who needed the mounting block to reach my mane, Claire now stands eye to eye with me.

Those days when Claire comes home fill me with joy! Claire still tacks me up in the same way she has done for what must be ten years now, for the new dentist recently observed that I am in my early thirties. In the ring, Claire guides me surely through my paces, keeping her calves tight on me, holding me up, and guiding me on. She likes to reassure me, "I've got you, Chancey. I've got you." Then, together, we pop over a tiny fence; it still feels as if we are each other's wings.

After warming up in the ring, Claire asks me, "Whaddya say, Chance? Are you up for a nice gallop through the mountains?" She does not wait for me to nicker, though I always do. Claire takes off the saddle and rides me bareback across the Maury River, up the right bank, and into the blue mountains. When I feel her ask for the canter with a light squeeze, I wait until Claire whispers two words before giving in.

"Yah, boy," she tells me softly. "Yah, boy!" she yells into the wind.

Though I can no longer see any of the trail before me, the eye of my heart sees perfectly well—just as clearly as if I had never been marked by this cancer. I can see Claire in her overalls, tenderly reaching the mask around my eyes to protect them from the sun. I can see the moment that changed me—forever.

Shortly after my arrival at the Maury River Stables, Claire had reached out to touch my marred face. I stood before her. I was malnourished, soiled, and nearly used up. I had wanted to save her from loving me and being disappointed. I know now that Claire loved me the very second that I loved her, and so she already knew everything about me that she needed to know. What she did not yet know she would come to accept with a greater compassion toward me than I ever thought possible, except, perhaps, from my own dam. Claire would not leave me to feel sorry for myself; Claire would continue to love me.

She never saw me as the castoff that I had become, abandoned in a field. Instead, she saw the horse that I was born to be, the great horse that the stars foretold on the night of my birth. Yet more than the stars could ever have predicted, I know that if I have been made great, at all, it is due entirely to the prayers of Dam and the love of Claire. So here I will stand, facing Saddle Mountain, listening for the whisper of Claire's return, and offering back all that I am now able, an infinite thanksgiving for this truly blessed life I have lived.

ACKNOWLEDGMENTS

Thanks, Lance, for not shooting the albino buck in Cartersville. Thank you, Penny Ross, the Glenmore Hunt, Rhodes Farm at Wintergreen, the Stables at the Homestead, and Deb Sensabaugh of Virginia Mountain Outfitters for offering breathtaking hacks through the Blue Ridge and Allegheny Mountains. Thanks to Kathy, Judith, Elizabeth, and Rebecca for taking me on my first hunter pace and encouraging me to let Albert run. JEA, here's to our pretty fourth-place ribbon! Never has research been so invigorating! For teaching me about therapeutic riding: Kathy Pitt of Smooth Moves in Powhatan, Virginia, and Sue Alvis of Ride On in Glen Allen. Small programs like these, all over the country, perform miracles every day with incredibly dedicated volunteers and devoted horses.

Thank you to the brilliant horsewomen—Judith Amateau, Gail Bird Necklace, Kate Fletcher, Beth Lindsay, and Jennifer Wright, DVM—and brilliant readers—Leigh Amateau, Deanna Boehm, Cindy Ford, Mary Ellis Gregg, Mary Kiger, Maggie Menard, Betty Sanderson, and Amy Strite—who read, and improved on, an early manuscript. Thank you to Mrs. Ford, librarian, and the talented writers of the Guild of Youth Authors at Midlothian Middle School in Midlothian, Virginia. Thank you to the Irvine/Grue family of House Mountain Inn in Lexington, Virginia, for their hospitality and mountain retreat, perfect for imagining Chancey and Claire.

Thank you, my agent, Leigh Feldman, of Darhansoff, Verrill, & Feldman, who made me promise never to write "Neigh!" (Did I keep the promise? Yes!) Always, thank you to my Key West godparents: Judy, David, and Mark, for their gracious, generous time and friendship.

Candlewick Press rocks! I love all y'all: Brittany Duncan, Kate Fletcher, Sherry Fatla, Sharon Hancock, Anne Irza-Leggatt, Caroline Lawrence, Tracy Miracle, Chris Paul, Nicole Raymond, Jennifer Roberts, Charlie Schroder, Elise Supovitz, Ginny Wallace (hi, Ginny!), and most especially, Karen Lotz, collaborator extraordinaire. K—every second with you and this book has been exactly, perfectly wonderful. I had so much fun—thank you! (Also, very important: Karen, I just don't think I would have met *my boy* Ray had it not been for you. SI.)

I give major props to Bubba—my best friend, my true love—for supporting Judith's and my passion for all things equine. Back at you on all things bovine, baby!

Most of all thank you to King Albert, our albino Appaloosa witch, and my daughter, Judith, a truly gifted writer and creative partner. I love you.